Lecture Notes in Bioinformatics 9162

Subseries of Lecture Notes in Computer Science

More information about this series at http://www.springer.com/series/5381

Naveen Ashish · Jose-Luis Ambite (Eds.)

Data Integration in the Life Sciences

11th International Conference, DILS 2015
Los Angeles, CA, USA, July 9–10, 2015
Proceedings

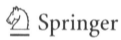 Springer

Editors
Naveen Ashish
USC Stevens Neuroimaging and Informatics
   Institute
Los Angeles, CA
USA

Jose-Luis Ambite
USC Information Sciences Institute
Marina del Rey, CA
USA

ISSN 0302-9743   ISSN 1611-3349 (electronic)
Lecture Notes in Bioinformatics
ISBN 978-3-319-21842-7   ISBN 978-3-319-21843-4 (eBook)
DOI 10.1007/978-3-319-21843-4

Library of Congress Control Number: 2015944436

LNCS Sublibrary: SL8 – Bioinformatics

Springer Cham Heidelberg New York Dordrecht London
© Springer International Publishing Switzerland 2015

Printed on acid-free paper

Springer International Publishing AG Switzerland is part of Springer Science+Business Media
(www.springer.com)

Preface

The 2015 Data Integration in the Life Sciences (DILS 2015) conference was the 11th conference in this international conference series on biomedical data integration. The focus of interest this year included topics such as data integration technologies, knowledge engineering and ontologies, data standards and coding, and novel applications in biomedical research. This year we also added new topics such as virtual appliances for data analysis.

The call for papers attracted many submissions on the workshop topics. After a careful reviewing process the international Program Committee accepted 21 research papers and four graduate student consortium abstracts. DILS 2015 also featured two keynote presentations by Dr. Arthur W. Toga of the USC Stevens Neuroimaging and Informatics Institute and Dr. Dan M. Cooper of the University of California Irvine.

As the program chairs and editors of this volume, we would like to thank all authors who submitted papers, as well as the Program Committee members and additional reviewers for their excellent work in evaluating the submissions. Special thanks to the Information Sciences Institute of the University of Southern California for providing the facilities to host the conference. Finally, we would like to thank Alfred Hofmann and his team at Springer for their cooperation and help in putting this volume together.

June 2015

Naveen Ashish
Jose-Luis Ambite

Organization

Program Committee Chairs

Naveen Ashish   Keck School of Medicine, University of Southern California, USA
Jose-Luis Ambite   USC Information Sciences Institute, USA

Program Committee

Sivaram Arabandi   Ontopro
Aziz Boxwala   Meliorix
Lisa Dahm   University of California Irvine, USA
Greg Farber   NIH, USA
Helena Galhardas   University of Lisbon, Portugal
Satrajit Ghosh   MIT, USA
Paul Groth   VU University Amsterdam, The Netherlands
Vasant Honavar   Penn State University, USA
Ramakanth Kavuluru   University of Kentucky, USA
Craig Knoblock   USC Information Sciences Institute, USA
Peter Mork   Noblis
Norman Paton   Manchester University, UK
Cartic Ramakrishnan   IBM Almaden Research Center, USA
Alan Ruttenberg   University at Buffalo, USA
Satya Sahoo   Case Western Reserve University, USA
Michael Schroeder   TU Dresden, Germany
Ajay Shah   City of Hope
Biplav Srivastava   IBM India Research Lab, India
Paul Thompson   Keck School of Medicine, University of Southern California, USA
Arthur Toga   Keck School of Medicine, University of Southern California, USA
Jessica Turner   Georgia State University, USA

General Chair

Carl Kesselman   USC Information Sciences Institute, USA

Student Research Consortium Chair

Ashutosh Jadhav   Wright State University, USA

Steering Committee

Naveen Ashish	Keck School of Medicine, University of Southern California, USA
Jose-Luis Ambite	USC Information Sciences Institute, USA
Carl Kesselman	USC Information Sciences Institute, USA
Louiqa Raschid	University of Maryland, USA

Contents

Biomedical Data Standards and Coding

Medical Research Applications

Graduate Student Consortium

Data Integration Technologies

Combining Multiple Knowledge Sources: A Case Study of Drug Induced Liver Injury

Casey L. Overby[2], Alejandro Flores[1], Guillermo Palma[1], Maria-Esther Vidal[1], Elena Zotkina[2], and Louiqa Raschid[2(✉)]

[1] Universidad Simón Bolívar, Caracas, Venezuela
{aflores,gpalma,mvidal}@ldc.usb.ve
[2] University of Maryland, College Park, USA
coverby@medicine.umaryland.edu
{ezotkina,louiqa}@umiacs.umd.edu

Abstract. Many classes of drugs, their interaction pathways and gene targets are known to play a role in drug induced liver injury (DILI). Pharmacogenomics research to understand the impact of genetic variation on how patients respond to drugs may help explain some of the variability observed in the occurrence of adverse drug reactions (ADR) such as DILI. The goal of this project is to combine rich genotype and phenotype data to better understand these scenarios. We consider similarities between drugs, similarities between drug targets, drug-pathway-gene interactions, etc. Links to the patients will include patient drug usage, ADR, disease outcomes, etc. We will develop appropriate protocols to create these rich datasets and methods to identify patterns in graphs for explanation and prediction.

1 Introduction

The proliferation of Linked Data has lead to many research efforts on learning and prediction with drug and gene target datasets. One of the most successful examples has been in drug re-purposing and involves drug to gene-target interaction prediction [4–6]. Since much of this data is networked data, methods have included clustering, ranking and learning based on shared neighbors [5]. The state-of-the-art is represented by examples that include a method based on PSL [6] that performs relational learning using structured features. More recent access to clinical Big Data has also lead to several successful research efforts. e.g., to mine patient records to identify adverse drug reactions (ADRs) [9,11].

This paper presents an ongoing effort to build upon these past successes and aims to benefit from combining datasets including knowledge of associations between genotypes and phenotypes relevant to drug treatment. The motivating example will be a case study around drugs known to lead to unpredictable ("idiosyncratic") adverse drug reactions (ADRs) in susceptible individuals. Identifying genetic risk factors associated with idiosyncratic ADRs has the potential to facilitate detection of "at risk" patients prior to choosing a course of treatment, or to

© Springer International Publishing Switzerland 2015
N. Ashish and J.-L. Ambite (Eds.): DILS 2015, LNBI 9162, pp. 3–12, 2015.
DOI: 10.1007/978-3-319-21843-4_1

determine contributing factors once an ADR occurs, and to determine the subsequent choice of an appropriate course of treatment. Drug-induced liver injury (DILI) is one ADR for which the associated genetic factors have been studied since the 1980s. It is a rare, but potentially serious, ADR associated with treatment with certain commonly used drugs. The drugs that lead to this toxicity are structurally diverse and belong to a number of different therapeutic classes. A comprehensive review of the genetic basis of DILI and its mechanisms can be found in [23,26]. For our initial study, we choose the following three medications that have been implicated in patients experiencing DILI: simvastatin, atorvastatin, and zileuton.

This paper is organized as follows: Sect. 2 will discuss our proposed work including potential datasets and ontologies that will be used to exploit semantic knowledge and to create (layered) knowledge graphs. A simple representation informed by the V-Model [21] will model temporal clinical events. We also discuss protocols to apply text analytics to extract patient phenotype data from clinical records. Section 3 will present our current methodology - semantics based edge partitioning (semEP)-to identify patterns in layered graphs; semEP currently can process bipartite graphs with 2 layers [1,20]. Section 4 will outline a case study on DILI.

2   Knowledge Graphs and Datasets and Ontologies

Figure 1 is a representation of the complex and heterogeneous knowledge that will be used to study DILI. The V-Model [21] represents temporal clinical events and provides a framework for clinical problem-action relationships. Temporal clinical events informed by the V-Model, coupled with information from the PharmGKB [28] knowledge graph, is illustrated in Fig. 1. It will provide information for temporal reasoning in order to propose possible drugs (actions) causing an ADR (problems) (Fig. 1, questions 1–3). The questions are as follows:

- What problems indicate the ADR?
- What encounter occurred prior to the ADR?
- What actions could have caused the ADR?

Resources including DrugBank [17], PharmGKB [28], the Human Phenotype Ontology [16,22], and the Disease Ontology [15,25] all capture semantic knowledge around the concepts of drugs, biological pathways, gene-targets, diseases, and phenotypes. They facilitate inferring potential causal relationships between drugs and ADRs (Fig. 1, question 4), namely, *Is the ADR due to a drug?*

We briefly summarize the semantic knowledge that will be applied to our case study as follows:

- We will consider similarities between pairs of drugs and between pairs of gene targets.
- We will consider shared pathways and interactions between pairs of drugs; this may also lead to adverse drug reactions (ADRs).
- We will consider more complex interactions in pathways of drug targets, metabolizing enzymes, transporters, etc.

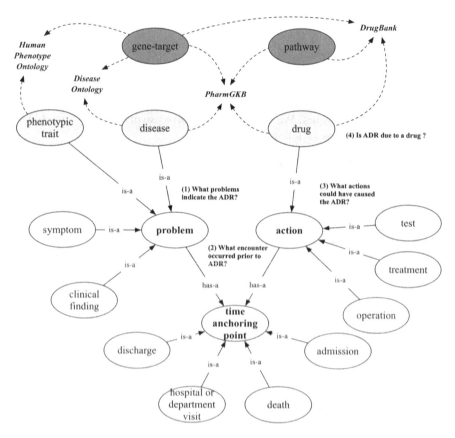

Fig. 1. V-Model Representation of clinical events and the PharmGKB Knowledge Graph for pharmacogenomic data.

– For a drug in use, we will consider interactions between (a) phenotypes or diagnoses associated with an ADR exhibited by the patient and (b) gene targets involved in drug mechanisms. This will provide evidence for or against the drug in question being a causal factor of a given ADR.

Layered Graphs. As will be discussed in the next section, our methodology to discover patterns will focus on typed graphs, i.e., where all nodes and edges are associated with a type. We focus on labeled bipartite graphs, $BG = (D \cup T, WE)$, e.g., D represents a set of drugs, T represents gene-targets, and WE represents interactions between a drug and gene-target pair. We also use the notation $WE(D, T)$ for a bipartite graph. We consider an extension to layered graphs, i.e., a concatenation of two or more bipartite graphs through the concatenation of a pair of edges that are incident on the same node in both graphs. Example layered graphs include the following, where we use the symbol & to represent the concatenation of the individual bipartite graphs:

- Drug-Usage(Patient, Drug) & Interacts(Drug, Pathway) & Interacts(Pathway, Gene-Target).
- Interacts(Drug, Pathway) & Interacts(Pathway, Phenotype-Disease).

We note that we can define the concatenation operator in the spirit of an outer join operator so that edges in the individual bipartite graphs can be retained.

Datasets and Ontologies. We will make extensive use of existing Linked Data resources and ontologies as follows:

- Associations between phenotypes or diseases, time anchoring points and interventions (drugs or treatments) will be extracted from the electronic clinical records of patients taking medications implicated in DILI, including those identified in the LiverTox database [10]:
    http://livertox.nih.gov.
- Drug-target interactions from the following sources: [4,5].
- Drug-drug interactions and ADRs from the ADEpedia portal [12,13]:
    http://informatics.mayo.edu/adepedia/index.php/Main_Page.
- We will use PharmGKB and DrugBank to annotate biological datasets and Unified Medical Language System (UMLS), Human Phenotype Ontology (HPO), and Disease Ontology (DO) to annotate biomedical datasets.
- For drugs, PubChem provides chemical similarity:
    http://pubchem.ncbi.nlm.nih.gov/.
    We will also use similarity values computed from the SMILES chemical representation using SIMCOMP [8].

Protocols to Extract Phenotype from Clinical Records. We will map clinical data into our representation of temporal clinical events (Fig. 1, solid lines). Relevant clinical data will be extracted for known DILI patients using previous approaches [19]. We will consider datasets from environments in which there is an electronic health record systems (EHR) with computerized provider order entry (CPOE) in order to facilitate running queries of temporal data including patient encounters, e.g., visits, and medication orders. Some phenotypes and diagnoses can also be identified using billing codes, e.g., ICD-9 code for "Acute Liver Injury". Many phenotypes relevant to liver injury, however, are captured primarily in clinical notes and will require Natural Language Processing (NLP) and Information Extraction (IE) techniques to find and extract those terms. We will explore the use of existing programs to map biomedical text to concepts in a range of knowledge bases containing disease and phenotype information, including MetaMap [2], Apache cTAKES [24], and the NCBO annotator [14].

3   semEP Methodology to Identify Patterns in Layered Graphs

Our methodology to find patterns in graphs relies on a semantics based edge partitioning (semEP) solution; semEP is a variant of community detection. Details of semEP are in [20]. For ease of understanding, we skip the technical details and use

Fig. 2 to illustrate applying semEP to a bipartite graph between a set of drugs, a set of gene targets, and with drug-to-target interaction edges.

In this example, the semantics are represented by similarity scores between a pair of drugs, as well as between a pair of gene targets. The hypothesis underlying most drug re-purposing solutions is that similar drugs interact with the same targets, and similar targets interact with the same drugs. Thus the similarity scores will be used by semEP for community detection and groups of similar drugs that interact with groups of similar targets will be placed within a cluster.

Further, a drug may be complex in its behavior. Hence, a drug d_j may be similar to another drug d_i based on shared pathways, but it may be more similar to d_k based on chemical structure. To support this, semEP performs an edge partitioning that allows a drug to participate in multiple clusters of communities. In the above case, drug d_j may participate with d_i in one community but may also participate in d_k in another community that does not include d_i.

We summarize the objectives of semEP as follows:

- An edge partitioning that allows the overlap of nodes in multiple clusters; this matches the semantics of complex functions associated with drugs.
- Create clusters with high cluster quality. We have studied a number of metrics including the use of similarity scores and cluster density.
- Exploit semantic knowledge such as edge constraints during edge partitioning.
- Balance these competing objectives by creating a minimal number of clusters, each of which has maximal cluster density (or other metric for cluster quality).

The quality of a cluster is specific to the semantic knowledge encoded in the graph; in this example the quality would be specific to drug-target interactions. A high quality cluster could thus lead to more accurate predictions of previously unknown drug to gene-target interactions. In Fig. 2, known positive interaction edges are black solid edges while predicted edges are red broken edges.

We illustrate the impact of these competing objectives on cluster quality and drug-target interaction prediction accuracy using the two edge partitions A and B in Fig. 2. Consider the following drug-drug and target-target similarity scores: $s_d(d_1, d_3) = s_d(d_2, d_3) = s_t(t_1, t_3) = s_t(t_2, t_3) = 0.1$, and $s_d(d_1, d_2) = s_t(t_1, t_2) = 0.4$. Both partitions have the same cluster density of 0.47; see [20] for details. However, partition A includes four prediction edges while B only includes one prediction edge. Assuming that these are all true positive predictions, then partition A, which satisfies the two semEP objectives of maximum aggregate cluster density and minimal number of clusters, has the same precision and greater recall, compared to partition B. However, there may be a much higher probability that some of the predicted interaction edges are false positives; in this case, partition B may have higher precision and higher accuracy with lower recall.

In the example of Fig. 2, we used drug-drug and target-target similarity to capture semantic knowledge. For DILI, we plan to include additional knowledge, e.g., the type of pathway or the class of drugs.

There are several possible options to extend semEP to layered graphs.

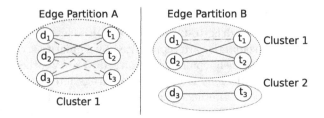

Fig. 2. Two partitions with the same cluster density [20]; solid edges are known positive interactions and red broken edges are predicted interactions

- For the layered graph Drug-Usage(Patient, Drug) & Interacts(Drug, Pathway), we can apply semEP to the two independent bipartite graphs. We can then merge the clusters of Drug-Usage(Patient, Drug) and Interacts(Drug, Pathway) based on the overlap of drugs in these clusters.
- As an alternative, we can choose an order, e.g., Drug-Usage followed by Interactions. Then we first apply semEP to the bipartite graph Drug-Usage(Patient, Drug). The grouping of drugs in these clusters will provide additional constraints that will be used as we next apply semEP to the bipartite graph Interacts(Drug, Pathway).
- A final alternative would be to first apply the concatenation operator to pairs of edges to create a new bipartite graph Drug-UsageANDInteracts(Patient, Pathway). semEP can then be applied to this bipartite graph. The disadvantage is that we may not be able to apply the semantics associated with the two independent bipartite graphs. An additional disadvantage is that this will exclude edges in the original bipartite graphs that do not participate in paths.

4   A Case Study of Drug Induced Liver Injury (DILI)

We report on preliminary results of applying semEP to a bipartite graph of drug to gene-target interactions. We note that our current dataset [4,5] was created with a focus on interactions where a drug *binds* to a specific target. It may not include interaction pathways that reveal how a drug is metabolized or broken down and processed. It is these latter interactions that are most relevant to DILI.

Clusters 1, 3, and 4 in Fig. 3 are associated with simvastatin and/or atorvastatin. Statins inhibit endogenous cholesterol production by inhibiting HMG-CoA reductase (HMGCR). They can be associated with severe outcomes such as liver failure, transplantation and death. One large study analyzing data reported to the Swedish Adverse Drug Reactions Advisory Committee during 1988–2010 found that of 73 suspected DILI cases, 41 % and 38 % were atorvastatin-induced and simvastatin-induced DILI cases, respectively. Two patients died of acute liver failure, one underwent liver transplantation, and three patients were *rechallenged* with the same statin which produced a similar pattern of liver injury [3]. While the cause of hepatic injury from simvastatin[1] and atovastatin[2] is unknown, they

---

[1] http://livertox.nlm.nih.gov/Simvastatin.htm.
[2] http://livertox.nlm.nih.gov/Atorvastatin.htm.

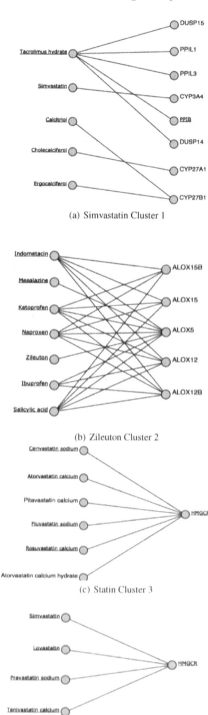

(a) Simvastatin Cluster 1

(b) Zileuton Cluster 2

(c) Statin Cluster 3

(d) Statin Cluster 4

Fig. 3. Four clusters (matching simvastatin, atorvastatin, and zileuton) retrieved from a drug to gene-target interaction dataset [4,5].

are both metabolized in part in the liver by CYP3A4 and are excreted in bile. Statin-induced muscle toxicity such as myalgia, myopathy, myositis and rhabdomyolysis [18] are also relevant ADRs. Candidate gene polymorphisms have been associated with CK elevation (as a marker for muscle toxicity) for simvastatin and atrovastin (ABCB1 [7] and CYP3A5 [29], respectively).

Cluster 1 indicates a direct connection between simvastatin and CYP3A4 which supports existing knowledge of CYP3A4 metabolizing simvastatin in the liver. Another drug that appears in Cluster 1, tacrolimus, is also known to have hepatic metabolism mediated by CYP3A4. Three other drugs, calcitriol, ergocalciferol, and cholecalciferol are used to treat vitamin D deficiency, refractory rickets, familial hypophospatemia and hypoparathyroidism, and hypocalcemia and renal osteodystrophy.

Clusters 3 and 4 support that HMGCR is a relevant enzyme for simvastatin and atorvastatin, respectively. Clusters 3 and 4 together include other statins including cerivastatin, pitavastatin, fluvastatin, rosuvastin, lovastatin, pravastatin, and tenivastatin preparations. Given HMGCR is a drug target for statins broadly, these results are expected and provided confirmatory evidence of the semEP methodology.

Cluster 2 was generated with zileuton as the input medication. zileuton is an anti-inflammatory leukotriene pathway inhibitor that acts by inhibiting the 5-lipoxygenase enzyme (LOX-5). It has been linked to several cases of DILI. In one study with more than 2,000 patients treated with zileuton, it was estimated that less than 0.1 % of patients experienced liver injury [27]. While the mechanism of liver injury due to zileuton is unclear, it most likely occurs through reactive intermediates of metabolism[3].

Cluster 2 indicates that ALOX5 is relevant. This is appropriate given mutations in the promotor region of ALOX5 lead to diminished response to anitleukotriene drugs such as zileuton. Several non-steroidal anti-inflammatory (NSAID) drugs including ibuprofen, naproxen and ketoprofen were also included in Cluster 2. All three medications rarely cause serious acute liver injury. While the mechanisms for liver injury is not well known, heptotoxicity is likely due to an idiosyncratic reaction in a metabolic process for ibuprofen[4], naproxen[5], and ketoprofen[6], and ibuprofen specifically may involve an immuno-allergic reaction.

5   Summary

The paper provides an outline of an ongoing study of drug induced liver injury (DILI) associated with three drugs, simvastatin, atorvastatin, and zileuton. The study will combine genotype, phenotype and pharmacogenomic knowledge and datasets. A simple representation of temporal clinical events informed by the

---

[3] http://livertox.nlm.nih.gov/Zileuton.htm.
[4] http://livertox.nlm.nih.gov/Ibuprofen.htm.
[5] http://livertox.nlm.nih.gov/Naproxen.htm.
[6] http://livertox.nlm.nih.gov/Ketoprofen.htm.

V-Model [21] models temporal clinical events and provides a framework to connect clinical problem-action relationships. A methodology based on semEP - semantics based edge partitioning to create communities - will be extended to find patterns in layered graphs. The results of a preliminary analysis of drug to gene-target *binding* interactions was presented.

References

1. Anderson, P., Thor, A., Benik, J., Raschid, L., Vidal, M.E.: Pang - finding patterns in annotation graphs. In: Proceedings of the ACM Conference on the Management of Data (SIGMOD) (2012)
2. Aronson, A.R., Lang, F.-M.: An overview of metamap: historical perspective and recent advances. J. Am. Med. Inform. Assoc. **17**(3), 229–236 (2010)
3. Björnsson, E., Jacobsen, E.I., Kalaitzakis, E.: Hepatotoxicity associated with statins: reports of idiosyncratic liver injury post-marketing. J. Hepatol. **56**(2), 374–380 (2012)
4. Bleakley, K., Yamanishi, Y.: Supervised prediction of drug-target interactions using bipartite local models. Bioinformatics **25**(18), 2397–2403 (2009)
5. Ding, H., Takigawa, I., Mamitsuka, H., Zhu, S.: Similarity-based machine learning methods for predicting drug-target interactions: a brief review. Briefings Bioinfor. **15**, 734–747 (2013)
6. Fakhraei, S., Huang, B., Raschid, L., Getoor, L.: Network-based drug-target interaction prediction with probabilistic soft logic. IEEE/ACM Trans. Comput. Biol. Bioinfor. **11**, 775–787 (2014)
7. Fiegenbaum, M., Silveira, F.R., Van der Sand, C.R., Van der Sand, L.C., Ferreira, M.E., Pires, R.C., Hutz, M.H.: The role of common variants of abcb1, cyp3a4, and cyp3a5 genes in lipid-lowering efficacy and safety of simvastatin treatment. Clin. Pharmacol. Ther. **78**(5), 551–558 (2005)
8. Hattori, M., Okuno, Y., Goto, S., et al.: Development of a chemical structure comparison method for integrated analysis of chemical and genomic information in metabolic pathways. J. Am. Chem. Soc. **125**(39), 1853–1865 (2003)
9. Ho, J., Ghosh, J., Steinhubl, S., Stewart, W., Denny, J., Malin, B., Sun, J.: Limestone: high-throughput candidate phenotype generation via tensor factorization. J. Biomed. Inform. **52**, 199–211 (2014)
10. Hoofnagle, J.H., Serrano, J., Knoben, J.E., Navarro, V.J.: Livertox: a website on drug-induced liver injury. Hepatology **57**(3), 873–874 (2013)
11. Iyer, S., Harpaz, R., LePendu, P., Bauer-Mehren, A., Shah, N.: Mining clinical text for signals of adverse drug-drug interactions. JAMIA **21**(2), 353–362 (2014)
12. Jiang, G., Liu, H., Solbrig, H., Chute, C.: Adepedia 2.0: integration of normalized adverse drug events (ades) knowledge from the UMLS. In: Proceedings of the AMIA Joint Summits on Translational Science, pp. 100–104 (2013)
13. Jiang, G., Wang, L., Liu, H., Solbrig, H., Chute, C.: Building a knowledge base of severe adverse drug events based on aers reporting data using semantic web technologies. Stud. Health Technol. Inform. **192**, 496–500 (2013)
14. Jonquet, C., Shah, N., Youn, C., Callendar, C., Storey, M.-A., Musen, M.: Ncbo annotator: semantic annotation of biomedical data. In: International Semantic Web Conference (2009)

15. Kibbe, W.A., Arze, C., Felix, V., Mitraka, E., Bolton, E., Fu, G., Mungall, C.J., Binder, J.X., Malone, J., Vasant, D. et al.: Disease ontology 2015 update: an expanded and updated database of human diseases for linking biomedical knowledge through disease data. Nucleic Acids Res. D1071–D1078 (2014)

16. Köhler, S., Doelken, S.C., Mungall, C.J., Bauer, S., Firth, H.V., Bailleul-Forestier, I., Black, G.C., Brown, D.L., Brudno, M., Campbell, J., et al.: The human phenotype ontology project: linking molecular biology and disease through phenotype data. Nucleic Acids Res. 1–9 (2013)

17. Law, V., Knox, C., Djoumbou, Y., Jewison, T., Guo, A.C., Liu, Y., Maciejewski, A., Arndt, D., Wilson, M., Neveu, V., et al.: Drugbank 4.0: shedding new light on drug metabolism. Nucleic Acids Res. **42**(D1), D1091–D1097 (2014)

18. McKenney, J.M., Davidson, M.H., Jacobson, T.A., Guyton, J.R.: Final conclusions and recommendations of the national lipid association statin safety assessment task force. Am. J. Cardiol. **97**(8), S89–S94 (2006)

19. Overby, C.L., Pathak, J., Gottesman, O., Haerian, K., Perotte, A., Murphy, S., Bruce, K., Johnson, S., Talwalkar, J., Shen, Y., et al.: A collaborative approach to developing an electronic health record phenotyping algorithm for drug-induced liver injury. J. Am. Med. Inform. Assoc. pages amiajnl-2013 E243–E252 (2013)

20. Palma, G., Vidal, M.-E., Raschid, L.: Drug-target interaction prediction using semantic similarity and edge partitioning. In: Mika, P., Tudorache, T., Bernstein, A., Welty, C., Knoblock, C., Vrandečić, D., Groth, P., Noy, N., Janowicz, K., Goble, C. (eds.) ISWC 2014, Part I. LNCS, vol. 8796, pp. 131–146. Springer, Heidelberg (2014)

21. Park, H., Choi, J.: V-model: a new perspective for EHR-phenotyping. BMC Medical Informatics and Decision Making, 14(90) (2014)

22. Robinson, P.N., Mundlos, S.: The human phenotype ontology. Clin. Genet. **77**(6), 525–534 (2010)

23. Russmann, S., Jetter, A., Kullak-Ublick, G.: Pharmacogenomics of drug-induced liver injury. Heptology **52**(2), 748–761 (2010)

24. Savova, G.K., Masanz, J.J., Ogren, P.V., Zheng, J., Sohn, S., Kipper-Schuler, K.C., Chute, C.G.: Mayo clinical text analysis and knowledge extraction system (ctakes): architecture, component evaluation and applications. J. Am. Med. Inform. Assoc. **17**(5), 507–513 (2010)

25. Schriml, L.M., Arze, C., Nadendla, S., Chang, Y.-W.W., Mazaitis, M., Felix, V., Feng, G., Kibbe, W.A.: Disease ontology: a backbone for disease semantic integration. Nucleic Acids Res. **40**(D1), D940–D946 (2012)

26. Urban, T., Daly, A., Aithal, G.: Genetic basis of drug-induced liver injury: present and future. Semin. Liver Inj. **34**(2), 123–133 (2014)

27. Watkins, P.B., Dube, L.M., Walton-Bowen, K., Cameron, C.M., Kasten, L.E.: Clinical pattern of zileuton-associated liver injury. Drug Saf. **30**(9), 805–815 (2007)

28. Whirl-Carrillo, M., McDonagh, E., Hebert, J., Gong, L., Sangkuhl, K., Thorn, C., Altman, R., Klein, T.E.: Pharmacogenomics knowledge for personalized medicine. Clin. Pharmacol. Ther. **92**(4), 414–417 (2012)

29. Wilke, R.A., Moore, J.H., Burmester, J.K.: Relative impact of cyp3a genotype and concomitant medication on the severity of atorvastatin-induced muscle damage. Pharmacogenet. Genomics **15**(6), 415–421 (2005)

GEM: The GAAIN Entity Mapper

Naveen Ashish[1(✉)], Peehoo Dewan[1], Jose-Luis Ambite[2], and Arthur W. Toga[1]

[1] Laboratory of NeuroImaging, Keck School of Medicine of USC, USC Stevens Neuroimaging
and Informatics Institute, University of Southern California, 2001 N Soto Street,
Los Angeles, USA
{nashish,pdewan,toga}@loni.usc.edu
[2] Information Sciences Institute, University of Southern California,
4676 Admiralty Way, Marina del Rey, Los Angeles, CA 90292, USA
ambite@isi.edu

Abstract. We present a software system solution that significantly simplifies data sharing of medical data. This system, called GEM (for the GAAIN Entity Mapper), harmonizes medical data. Harmonization is the process of unifying information across multiple disparate datasets needed to share and aggregate medical data. Specifically, our system automates the task of finding corresponding elements across different independently created (medical) datasets of related data. We present our overall approach, detailed technical architecture, and experimental evaluations demonstrating the effectiveness of our approach.

1 Introduction

This paper describes a software solution for medical data *harmonization*. Our work is in the context of the "GAAIN" project in the domain of Alzheimer's disease data. However, this solution is applicable to any medical and clinical data harmonization in general. GAAIN stands for the Global Alzheimer's Association Interactive Network[1], a data sharing federated network of Alzheimer's disease datasets from around the globe. The aim of GAAIN is to create a network of Alzheimer's disease data, researchers, analytical tools and computational resources to better our understanding of this disease. A key capability of this network is also to provide investigators with access to harmonized data across multiple, independently created Alzheimer's datasets.

Our primary interest is in medical data sharing and specifically data that is harmonized in the process of sharing. Harmonized data from multiple data providers has been curated to a unified representation after reconciling the different formats, representation, and terminology from which it was derived [7, 16]. The process of data harmonization can be resource intensive and time consuming and our work is a software solution to significantly automate that process. Data harmonization is fundamentally about data alignment - which is to establish correspondence of related or identical data elements across different datasets. Consider the very simple example of a data element capturing the gender of a subject that is defined as 'SEX' in one dataset, 'GENDER' in another

---

[1] http://www.gaain.org.

© Springer International Publishing Switzerland 2015
N. Ashish and J.-L. Ambite (Eds.): DILS 2015, LNBI 9162, pp. 13–27, 2015.
DOI: 10.1007/978-3-319-21843-4_2

and 'M/F' in yet another. When harmonizing data, a unified element is needed to capture this gender concept and to link (align) the individual elements in different datasets with this unified element.

The data mapping problem can be solved in two ways. We could map elements across two datasets, for instance match the element 'GENDER' from one data source (DATA SOURCE 1) to the element 'SEX' in a second source (DATA SOURCE 2). We could also map elements from one dataset to elements from a *common data model*. A common data model [7] is a uniform representation which all data sources or providers in a data sharing network agree to adopt. The fundamental mapping task is the same in both. Also, the task of data alignment is inevitable regardless of the data sharing model one employs. In a *centralized data sharing* model [15], where we create a single unified store of data from multiple data sources, the data from any data source must be mapped and trans-formed to the unified representation of the central repository. In *federated* or *mediated* approaches to data sharing [7] individual data sources (such as databases) have to be mapped to a "global" unified model through mapping rules [1]. The common data model approach, which is also the GAAIN approach, also requires us to map and transform every dataset to the (GAAIN) common data model. This kind of data alignment or mapping can be a multi-month effort *per dataset* in medical and clinical data integration case studies [1]. A single dataset typically has thousands of distinct data elements of which a large subset needs to be accurately mapped. On the other hand it is well acknowledged that data sharing and integration processes need to be simplified and made less resource intensive for data sharing in the medical and clinical domains [1, 7]) as well as the more general enterprise information integration domain [10]. The GEM system is built to achieve this by providing automated assistance to developers for such data alignment or mapping.

The GEM data mapping approach is centered on exploiting the information in the data documentation, typically in the form of *data dictionaries* associated with the data. The importance of data dictionary documentation, and for Alzheimer's data in particular, has been articulated in (Morris et al., 2006). These data dictionaries contain detailed descriptive information and metadata about each data element in the dataset. The rest of this paper is organized as follows. In the next section (Sect. 2) we review the work and available industrial or open-source software tools that are related to data mapping. This is followed by a detailed description of the GEM system. In Sect. 4 we present experimental results evaluating the efficacy of the GEM system and also a detailed comparison with related data mapping systems. Finally we propose further work and provide a conclusion.

2   Related Technologies

Data mapping is often done manually based on data dictionaries, on any other informa-tion such as database design diagrams [9], and in consultation with the original dataset creators and/or administrators. Data mapping is well understood (Halevy et al., 2005) and there are a number of software tools that have been developed in the past years that relate to it. We first examine existing software tools to (1) determine their applicability to our domain, (2) understand what functions are still needed in the GEM system.

Existing tools can be categorized as metadata visualization tools, Extract-Transform-Load (ETL), and schema-mapping tools. *Metadata visualization tools* are those that create a visual representation of the design of a database by examining the database itself. For instance SchemaSpy[2] provides functionality of "reverse engineering" to create a graphical representation of metadata, such as an "ER" (Entity-Relationship) diagram [9] from the database metadata. Altova[3] is a tool for analyzing and managing relationships among data in data files in XML. These tools are relevant to our task as they can be employed to examine the data and/or metadata of a new dataset that we have to map. *Extract-Transform-Load (ETL)* tools provide support for data schema mapping. However the mappings are not automated and have to be created by hand using a graphical user interface (GUI). Tools in this category include Talend[4], Informatica[5] and Clio (Haas et al., 2000). The category most relevant to our data mapping problem is *Schema-Mapping* which provides automated mapping of data elements from two different database or ontology schemas. These tools take as input the data definition language or "DDL" [9] associated with a dataset (database) and are able to match elements across two database schemas based on the DDL information. Prominent examples in this category include the Harmony schema-mapping tool[6] from the Open Information Integration or OpenII initiative and Coma++ (Rahm et al., 2012). There are also schema-mapping tools that are based on "learning-from-examples" i.e., the system is trained to recognize data element mappings from a tagged corpus of element matches (from the domain of interest). LSD [8] is an example in this category. Another tool is KARMA[7] which actually has more of an ontology alignment focus as opposed to data (element) mapping. Finally, PhenoExplorer [8], is an online tool that allows researchers to identify research studies of interest. Specifically, a researcher can search for studies along a set of dimensions, including race/ethnicity, sex, study design, type of genetic data, genotype platform, and diseases studied and the system determines the relevance of a study by mapping data elements in a study to dimensions specified by a researcher.

Our work was motivated by the observation that the rich metadata available in data dictionaries of medical datasets can be leveraged towards a significantly more automated approach to schema-mapping than could be done with existing tools. The next section describes the details of our approach.

3   Methods

This section describes our approach and the technical details of the GEM system. We begin with enumerating the particular data characteristics of Alzheimer's disease and

---

[2] http://schemaspy.sourceforge.net.
[3] http://www.altova.com.
[4] http://www.talend.com.
[5] http://www.informatica.com.
[6] http://openii.sourceforge.net.
[7] http://www.isi.edu/integration/karma/.

medical data schemas as they bear upon the data mapping approach. We also describe the metadata detail that is typically present in medical data dictionaries that can be accommodated. We then present the GEM architecture and description of the algorithms.

3.1   Medical Data Characteristics

Medical data and associated data schemas have the following characteristics that are relevant to the schema mapping problem:

(i)   **Availability of Metadata but not Data**. Overall, data providers may be more willing to make metadata (dictionaries) available during harmonization but the not the actual data. Alzheimer's and other medical research data are highly sensitive and data providers are typically willing to share their metadata (such as data dictionaries) but actual access to data may be restricted. In fact many data sharing and exploration networks help users to locate relevant data and cohorts but actual data must be obtained directly from data providers (Mandel et al., 2012). The data harmonization and thus the data mapping process must work with the metadata (only), and not assume the availability of actual data. This is an important distinction as some schema mapping tools, such as Coma ++, expect the availability of actual data (as well) to generate mappings.

(ii)   **Element Names and Element Descriptions.** Data elements often have cryptic names in medical datasets. An example is 'TR1S1' which is ill defined and difficult to infer. The element names can also be *composite*. Essentially, a data element may be one of an entire family of elements. For instance an element named 'MOMDEMYR1' has 3 sub-elements in the name which are MOM (for mother), DEM (for dementia) and YR1 for year 1. Element names thus are of limited utility in determining element mappings in this domain. On the other hand the element descriptions are often rather clear and detailed for each data element and we leverage that for mapping.

(iii)   **Presence of Special "Ubiquitous" Data Elements.** There are elements such as the subject identifier, date and timestamp fields, or subject visit number fields that are present in *every* database table in a database. Such elements must be pre-identified and filtered before matching, as they are not candidate matches for other "regular" data elements we seek to match.

3.2   Element Metadata

Relative to other domains such as enterprise data, medical metadata is richer in terms of element descriptions and also accompanying information about the element data type and constraints on values. The detailed metadata that can be extracted or derived from the dictionary information is as follows:

(i)   Element Description. We usually have a text description of what the element fundamentally is. In the example in Fig. 1 this is the text under the 'Short

Descriptor' and 'UDS Question sections' (UDS refers to the Uniform Data Set of clinical and cognitive variables in Alzheimer's disease data). The description is usually comprehensive and verbose to the extent required, as opposed to data schemas in other domains where the element (database column) descriptive information (the 'COMMENT' in a DDL) is simply absent or is typically terse.

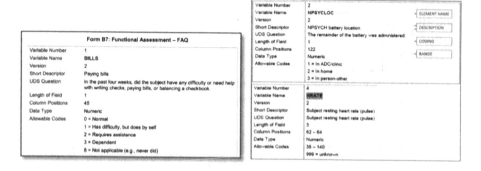

Fig. 1. Element metadata from data dictionary

- Data value constraints. For a majority of data elements, the metadata also contains constraints on the actual values they can take. This information is of two types:
- Coding legend information. The coding legend provided under 'Allowable Codes' tells us the interpretation of various codes, which is the set of possible values that element can take. We can also derive the number of distinct possible values for that element, which is 5 values (0,1,2,3,8) in this example.

(ii)   The Range of Values. For many numerical elements, the metadata provides the explicit range of allowable values, for instance the range 0–30 for 'MMSE' scores, etc. MMSE stands for the Mini-Mental State Examination and is commonly used to measure cognitive impairment (Escobar et al., 1986).

(iii) The Element *Category*. Elements can be divided into a few distinct categories based on the kind of values they can take. For instance the element may take one of small set of prefixed codes as values (as in Fig. 1), or take a numerical value such as the (actual) heart rate, etc., This category can be derived from the metadata and is described in more detail below.

All of the above element information is utilized during data mappings, as we describe.

3.3   System

Before describing the system we clarify some terminology and definitions. A dataset is a *source* of data. For instance a dataset provided by ADNI would be a source. A *data dictionary* is the document associated with a dataset, which defines the terms used in the dataset. A *data element* is an individual 'atomic' unit of information in a dataset, for instance a field or a column in a table in a database or in a spreadsheet. The documentation for each data element in a data dictionary is called *element metadata* or *element information*. A *mapping* or element mapping is a one-to-one relationship across two data elements, coming from different sources. Mappings are created across two distinct sources. The element that we seek to match is called the *query element*. The source we must find matches *from* is called the *target source* and the source of the query element is called the *query source*. Note that a common data model may also be treated as a target source.

The key task of the GEM system is to find element mappings with a "match" operation. "match" is an operation which takes as input (i) a query element, (ii) a target source, and (ii) a matching threshold. It returns a set of elements, from the target source, that match the source element and with a match confidence score associated with each matched element.

Figure 2 illustrates the high level steps of the system. The first step is the *metadata ingestion* step where we start from data dictionaries, extract and synthesize detailed metadata from the data dictionaries for each data element, and store the synthesized metadata in a database. This database is called the *metadata database*. The second step is the *element matching* step where matching algorithms find matches for data elements based on the information in the metadata database.

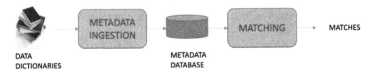

Fig. 2. System phases

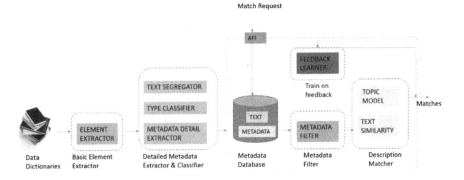

Fig. 3. System architecture

Figure 3 illustrates the architecture and key modules in more detail.

3.3.1 Metadata Ingestion

This part of the pipeline is comprised of two modules. One is for basic individual element metadata extraction from the data dictionary. The other synthesizes detailed metadata per data element.

Basic Element Extractor. The element extractor identifies the description and metadata per data element. In many cases the data dictionary is available in a structured format, such as a spreadsheet, with various components such as the data element name, any (text) descriptions(s) of the field, and other information such the allowable values for the data element etc., clearly delineated. If structured metadata is available this step is not required, however there are instances when data dictionaries are available only as Word or PDF documents. We have developed element extractors for Word and PDF formats to work with these semi-structured documents and extract the per element metadata.

Detailed Metadata Synthesizer. The detailed metadata synthesizer has three components. (1) The first segregates the various important portions of the element overall metadata. (2) The second classifies the data element into a distinct category. (3) The final component extracts specific data constraints that may have been specified for the data element. We describe these.

Segregator: As illustrated in Fig. 1, we model the element information comprised of 4 segments, namely:

(i)   The element or field **name**.
(ii) The text **description** of the element, which is the "Short Descriptor" as well as "UDS Question" in the above example data dictionary.
(iii) The value **coding legend**, for applicable elements.
(iv) The value **numerical range** (if any) for a numerical element.

For many data dictionaries segmentation is already complete if the data dictionary itself is structured with various segments in segregated fields. For other formats, such as the example in Fig. 1 (which is a PDF document) we use simple semi-structured data extraction techniques exploiting the labels for the various segments.

Category classifier: The type information of an element (Data Type') illustrated in Fig. 2 is usually provided. We categorize a data element based on the kinds of values it can take. Data elements fall into one of the below categories:

(i)   **Coded** elements i.e., where the data values are specific codes for a small finite set of values. Coded elements can be:
   a.   **Binary** coded elements i.e., elements that take a Yes/No value
   b.   **Other** coded elements
(ii) **Numerical** elements that take a non-coded, actual numerical value. Examples are elements such blood pressure or heart rate.
(iii) **Text** elements that take an actual text value.

We developed an element category classifier that is driven by heuristics as follows:

- Coded elements can be identified by the presence of a coding legend in the element metadata.
- Coded elements can further be classified as Binary Coded elements if they contain legend values such as Yes/No, Present/Absent, 0/1, Normal/Abnormal etc.,
- Numerical elements have a (data) type for numbers (such as integer, float etc.). Also a range is usually specified for numerical elements.
- Text elements have a data type for text strings.
- Special elements
- Elements for date or timestamps are identified by appropriate regular expression patterns
- (Subject) identifier elements are identified by the element name, usually having indicators such as 'ID' in the name.

Metadata Detail Extractor: Here we extract and synthesize the metadata details, specifically, (i) The element cardinality (number of distinct possible data values) from the coding legend, and (ii) The range (minimum and maximum permissible values) for numerical values. This extraction and derivation (for cardinality) is performed using simple regular expression based extraction patterns, and label information.

3.3.2   Metadata Database
The metadata database is a uniform, detailed repository of the extracted metadata. This metadata database powers the various matching algorithms in the matching phase.

3.3.3   Matching
The matching step has two sub-steps as follows:

(1) A *candidate elimination* or *blocking* sub-step, where for a given data element we eliminate *incompatible* candidate elements from consideration. The incompatibility is determined using some metadata details. This step is analogous to *blocking* in record linkage where incompatible or improbable candidates are eliminated in a filtering step (Minton et al., 2005).
(2) A *similarity matching* sub-step, where we determine similarity among compatible candidate elements (to the original element we are seeking a match for) based on the element description.

Incompatible Candidate Blocking. Incompatible candidates can be identified in different ways. The first, applicable to all data elements, is if the original element and the candidate match element have incongruent (different) categories. So essentially all candidates with element category other than that of the original element are incompatible. Candidates can then further be eliminated based on the other metadata constraints, specifically cardinality or range. The cardinality of an element applies to elements where the data values take one of a fixed and finite set of values, typically the set of values is small. The cardinality of the element is then the number of possible such data values it can take. The cardinalities of two matching elements need to be "close" but not necessarily exactly equal. For instance one data source may have a GENDER element with cardinality of 3 (taking values 'M', 'F', or 'U' for unknown) whereas another source may have a corresponding (gender) element with cardinality of 4 (say 1 each for male and female, 1 for unknown, and 1 for error). For a given element with cardinality O we assume that the cardinalities of any corresponding elements are distributed *normally* with O as the mean and a standard deviation of 1. For a candidate element, with cardinality O', we compute the probability that O' belongs to the normal distribution with $\mu = O$ and $\sigma = 1$. Candidates with this probability below a certain threshold are eliminated.

Candidates in the numerical category can be eliminated based on a range of values. Certain elements have a strict fixed range, by definition, in any dataset. For instance the MMSE score element by definition takes values 0–30 (only). On the other hand an element for heart rate may have a range specified as 35–140 in one dataset and 30–150 in another, both being "reasonable" range bounds for the values. We employ a *range match score* (RMS) that is defined as follows:

$$RMS\,(e1, e2) = \frac{|\min\,(U1, U2) - \max\,(L1, L2)|}{\max\,(U1 - L1, U2 - L2)}$$

This RMS score is measure of the overlap of the range of values across two elements. Candidates with an RMS score below a certain threshold are eliminated.

Similarity Matching. After candidate elimination based on metadata constraints we compute an element similarity match based on the similarity of the element text descriptions. We mentioned that the element (text) description is relatively more comprehensive and verbose in medical data dictionaries and this is the reason we have explored and utilized more sophisticated approaches to determine element description similarity across two elements. Our approach employs *topic modeling* on the element descriptions. Topic modeling (Blei 2012) is an unsupervised machine learning approach, which is used for discovering the abstract "topics" that occur in a collection of documents (data dictionaries). The underlying hypothesis is that a document is a mixture of various topics and that each word in the document is attributable to one of the document's topics. We formally define a topic to be a probability distribution over the unique words in the collection. Topic modeling is a generative statistical modeling technique which defines a joint probability over both observed and hidden random variables. This joint probability is used to calculate the conditional distribution of the hidden variables given the observed variables. In our case, the documents in the collection are the observed variables whereas the topic structure which includes both the topic distribution per document and the word distribution per topic is latent or hidden.

In our approach, each column from the source is considered as a document, with the column name as the document name and the column description as the content of the document. After formatting our input in this way and generating a topic model, we receive a document distribution probability matrix where each row represents a document, each column represents a topic, and each particular document topic cell contains the probability that the particular document belongs to that particular topic. Thus we have for each document i.e., element description, a probability distribution over the set of topics. The similarity between two element descriptions is the cosine similarity or dot product [18] of the topic probability distribution vectors associated with the two element descriptions. The description similarity (DS) is defined as:

$$DS(e1, e2) = TPV(e1.description) \cdot TPV(e2.description)$$

where TPV = Topic Probability Vector (associated with an element description).

4   Results

We conducted a series of experimental evaluations with the GEM system which are centered on evaluating the mapping accuracy of GEM with various data schema pairs. Specifically, we determined (i) The optimal configuration for the GEM system that results in high mapping accuracy, (ii) The actual data mapping accuracy that can be achieved by GEM for various GAAIN dataset pairs, and (iii) Comparison of mapping accuracy of GEM with that of other schema-mapping systems.

Experimental Setup. We used six of the data sources of Alzheimer's disease data that we have in GAAIN namely (1) the Alzheimer's Disease Neuroimaging Initiative (ADNI) [17], (2) the National Alzheimer's Coordinating Center database (NACC) [3], (3) the Dominantly Inherited Alzheimer Network database (DIAN) [13], (4) the Integrated Neurogenerative Disease Database (INDD) [21], (5) the Layton Aging and Alzheimer's Disease Center database [20] and (6) the Canadian Longitudinal Study of Aging (CLSA)[8]. The original data provider provided the data dictionaries for each source. We conducted multiple data mappings using GEM, for various pairs of the six datasets as well from the datasets (one at a time) to the GAAIN common model. We also conducted data mappings for some of these dataset pairs using the Harmony system, for comparison. We manually created truth sets of data mappings across these dataset pairs, which are used as the gold standard against which GEM generated mappings are evaluated.

Mapping Accuracy Evaluations. The GEM system provides multiple alternatives as suggested matches for a given data element. The (maximum) number of alternatives provided is configurable. We present results showing data mapping accuracy as a function of the number of alternatives for a set of evaluations below.

Topic modeling vs TFIDF. The first set of evaluations is to determine the effectiveness of topic modeling based text description by evaluating the impact of the text description match algorithm on the mapping accuracy. In addition to topic modeling based text match we also employed a TF-IDF Cosine similarity (Tata and Patel, 2007) algorithm for matching text descriptions. The mapping accuracies for various schema pairs are shown in Fig. 4.

---

[8] http://www.cihr-irsc.gc.ca.

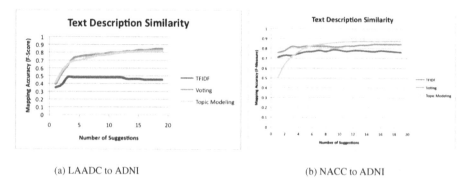

(a) LAADC to ADNI   (b) NACC to ADNI

Fig. 4. Text description similarity algorithm impact

Our results with various pairs of schemas, of which the three pairs illustrated in Fig. 4 are a subset, show that in most cases the mapping accuracy achieved with topic modeling based text description matching is superior to that achieved with TFIDF based text matching. This is however not the case universally as in the INDD to ADNI mapping (not illustrated) TFIDF based mapping outperformed that based on topic modeling. Our observation is that topic modeling based text matching works better when the two sources (being matched) have comprehensive data dictionaries with verbose text descriptions for data elements. On the other hand TFIDF appears to work better when one or both data sources have dictionaries with brief or succinct element text descriptions. While not obvious, this result is not surprising given that the underlying topic model generation algorithm, Latent Dirichlet Allocation (LDA), works by finding cohesive themes in large collections of unstructured data (Blei 2012). More elaborate element text descriptions provide a better basis for this algorithm to discover themes in the corpus of all descriptions. In Fig. 4 also show results for an approach that combines TFIDF and topic modeling text match. We use a voting algorithm that considers, for a specific matching instance, either one of topic modeling or TFIDF for determining the text similarity based on which of the two text matching approaches has a higher text match similarity score. The text match similarity score is in the range 0–1 for both approaches. A more principled way to address this however would be to assess the probabilistic confidence that a pair of elements match, given the match similarity scores from both TFIDF and topic modeling approaches. We propose to add this as part of the larger effort of incorporating machine-learning techniques into the system that we discuss in the Conclusions section.

Impact of Blocking Based on Metadata Constraints. Figure 5 illustrates the impact of employing metadata data constraint based filtering or blocking on mapping where we evaluate mapping accuracy with and without the metadata based blocking step.

We see that using metadata constraint based blocking indeed provides an improvement in mapping accuracy. The improvement is about 5 % on average and as high as 10 % in some cases as evaluated by mapping across various schema pairs.

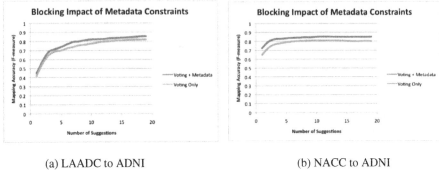

(a) LAADC to ADNI   (b) NACC to ADNI

Fig. 5. Impact of metadata Constraint Based Blocking

Comparison with Other Systems. We also compared our system with related systems to the extent we could, given limitations of other systems. Our aim was to compare the mapping accuracy of various schema pairs provided to GEM as well as to systems with identical functionality namely Harmony and Coma++. For Harmony, we could complete this comparison for only one of the schema pairs as the system could not work with other schema pairs, given its limitations in terms of the total number of database tables and columns it can reason with. That comparison, NACC to ADNI, is provided in Fig. 6(a) where GEM was significantly superior (around 12–15 % better) than Harmony in mapping this dataset pair. With Coma++, the mapping accuracies for all dataset pairs were less than an F-Measure of 0.3 and we do not report these results. Coma ++ is not designed to consider element text descriptions in schema mapping and the focus is more on matching ontology and XML schemas based on structural information (Bosch et al., 2011).

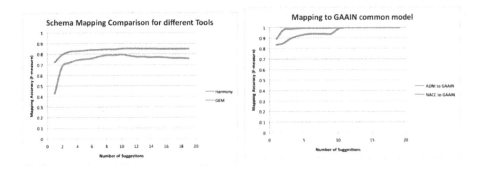

(a)   Comparison with Harmony   (b) Common Model Mapping

Fig. 6. Comparison, and mapping to GAAIN common model

Mapping to GAAIN Common Model. Finally, we evaluated the mapping accuracy of GEM to the current GAAIN common data model. The GAAIN common data model currently comprises of 24 data elements of key subject data elements that include demographic elements such as age and gender and also select patient assessments and scores. We represented the common model as (just) another data schema. The results of the mapping from ADNI to GAAIN and NACC to GAAIN are shown in Fig. 6(b).

4.1 Conclusions from Results

The experimental results provide several important conclusions regarding the performance and the configuration of GEM. The GEM system provides high mapping accuracy, in the range of 85 % or above F-Measure for GAAIN datasets and the common model, and for reasonable result window sizes of 6 to 8 result alternatives. The system performs better than existing systems such as Harmony, in terms of both scalability in handling large data schemas as well as mapping accuracy. From a system configuration perspective we can conclude that it is indeed beneficial to determine element text description similarity using a sophisticated topic modeling based approach. This generally results in higher schema mapping accuracies, compared to using existing text similarity techniques. Further, it is advantageous to train the topic model used for text matching, on element text descriptions from a large number of data sources. Finally, metadata constraint based blocking is beneficial in achieving higher accuracy of mapping.

5 Conclusion

We described and evaluated the GEM system in this paper. Compared to existing schema mapping approaches, the GEM system is better optimized for medical data mapping such as in Alzheimer's disease research. Our experimental evaluations demonstrate significant mapping accuracy improvements that have been obtained with our approach, particularly by leveraging the detailed information synthesized from data dictionaries.

Currently we are integrating the GEM system with the overall GAAIN data transformation platform so that developers can operationally use the mapping capabilities to integrate new datasets. We are also enhancing the system with machine-learning based classification for schema mapping. This will enable us to systematically combine various match indicators such as text similarity using multiple approaches such as topic modeling and TFIDF cosine similarity, and also features based on data element name similarity. We are also developing an active learning capability (Rubens, Kaplan and Sugiyama, 2011) where developers can vet or correct GEM system mappings and the system is able to learn and improve from such feedback.

References

1. Ashish, N., Ambite, J.L., Muslea, M., Turner, J.A.: Neuroscience data integration through mediation: an (F)BIRN case study. Front. Neuroinform. 4:118 (2010). doi: 10.3389/fninf. 2010.00118. PUBMED PMID: 21228907 PMCID: PMC3017358

2. Aumueller, D., Do, H.H., Massmann, S., Rahm, E.: Schema and ontology matching with COMA++. In: Proceedings of the 2005 ACM SIGMOD International Conference on Management of Data, pp. 906–908. ACM, June 2005

3. Beekly, D.L., Ramos, E.M., Lee, W.W., et al.: The National Alzheimer's Coordinating Center (NACC) database: the uniform data set. Alzheimer Dis. Assoc. Disord. **21**, 249–258 (2007)

4. Blei, D.M.: Probabilistic topic models. Commun. ACM **55**(4), 77–84 (2012). doi: 10.1145/2133806.2133826. http://doi.acm.org/10.1145/2133806.2133826

5. Bosch, T., Mathiak, B.: Generic multilevel approach designing domain ontologies based on XML schemas. In: Workshop Ontologies Come of Age in the Semantic Web, pp. 1–12 (2011)

6. Do, H.H., Melnik, S., Rahm, E.: Comparison of schema matching evaluations. In: Chaudhri, A.B., Jeckle, M., Rahm, E., Unland, R. (eds.) Web, Web-Services, and Database Systems 2002. LNCS, vol. 2593, pp. 221–237. Springer, Heidelberg (2003)

7. Doan, A., Halevy, A., Ives, Z.: Principles of Data Integration. Elsevier, Amsterdam (2012)

8. Doan, A., Domingos, P., Halevy, A.Y.: Reconciling schemas of disparate data sources: a machine-learning approach. In: ACM Sigmod Record, vol. 30, no. 2, pp. 509–520. ACM, May 2001

9. Garcia-Molina, H.: Database Systems: The Complete Book. Pearson Education, India (2008)

10. Halevy, A.Y., Ashish, N., Bitton, D., Carey, M., Draper, D., Pollock, J., Sikka, V.: Enterprise information integration: successes, challenges and controversies. In: Proceedings of the 2005 ACM SIGMOD International Conference on Management of Data, pp. 778–787. ACM, June, 2005

11. Karlawish, J., Siderowf, A., Hurtig, H., Elman, L., McCluskey, L., Van Deerlin, V., Lee, V.M., Trojanowski, J.Q.: Building an integrated neurodegenerative disease database at an academic health center. Alzheimer's Dement. **7**, e84–e93 (2011). doi: 10.1016/j.jalz.2010.08

12. Mandel, A.J., Kamerick, M., Berman, D., Dahm, L.: University of California Research eXchange (UCReX): a federated cohort discovery system. In: 2012 IEEE International Conference on Healthcare Informatics, Imaging and Systems Biology, p. 146 (2012)

13. Morris, J.C., Weintraub, S., Chui, H.C., Cummings, J., DeCarli, C., Ferris, S., Foster, N.L., Galasko, D., Graff-Radford, N., Peskind, E.R., Beekly, D., Ramos, E.M., Kukull, W.A.: The Uniform Data Set (UDS): clinical and cognitive variables and descriptive data from Alzheimer Disease Centers. Alzheimer Dis. Assoc. Disord. **20**(4), 210–216 (2006)

14. Morris, J.C., et al.: Developing an international network for Alzheimer's research: the Dominantly Inherited Alzheimer Network. Clin. Invest. (Lond) **2**(10), 975–984 (2012). PMCID: PMC3489185

15. NDAR: National Database of Autism Research (2014). Web: http://ndar.nih.gov

16. Ohmann, C., Kuchinke, W.: Future developments of medical informatics from the viewpoint of networked clinical research. Methods Inf. Med. **48**(1), 45–54 (2009)

17. Shen, L., Thompson, P.M., Potkin, S.G., Bertram, L., Farrer, L.A., Foroud, T.M., Green, R.C., Hu, X., Huentelman, M.J., Kim, S., Kauwe, J.S., Li, Q., Liu, E., Macciardi, F., Moore, J.H., Munsie, L., Nho, K., Ramanan, V.K., Risacher, S.L., Stone, D.J., Swaminathan, S., Toga, A.W., Weiner, M.W., Saykin, A.J.: Generic analysis of quantitative phenotypes in AD and MCI: imaging, cognition and biomarkers. Brain Imaging Behav. **8**(2), 183–207 (2014)

18. Sidorov, G., Gelbukh, A., Gómez-Adorno, H., Pinto, D.: Soft similarity and soft cosine measure: similarity of features in vector space model. Computación y Sistemas **18**(3), 491–504 (2014). doi: 10.13053/CyS-18-3-2043. Accessed 7 October 2014

19. Tata, S., Patel, J.: Estimating the selectivity of tf-idf based cosine similarity predicates. SIGMOD Rec. **36**(2), 75–80 (2007)

20. Wu, X., Li, J., Ayutyanont, N., Protas, H., Jagust, W., Fleisher, A., Reiman, E., Yao, L., Chen, K.: The receiver operational characteristic for binary classification with multiple indices and its application to the neuroimaging study of Alzheimer's disease. IEEE/ACM Trans. Comput. Biol. Bioinf. **10**, 173–180 (2013)
21. Xie, S.X., Baek, Y., Grossman, M., Arnold, M.S., Weiner, M.W., Thal, L.J., Peterson, R.C., Jack, C., Jagust, W., Trojanowski, J.Q., Toga, A.W., Beckett, L.: Alzheimer's disease neuroimaging initiative. Neuroimaging Clin. N. Am. **15**(4), 869–877 (2008)

Data Integration in the Human Brain Project

Tassos Venetis[✉] and Vasilis Vassalos

Department of Informatics, Athens University of Economics and Business,
Patision 76, 10434 Athens, Greece
`avenet@aueb.gr`

Abstract. The Medical Informatics Platform of the Human Brain Project has the challenging task of organizing and presenting to its users a variety of data originating from different hospitals and hospital systems in a unified way, while protecting patients privacy as imposed by national legislation and institutional ethics. In this paper we view these challenges under the scope of data integration and analyze preliminary steps taken towards realizing the Medical Informatics Platform.

Keywords: Data integration · Standardization · Medical data

1 Introduction

Understanding the brain is one of the greatest challenges facing 21st century science. Gaining profound insights into what makes us human, developing new treatments for brain diseases and building revolutionary new computation technologies is the main goal of the Human Brain Project (HBP), a 10-year EU flagship project with 135 partner institutions in 26 countries. HBP will achieve its objective through the development of six ICT platforms dedicated to Neuroinformatics, Brain Simulation, High Performance Computing, Medical Informatics, Neuromorphic Computing and Neurorobotics, whose names are self-explanatory.

The goal of the Medical Informatics Platform (MIP) is to federate clinical data, such as genetics, imaging, and other, currently locked in hospital and research archives and make them available to relevant research communities, while guaranteeing protection for sensitive patient information as imposed by national legislation and institutional ethics. Subsequently, these data will be used with the aid of sophisticated Data Mining algorithms and techniques in order to identify biological signatures of diseases, mostly related to brain, as well as predict features of the brain that are difficult or even impossible to measure experimentally. The overall results will be used for diagnosis, more accurate prognosis and new types of drug discovery for the development of new medicines.

MIP similar projects are VPH-share,[1] p-medical,[2] and @neurIST.[3] VPH-Share system is an infrastructure which provides services for sharing and access

---

[1] http://www.vph-share.eu/.
[2] http://p-medicine.eu/.
[3] http://www.aneurist.org/.

© Springer International Publishing Switzerland 2015
N. Ashish and J.-L. Ambite (Eds.): DILS 2015, LNBI 9162, pp. 28–36, 2015.
DOI: 10.1007/978-3-319-21843-4_3

to data and tools for biomedical research and modeling, that however, has no control over the models, tools and data that are shared through its services. It cannot provide any assurances as to the quality of the material that is made available by external contributors, which constitutes a major difference comparing to MIP, where data quality is a significant consideration. In contrast, p-medicine, is much more tightly controlled. It focuses on specific communities in the cancer domain and on developing new tools, IT infrastructure and (Virtual Physiological Human) VPH models to accelerate personalized medicine. It has strong focus on data quality, curation and integration as well as data security. Finally, @neurIST is an initiative that integrates biomedical informatics in the management of cerebral aneurysms and has created a secure system that shares privacy preserving data from hospitals across Europe, in a same manner as planned for MIP.

MIP is composed of three different layers, as shown in Fig. 1. The first one, called the Web Portal, is the user interface of the platform, where users depending on their access rights will be able to perform epidemiological exploration queries, interactive analysis queries as well as complex data mining tasks, on the available data. The second layer, called the Federation Layer is responsible for translating

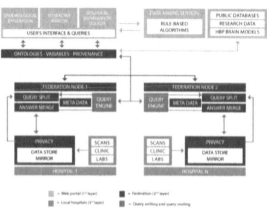

Fig. 1. The medical informatics platform

queries posed over the Web Portal to proper queries that can be answered from each individual hospital. Additionally, it is responsible for collecting responses from individual hospitals and merging their results. Finally, the Local Layer is responsible for collecting disparate (raw) hospital data and making them available in a unified manner. Such data are images (MRIs), CSV files or even raw text, output of proprietary medical systems, as well as relational databases; either commercial or open source.

It is obvious that the challenges MIP is confronted with are mainly data integration challenges. Data Integration has gained a lot of attention in life sciences as the explosion of data in the biomedical research and in the healthcare systems demands urgent solutions for data management [3,9,10,16]. Data integration is the key to interoperable access, hence a key objective of the MIP.

In this paper, we show how data integration theory binds with the needs of each layer of the architecture of MIP. We present a preliminary approach to the proposed solutions that involves the exchange of data, the use of ontologies/terminologies for standardization, as well as (distributed) query answering, while protecting sensitive patient information.

2 Data Integration

The goal of Data Integration [5,8,11,14,18,20] is to provide users with uniform access over a set of disparate data sources that have been created and stored autonomously. A variety of possible architectures exist, however they all fall somewhere in the spectrum between *warehousing* and *virtual integration.*

In warehousing, data from individual data sources are subject to complex transformation processes, which may include cleaning, value transformations and aggregation, and then are loaded into a target database, accessible to users. When those complex transformations are defined by declarative (schema) mappings and performed through a chase procedure [1] the process is called *data exchange* [6]. On the other hand, in virtual integration no physical database is created. Instead, users interact with the data integration system through a single target logical schema, called global, that provides the unified view of the whole system and does not contain stored data. In this setting the data reside in the data sources, where they were originally stored, and are accessed, with the aid of declarative (schema) mappings, at query time.

The formalism used to express schema mappings, in both data exchange and virtual integration, is Tuple Generating Dependencies (TGDs) [1], that can also be used to express constraints in a database schema. In our setting we consider s-t TGDs, a subset of TGDs whose body (head) contains only source (target) predicates to express schema mappings, and weakly acyclic TGDS, to express target constraints, that offer PTIME data and EXPTIME combined complexity [6]. For example, the following formula is a (s-t) TGD (that also contains user defined functions) that joins tuples of tables *hbp_diags* and *hbp_patients* on the *hid* attribute/variable and populates the *diagnostic* table with values of the *pid*, *code*, *type*, and *date* variables. Moreover "$CHUV$" is a constant, while newID is a function that produces a unique identification number for each tuple.

$$hbp\_diags(hid, \textbf{date}, \textbf{code}, \ descr, \textbf{type}), hbp\_patients(hid, \textbf{pid}, \ldots) \rightarrow$$
$$diagnostic(\textsf{newID}(), \textbf{pid}, \textbf{code}, \textbf{type}, \textbf{date}, "CHUV") \quad (1)$$

3 MIP Architecture and Data Integration

In this section we present a detailed bottom up analysis of the MIP architecture (Fig. 1) while at the same time we highlight the data integration challenges that each MIP layer faces, as well as the approaches towards addressing them.

3.1 Local Layer

Initially, the Local Layer is responsible for collecting hospital data and creating a Local Data Store Mirror (LDSM), for every participating hospital. This Mirror will be the access point of the MIP to the hospital data, through the RAW query engine [12], an in situ query processor that eliminates data loading by accessing data in its original format and location.

The original hospital data provided for the creation of the LDSM, include raw data, such as images (MRIs), CSV files that correspond to genetics and clinical data. They use divergent schemata and possibly different references to the same objects, hence we need to deal with syntactic, value and semantic heterogeneities and inconsistencies. All these challenges imply that the Local Layer addresses a data warehousing integration problem. To the time being the only hospital that participates in the MIP is the University Hospital of Lausanne (CHUV).

The first challenge addressed towards the creation of the LDSM for CHUV is the creation of its schema. At its current state, it consists of thirteen tables, that describe information regarding patients, diagnostics, diseases, laboratory examinations, genetic information as well as brain information. Additionally, these tables describe meta-data, such as annotations and provenance information. Schema creation is tightly connected with variable extraction, a collaborative effort between computer scientists and medical experts identifying variables that play a prominent role in the supported MIP services. Moreover, an effort is undertaken for the schemata of the local hospitals to be similar to each other and to that of the Web Portal. An efficient way to achieve this is by using standardized schema variables. So, another challenge is the standardization of the extracted variables and their values. These challenges are also addressed at the Web Portal.

Our approach, regarding (data and query) standardization, concerns using variables (query terms) from the Logical Observation Identifier Names and Codes (LOINC) [7] ontology. LOINC provides a universal code system for reporting laboratory and other clinical observations and contains more than 30,000 different observations. For each observation the LOINC database includes a code, a long formal name, a "short" name as well as synonyms. For example, the *diagnosis* variable is represented by code 52797-8, with a long (and short) name "Diagnosis ICD code", and synonyms "International Classification of Diseases", "DX ICD code" and other.

Additionally, in order to capture the MRI image processing pipelines we have followed the Cortical Labelling Protocol [13] atlas that identifies brain regions. Region examples are "Right Cerebellum Exterior", "Left Hippocampus" and others and corresponding values are estimated volumes in cc produced by a feature extraction process [2]. Moreover, regarding genetic data, we focus on Single Nucleotide Polymorphisms (SNPs) that represent the difference in a pair of nucleotides from the general population. SNPs are probably the most important category of genetic changes influencing common diseases, since they have been shown to influence disease risk, drug efficacy and side-effects, provide information about ancestry, and predict aspects of how humans look and even act. We follow rs names provided by dbSNP [19]. For example, rs2075650 is an example of an SNP found on gene TOMM40 of chromosome 19 associated with high risk of Alzheimer disease. Each SNP is represented by a value from the range of $\{0, 1, 2\}$, where 0 means that the two nucleotides are the same as the reference (healthy nucleotides), 1 means that one of them is different, while 2 that both are different.

While the above standards capture variables used when issuing a query, standardization is also needed to provide query constant values as well as to capture answers of queries. Therefore, our approach incorporates International

Classification of Diseases ICD-10 codes [17] that refer to classification of mental and behavioural disorders. For example, *Alzheimer disease with early onset*, represented by code G30.1, is a subcategory of *Alzheimer disease*, represented by code G30.

In order to populate the LDSM with metadata provided by standards TGDs are used. For example TGD

$$hbp\_SNP(\textbf{pid}, \textbf{rsName}, \textbf{rsValue}), dbSNP(\textbf{rsName}, \textbf{gene}, \textbf{chrom}, pos) \rightarrow$$
$$gene\_snp(\textbf{pid}, \textbf{rsName}, \textbf{rsValue}, \textbf{gene}, \textbf{chrom}, \text{date}()) \quad (2)$$

joins tables *hbp_SNP* and *dbSNP* on the *rsName* variable and creates tuples that are enriched with gene and chromosome information, beside the specific rs and its value. The same applies, in a similar manner, for every used standard.

Besides standardization TGDs are used in order to address another major challenge; the creation of schema mappings that ensure necessary transformations will be applied on the original CHUV data to translate them to a uniform coherent representation, i.e., the LDSM schema. These transformations will be performed to all but imaging data and include cleaning, normalizing and integrating/merging the input data. Use of declarative mappings is heavily based on the fact that mappings are formal, easily reusable, even by non computer experts and that chase engines can be highly efficient.

For the creation and execution of all these TGDs we have developed a visual mapping tool, called MIPMap (Fig. 2) that extends the open source mapping tool ++Spicy [15] in order to meet the needs of HBP. MIPMap, also includes an improved mapping execution engine to deal with the complexity and size of HBP data transformations. MIPMap supports the execution of s-t TGDs while allowing the target schema to contain weakly acyclic constraints.

The first batch of data available to populate the CHUV LDSM involves patient information as well as diagnostics for patients over eighteen years old that have undergone imaging examinations. More precisely, tables *hbp_diags* and *hbp_patient* have been made available. The first one includes information about diagnostic examinations, while the second general information about these patients. Taking into account the schema created for the CHUV Local Data Store Mirror, shown in the right of Fig. 2, we have created a set of TGDs that are able to translate the input data to the schema of the Local Data Store Mirror. These TGDs are rules (1) and (3).

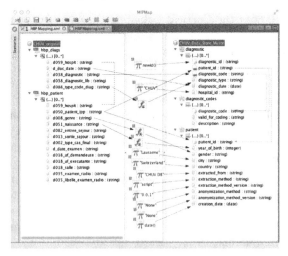

Fig. 2. MIPMap mapping tool.

Note that *hospitalid* and *patient_ipp* (presented as *hid* and *pid*, respectively, in the rules) values used are not the original hospital and patient identification numbers, but pseudo-identification numbers produced at the first stage of the anonymization process. Additionally, note that table *diagnostic_codes* (Fig. 2) is populated by ICD-10 codes and descriptions.

$$hbp\_patients(hid, \textbf{pid}, \textbf{gender}, \textbf{dob}, entrD, extD, \ldots) \rightarrow$$

$$patient(\textbf{pid}, \textsf{yOB}(\textbf{dob}), \textsf{sel}(\textbf{gender}), \text{``}Lausanne\text{''}, \text{``}Switzerland\text{''}, \textsf{date}()) \quad (3)$$

Rule (3) uses the *pid*, *dob* (date of birth) and *gender* variables of table *hbp_patients* in order to populate table *patient*. *pid* values are copied, while *dob* and *gender* values undergo a pre-processing step. More precisely, function yOB is applied on the *dob* values to extract the year of birth. Subsequently, since the original CHUV data is in French, function *sel* reads the input gender (*homme* or *femme*) and selects its English equivalent. Finally, function date outputs the current date (date of translation), while also constant values *Lausanne* and *Switzerland* are used to populate the *patient* table. Hence, except for the direct translation of variable values, MIPMap also allows the use of functions that are performed on tuple's values and produce outputs that populate the target schema. Note, that MIPMap also supports the use of existential variables in the head of the TGDs.

Anonymization. Guaranteeing protection for sensitive patient information as imposed by national legislation and institutional ethics, is a key constraint for the development of MIP. This will be achieved through an anonymization process, that is separated in two stages.[4]

The first stage, concerns the anonymization of the original hospital data, that are going to be stored on the LDSM. More precisely, data exported by hospital systems will follow a anonymization process according to the Health Insurance Portability and Accountability Act (HIPAA) [4]. HIPAA provides 18 identifiers that should be removed from any dataset in order for the dataset to be safe and cannot be used to identify an individual. For the MIP the identifiers to be removed are names, social security numbers, medical record numbers and biometric identifiers. Regarding imaging data other approaches will also be employed such as performing data normalization, that will ensure that patients cannot be identified by MRIs. Hence, the LDSM will not contain information that can be used to identify individuals.

At the second stage, all the query results leaving the LDSM will be filtered for any personal identifiers left, such as headers of imaging data. Additionally, certain fields that could compromise the privacy of patients will be excluded by the queries of the Web Portal. Moreover, the LDSM shall respond to queries by only returning aggregated results and never individual patient details. Especially for cases where less than k values exist the MIP shall provide k-anonymity [21].

---

[4] CHUV anonymization will be performed by gnúbila, an external subcontractor.

3.2 Federation Layer

The Federation Layer hides from the users of the platform the distributed architecture, i.e., the fact that hospital data remain stored at each hospital.

Initially, it is responsible for forwarding analysis and data mining queries to the hospitals and collecting/merging their results. However, the sensitive patient information protection constraints of MIP imply a no move/no copy policy of individual patient data while allowing only aggregate information to leave each hospital (see also Sect. 3.1). This combined with the distributed storage of the data produce limitations in the way that the analyses and data mining algorithms can be performed. For example, analysis and data mining algorithms need to compute complex measures, such as entropy (for the ID3 algorithm), that are statistical measures performed on the overall dataset (all the hospitals). Since the information retrieved from each hospital cannot contain individual records but only aggregates (counts, sums, etc.) each algorithm will have to be implemented in a distributed manner taking into consideration these constraints. Hence, the Federation Layer will play a key role in pushing down to hospitals computations needed for each task, possibly in an iterative manner, following the privacy preserving limitations.

Additionally, even though an effort is undertaken for all hospital schemata to be identical, and hence for the Web Portal schema to also be identical to them, achieving this is highly unlikely. Therefore, the Federation Layer will be responsible, except for forwarding queries to the hospitals, to also reformulate them, i.e., translate them into terms and nomenclature that is used by each hospital. To achieve this declarative schema mappings need to be provided between the Web Portal and each hospital. To this end we have been developing a web based version of MIPMap, that will be responsible for semi-automatically creating mappings, through the implementation of various schema matching techniques and algorithms [5], as well as for applying query reformulation on issued queries and merging gathered hospital results.

4   Conclusion

In this paper we have presented the architecture of the Human Brain Project Medical Informatics Platform and have highlighted the significance of data integration challenges it faces. Additionally, we have presented the integration approaches we are undertaking towards realizing the goal of the MIP.

Acknowledgment. Tassos Venetis was funded by the Research Centre of the Athens University of Economics and Business, in the framework of "Research Funding at AUEB for Excellence and Extroversion" and Vasilis Vassalos has received funding from the European Union Seventh Framework Programme (FP7/2007–2013) under grant agreement no.604102 (Human Brain Project).

References

1. Abiteboul, S., Hull, R., Vianu, V.: Foundations of Databases. Addison-Wesley, Boston (1995)
2. Ashburner, J., Friston, K.J.: Diffeomorphic registration using geodesic shooting and Gauss-Newton optimisation. NeuroImage **55**(3), 954–967 (2011)
3. Davidson, S.B., Buneman, O.P., Crabtree, J., Tannen, V., Overton, G.C., Wong, L.: Biokleisli: integrating biomedical data and analysis packages. In: Letovsky, S. (ed.) Bioinformatics: Databases and systems, pp. 201–211. Springer, USA (1999)
4. Centers for Disease Control and Prevention and others: Hipaa privacy rule and public health. Guidance from CDC and the us department of health and human services. MMWR: Morbidity and Mortality Weekly Report, vol. 52, Suppl. 1, pp. 1–17 (2003)
5. Doan, A., Halevy, A.Y., Ives, Z.G.: Principles of Data Integration. Morgan Kaufmann, San Francisco (2012)
6. Fagin, R., Kolaitis, P.G., Miller, R.J., Popa, L.: Data exchange: semantics and query answering. Theoret. Comput. Sci. **336**(1), 89–124 (2005)
7. Forrey, A., et al.: Logical observation identifier names and codes (LOINC) database: a public use set of codes and names for electronic reporting of clinical laboratory test results. Clin. Chem. **42**(1), 81–90 (1996)
8. Garcia-Molina, H., Papakonstantinou, Y., Quass, D., Rajaraman, A., Sagiv, Y., Ullman, J., Vassalos, V., Widom, J.: The tsimmis approach to mediation: Data models and languages. J. Intell. Inf. Syst. **8**(2), 117–132 (1997)
9. Haas, L.M., Kodali, P., Rice, J.E., Schwarz, P.M., Swope, W.C.: Integrating life sciences data-with a little garlic. In: Proceedings IEEE International Symposium on Bio-Informatics and Biomedical Engineering, 2000, pp. 5–12. IEEE (2000)
10. Hernandez, T., Kambhampati, S.: Integration of biological sources: current systems and challenges ahead. ACM Sigmod Rec. **33**(3), 51–60 (2004)
11. Josifovski, V., Schwarz, P., Haas, L., Lin, E.: Garlic: a new flavor of federated query processing for db2. In: Proceedings of the 2002 ACM SIGMOD International Conference on Management of data, pp. 524–532. ACM (2002)
12. Karpathiotakis, M., Branco, M., Alagiannis, I., Ailamaki, A.: Adaptive query processing on RAW data. PVLDB **7**(12), 1119–1130 (2014)
13. Klein, A., Tourville, J.: 101 labeled brain images and a consistent human cortical labeling protocol. Front. Neurosci. **6**, 101 (2012)
14. Knoblock, C.A., Minton, S., Ambite, J.L., Ashish, N., Muslea, I., Philpot, A.G., Tejada, S.: The ariadne approach to web-based information integration. Int. J. Coop. Inf. Syst. **10**(01n02), 145–169 (2001)
15. Marnette, B., et al.: ++Spicy: an opensource tool for second-generation schema mapping and data exchange. PVLDB **4**(12), 1438–1441 (2011)
16. Merelli, I., Pérez-Sánchez, H., Gesing, S., D'Agostino, D.: Managing, analysing, and integrating big data in medical bioinformatics: open problems and future perspectives. BioMed Res. Int. **2014**, 13 (2014)
17. Organization, W.H., et al.: The ICD-10 Classification of Mental and Behavioural Disorders: Clinical Descriptions and Diagnostic Guidelines. World Health Organization, Geneva (1992)
18. Peim, M., Franconi, E., Paton, N.W., Goble, C.A.: Query processing with description logic ontologies over object-wrapped databases. In: Proceedings 14th International Conference on Scientific and Statistical Database Management, 2002, pp. 27–36. IEEE (2002)

19. Sherry, S.T., Ward, M., Sirotkin, K.: dbSNPdatabase for single nucleotide poly-morphisms and other classes of minor genetic variation. Genome Res. **9**(8), 677–679 (1999)
20. Stevens, R., Goble, C., Paton, N.W., Bechhofer, S., Ng, G., Baker, P., Brass, A.: Complex query formulation over diverse information sources in tambis. In: Lacroix, Z., Critchlow, T. (eds.) Bioinformatics: Managing Scientific Data. Morgan Kaufmann, San Francisco (2003)
21. Sweeney, L.: k-anonymity: A model for protecting privacy. Int. J. Uncertainty Fuzziness Knowl. Based Syst. **10**(05), 557–570 (2002)

SchizConnect: Virtual Data Integration in Neuroimaging

Jose Luis Ambite[1]([✉]), Marcelo Tallis[1], Kathryn Alpert[2],
David B. Keator[3], Margaret King[4], Drew Landis[4],
George Konstantinidis[1], Vince D. Calhoun[4,5], Steven G. Potkin[3],
Jessica A. Turner[4,6], and Lei Wang[2]

[1] University of Southern California, Los Angeles, CA, USA
{ambite,tallis,konstant}@isi.edu
[2] Northwestern University, Chicago, IL, USA
{k-alpert,leiwang1}@northwestern.edu
[3] University of California, Irvine, CA, USA
{dbkeator,sgpotkin}@uci.edu
[4] Mind Research Network, Albuquerque, NM, USA
{mking,dlandis,vdcalhoun}@mrn.org
[5] University of New Mexico, Albuquerque, NM, USA
[6] Georgia State University, Atlanta, GA, USA
jturner63@gsu.edu

Abstract. In many scientific domains, including neuroimaging studies, there is a need to obtain increasingly larger cohorts to achieve the desired statistical power for discovery. However, the economics of imaging studies make it unlikely that any single study or consortia can achieve the desired sample sizes. What is needed is an architecture that can easily incorporate additional studies as they become available. We present such architecture based on a virtual data integration approach, where data remains at the original sources, and is retrieved and harmonized in response to user queries. This is in contrast to approaches that move the data to a central warehouse. We implemented our approach in the SchizConnect system that integrates data from three neuroimaging consortia on Schizophrenia: FBIRN's Human Imaging Database (HID), MRN's Collaborative Imaging and Neuroinformatics System (COINS), and the NUSDAST project at XNAT Central. A portal providing harmonized access to these sources is publicly deployed at schizconnect.org.

Keywords: Data integration · Neuroimaging · Mediation · Schema mappings

1 Introduction

The study of complex diseases, such as Schizophrenia, requires the integration of data from multiple cohorts [1]. As a result, over the past decade we have witnessed the creation of many multi-site consortia, such as the Functional Biomedical Informatics Research Network (FBIRN) [2], the Mind Clinical Imaging Consortium (MCIC) [3], or

© Springer International Publishing Switzerland 2015
N. Ashish and J.-L. Ambite (Eds.): DILS 2015, LNBI 9162, pp. 37–51, 2015.
DOI: 10.1007/978-3-319-21843-4_4

the ENIGMA Network [4]. Within a consortium, researchers strive to harmonize the data. For example, FBIRN's Human Imaging Database (HID) [5] is a multi-site federated database where each site follows the same standard schema. However, across consortia harmonizing the data remains a challenge.

One approach to data integration, commonly called the *warehouse* approach, is to create a centralized repository with a uniform schema and data values. Data providers transform their data to the warehouse schema and formats, and move the data to the repository. An example of this approach within neuroscience is the National Database for Autism Research (NDAR) [6]. The warehouse approach is common in industry and in government and provides several advantages. The main ones are performance and stability. Since the data has been moved to a single repository, often a relational database, or other systems that allow for efficient query access, the performance of the system can be optimized by the addition of indices and restructuring of the data. Also, since the repository holds a copy of the original data, the life of the data can persist beyond the life of the original data generator. However, these strengths turn into disadvantages in more dynamic situations. First, the data in the warehouse is only as recent as the last update, so this approach may not be appropriate for data that is updated frequently. A more insidious problem is that once the schema of the warehouse has been defined and the data from the sources transformed and loaded under such schema, it becomes quite costly to evolve the warehouse if additional sources require changes to the schema.

An alternative approach to data integration, commonly called the *virtual data integration* or mediation approach, is to leave the data at the original sources, but map the source data to a harmonized virtual schema. These schema mappings are described declaratively by logical formulas. When the user specifies a query (expressed over the harmonized schema), the data integration system (also called a *mediator*) consults the schema mappings to identify the relevant data sources and to translate the query into the schemas used by each of the data sources. In addition, the system generates and optimizes a distributed query evaluation plan that accesses the sources and composes the answers to the user query. This approach has opposite advantages and disadvantages to the warehouse approach. The main advantages are data recency, ease of incorporation of new sources, and ease of restructuring the virtual schema. The user always gets the most recent data available since the answers to the user query are obtained live from the original data sources. Adding a new data source or changing the harmonized schema is accomplished by defining a set of declarative schema mappings. This process is often much simpler than reloading and/or restructuring a large warehouse. The fact that the schema mappings are a set of compact logical rules significantly lowers the cost of developing, maintaining and evolving the system. Conversely, a disadvantage of this system is that query performance generally cannot match that of a warehouse, since optimization options available in the centralized setting of a warehouse cannot be used in a distributed system. Nonetheless, as we will show in this paper, the virtual mediation approach can provide adequate performance.

Finally, the warehouse and the virtual data integration approaches are not mutually exclusive. The system can materialize the most stable data, but query in real time the data that changes more frequently.

For SchizConnect virtual data integration was preferable to data warehousing. First, it requires significantly less resources; essentially, just developing the web portal/query interface and hosting the mediator engine. There is no need for us to store and take care of large datasets locally. Second, it demands a minimum effort to integrate new data sources. In order to encourage data providers to participate in SchizConnect we required an approach that imposed minimum overhead to them. Finally, it does not require data providers to relinquish control of their data. Different data providers have different policies regarding data sharing and the virtual integration approach allows them to keep full control of who can access their data. Our mediator architecture allows for data sources to grant authorization to individual data requests based on the user's security credentials.

In this the paper we present how the virtual data integration approach has been applied to create the SchizConnect system, which is publicly available at www.schizconnect.org. First, we describe the data sources that have currently been integrated. Second, we present the behavior of the system from a user perspective, as an investigator interacting with the SchizConnect web portal. Third, we provide a technical description of the SchizConnect mediator process, including the definition of the harmonized schema, the schema mappings, the data value mappings, the query rewriting process, and the distributed query evaluation. Fourth, we provide some experimental results. Finally, we discuss related work, future work and conclusions.

2 Participating Data Sources

Currently, the SchizConnect system provides integrated access to the following sources of schizophrenia data, including demographics, cognitive and clinical assessments, and imaging data and metadata. These sources are also publicly available and have been extensively curated, documented, and subjected to quality assurance.

FBIRN Phase II @ UCI, http://fbirnbdr.nbirn.net:8080/BDR/ [2]. This study contains cross-sectional multisite data from 251 subjects, each with two visits. Data include structural and functional magnetic resonance imaging (sMRI, fMRI) scans collected on a variety of 1.5T and 3T scanners, including Sternberg Item Recognition Paradigm (SIRP) and Auditory Oddball paradigms, breath-hold and sensorimotor tasks. The data is stored in the HID system [5], which is powered by a PostgresSQL relational database located at the Univesity of California, Irvine. The SchizConnect mediator accesses HID using standard JDBC.

NUSDAST @ XNAT Central, central.xnat.org/REST/projects/NUDataSharing [7]. The Northwestern University Schizophrenia Data and Software Tool (NUSDAST) contains data from 368 subjects, the majority with longitudinal data (~ 2 years apart), include sMRI scans collected on a single Siemens 1.5T Vision scanner. The data is stored in XNAT central, a public repository of neuroimaging and clinical data, hosted at Washington University at Saint Louis. The site is built over the eXtensible Neuro-imaging Archiving Toolkit (XNAT), a popular framework for neuroimaging data [8]. XNAT provides a REST web service interface. The mediator uses the search API, which accepts queries in an XNAT-specific XML format and returns results as a XML document.

COBRE & MCICShare @ COINS Data Exchange, coins.mrn.org [9]. The Collaborative Imaging and Neuroinformatics System (COINS), contains data from 198 and 212 subjects from the COBRE and MCICShare projects, respectively. Data for COBRE include sMRI and rest-state fMRI scans collected on a single 3T scanner. Data for the multisite MCICShare include sMRI, rest-state fMRI and dMRI scans, collected on 1.5T and 3T scanners. COINS required special handling in SchizConnect because the native COINS architecture involves dynamic data packaging following the query, which does not allow for data to be immediately returned to the query engine. With permission from the COINS executive committee, we duplicated the COINS data relevant to SchizConnect in a relational MySQL database at USC/ISI.

SchizConnect is positioned to become the largest neuroimaging resource for Schizophrenia, currently providing access to over 21 K images for over 1 K subjects, and expected to significantly grow as new sources are federated into the system.

3   The SchizConnect Web Portal

To understand the SchizConnect approach, it is best to start with the user experience at its web portal, schizconnect.org. The portal provides an intuitive graphical interface for investigators to query schizophrenia data across sources.

Consider a query for "male subjects with schizophrenia with DTI scans and measures of executive function". An investigator constructs such query graphically by drag-and-drop of the main harmonized concepts into a canvas (Fig. 1(a)). Currently the supported concepts include Subject, MRI, Neuropsychiatric Assessments, and Clinical Assessments. Each concept has a number of attributes on which the user can make selections. Figure 1(b) shows the attributes of Subject, which include age, sex, and diagnosis, and a selection on the diagnosis attribute for subjects with schizophrenia in a broad sense. The values for diagnosis have a hierarchical structure and have been harmonized across the sources. In Sect. 4.3 we describe how the SchizConnect mediator classifies the subjects into these categories. Figure 1(c) shows the cognitive assessment concept (Neuropsych) and a selection on measures of executive function.

The results to this query appear in Figs. 2 and 3. The SchizConnect Portal shows the number of subjects, scans, and assessments that satisfy the query constraints, as well as a breakdown of the provenance of the data (Fig. 2). In this case, 117 images from 58 subjects come from the COBRE data source and 169 images from 82 subjects from MCICShare data source, for a total of 286 images and 6 distinct cognitive assessments of executive function for 140 subjects. Any investigator can obtain these

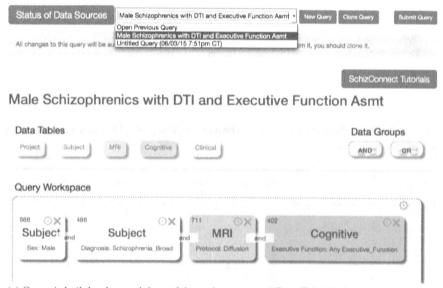

(a) Query is built by drag and drop of the main concepts ("Data Tables": Subject, MRI, Neuro-psychiatric assessments, etc) into a canvas ("Query Workspace"). The query asks for: "male subjects with schizophrenia, with DTI scans and measures of executive function".

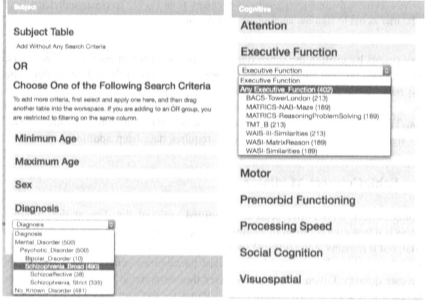

(b) Selecting Subjects with a diagnosis of Schizophrenia in a broad sense.

(c) Selecting subjects with cognitive assessments of executive function

Fig. 1. Schizconnect portal: sample query using the harmonized schema and terminology. Each concept presents different attributes, some of which take hierarchical values, according to the SchizConnect harmonized terminologies.

Your query returned 286 images and 6 assessments from 140 subjects. View My Query or Create New Query

- COBRE: 117 images and 3 assessments from 58 subjects
- MCICShare: 169 images and 3 assessments from 82 subjects

Note that some subjects have longidinal data, some visits contain multiple imaging sequences, and some scans have multiple formats.

To review your query, please use the View My Query link (the back button will take you to a blank query creation page).

To download images and assessments and/or view summary data, please Sign In or Sign Up.

Fig. 2. The results of the query from Fig. 1. The user can then proceed to request the data from the different repositories.

Provenance	Name	Subjectid	Age	Sex	Dx	Field_strength	Img_date	Dstauri	Msker	Model	Szn_protocol_hier	Assessment	Assessment_descrip
COINS	COBRE	A00038624	45	male	Schizophrenia_Strict	3	2013-01-01 00:00:00.0	2294526	Siemens	MIND TRIO 3.0T	Diffusion	WASI-Similarities	Wechsler Abbreviatec Scale of Intelligence Similarities
COINS	MCICShare	A00036106	21	male	Schizophrenia_Broad	1.5	2006-01-01 00:00:00.0	1926323	Siemens	MIC SMS SON 1.5T	Diffusion	TMT_B	Trail Making Test B
COINS	MCICShare	A00036106	21	male	Schizophrenia_Broad	1.5	2006-01-01 00:00:00.0	1926323	Siemens	MIC SMS SON 1.5T	Diffusion	TowerLondon	Tower of London
COINS	MCICShare	A00036106	21	male	Schizophrenia_Broad	1.5	2006-01-01 00:00:00.0	1926323	Siemens	MIC SMS SON 1.5T	Diffusion	WAIS-III-Similarities	Wechsler Adult Intelligence Scale-III Similarities

Fig. 3. An excerpt individual-level results of the query from Fig. 1. To obtain individual level results the user needs to sign the appropriate data sharing agreements.

summary counts by visiting the schizconnect.org portal. After an investigator registers, logs into the system, and signs the data sharing agreements of the data providers, she can also retrieve the individual-level data, which include summary tables (Fig. 3), as well as links to download the images and full cognitive assessments for the selected subjects. The system remembers previously signed agreements and asks the investigator to sign additional ones when her query requires data from additional sources.

4   The SchizConnect Mediator

The SchizConnect Web Portal presents a unified view of the data at the different sources, as if it was coming from in a single database. However, the data is not stored at the portal, but it remains at the original sources, structured under their original schemas. The SchizConnect mediator provides a *virtual* harmonized schema, over which the portal issues queries. Given a user query, over the harmonized schema, the mediator determines which sources have relevant data, translates the user query to the schemas of the sources, and constructs, optimizes, and executes a distributed query evaluation plan that computes the answers to the user query by accessing the data sources in real time. The SchizConnect mediator builds upon the BIRN Mediator [10]. In this section, we describe each of the components of the mediator that make this data harmonization and query processing possible.

4.1   SchizConnect Domain Schema

In order to integrate data from disparate sources, we need to understand the semantics of the data, and how different schema elements at different sources related to other elements. The common approach to specific such semantics is to map the schema of each source to a common harmonized schema (also called the target, or domain, or global schema) [11]. This common schema is a degree of freedom for the designer of the integration system.


```
project(provenance, name, projectid, description)
subject(provenance, subjectid, age, sex, dx)
in_project(provenance, subjectid, projectid)
imaging_protocol( provenance, subjectid, szc_protocol, img_date, notes,
                  datauri, maker, model, field_strength)
cognitive_assessment(provenance, study, subjectid, szc_assessment, description)
cognitive_assessment_data( provenance, study, subjectid, szc_assessment,
                  question_id, question_value)
clinical_assessment(provenance, study, subjectid, szc_assessment, description )
clinical_assessment_data( provenance, study, subjectid, szc_assessment,
                  question_id, question_value)
```

Fig. 4. SchizConnect current domain model.

It does not need to include every schema element present in the sources; just those elements useful for the purposes of the integration problem at hand. The design of the common schema is a balance between minimalism, that is, only include elements that exist in the sources and that are needed to answer the current query load, and generality, that is, a schema design that can easily be extended to model additional sources and query types. Our philosophy leans towards minimalism. Instead of attempting to model the neuroimaging domain wholesale, we build the common schema incrementally as we find sources that provide data for the desired concepts in the domain.

The current domain schema in SchizConnect follows the relational model and is composed of the following predicates (Fig. 4):

Project contains the name and description of the studies in the data sources.

Subject contains demographic and diagnostic information for individual participants, including "subject id", "age", "sex" and "diagnosis".

Imaging Protocol (MRI) contains information on MRIs a subject has, including the type of the scan and metadata about the scanner. The values of the protocol attribute are organized hierarchically (cf. Sect. 4.3).

Cognitive Assessment contains information on which subjects have which neuropsychological assessments. The values of the "assessment" attribute are also organized hierarchically (cf. Sect. 4.3).

Cognitive Assessment Data contains full information on the assessments including the values for each measure in each assessment for each subject.

Clinical Assessment and **Clinical Assessment Data** contain assessments for different symptoms in the subjects.

The first attribute in each of the domain predicates is "provenance", which records which source provided the data elements (see Fig. 3).

4.2 SchizConnect Schema Mappings

The SchizConnect domain predicates, shown in Fig. 4, provide a consistent view of the data available from the sources. However, the mediator does not pre-compute such data as in a warehouse, but obtains these data on-the-fly from the sources at query time. For this process, the mediator uses a set of declarative schema mappings, which define how predicates from the source schema relate to predicates in the domain schema. These mappings are usually logical implications of the form:

$$\forall \vec{X}, \vec{Y}, \Phi_S(\vec{X}, \vec{Y}) \rightarrow \exists \vec{Z}, \Psi_G(\vec{X}, \vec{Z})$$

with a conjunctive antecedent (Φ_S) over predicates from the source schemas (S), and a conjunctive consequent (Ψ_G) over predicates from the domain schema (G). These mappings are also known as source-to-target tuple-generating dependencies (st-tgds) in the database theory literature [12]. The SchizConnect mediator supports full conjunctive st-tgds (aka GLAV rules) [13], but so far the domain and schema mappings we have developed only needed to be Global-as-View (GAV) rules [11], which are st-tgds with a single predicate in the consequent.

Some sample schema mappings appear in Fig. 5. We use a logical syntax for the rules. We show domain predicates in bold (e.g., **subject**) and source predicates in italics (e.g., *HIDPSQLResource_nc_subjexperiment*). The first rule states that the source XNAT provides data for subjects. More precisely, that invoking the source predicate *XnatSubjectResource_xnat__subjectData*, and then joining the results with the *MappingsMySQLResource_dx_mappings* source predicate (which are located at different sources, XNAT and a MySQL db), yields the domain predicate **subject**. A shared variable in the antecedent of a rule (e.g., SRC_DX) denotes an equi-join condition. Other type of conditions can be included in antecedents by adding relational predicates (e.g., the selection 'nc_experiment_uniqueid = 9610' in the fourth rule). Variables in the consequent denote projections over data sources.

Rules with the same consequent denote *union*. For example, in Fig. 5 the domain predicate **subject** is obtained as the union of three rule, one for each data source (XNAT, COINS, and HID). Note how each of the rules includes a constant in the consequent to denote the provenance of the data (i.e., "XNAT").

Our mediator language allows for non-recursive logic programs. For example, the third rule in Fig. 5 states that the **subject** domain predicate for HID is constructed by the *join* of 3 domain predicates: **subject_age**, **subject_sex**, and **subject_dx**. The next two rules show how the diagnoses for the subjects (**subject_dx**) in the HID source are calculated based on specific values for the assessments as stored in the original HID tables. For example, a subject with values of 3 and 1 in questions P47 and P53 of the SCID assessment, resp., is assigned a diagnosis of schizophrenia in the strict sense.

Finally, the last two rules show how to obtain the **imaging_protocol** domain predicate for the HID and XNAT sources. Normalization of the imaging protocol and

subject("XNAT", SUBJECT_ID, AGE, SEX, DX) <-
  XnatSubjectResource_xnat__subjectData(project, SUBJECT_ID, AGE, SEX, SRC_DX, QS) ∧
  MappingsMySQLResource_dx_mappings(DX, "NUSDAST", 777, SRC_DX, id)

subject("COINS", SUBJECT_ID, AGE, SEX, DX) <-
  COINSMySQLResource_subjects_v(SUBJECT_ID, SEX, yob, SRC_DX, STUDY_ID, AGE) ∧
  MappingsMySQLResource_dx_mappings(DX, "COINS", STUDY_ID, SRC_DX, id)

subject("HID", SUBJECTID, AGE, SEX, DX) <-
  subject_age("HID", SUBJECTID, AGE) ∧ ***subject_sex***("HID", SUBJECTID, SEX) ∧
  subject_dx("HID", SUBJECTID, DX)

...

subject_dx("HID",SUBJECTID, 'No_Known_Disorder') <-
  HIDPSQLResource_nc_subjexperiment(uniqueid, tableid, owner, modtime, moduser,
       nc_experiment_uniqueid, SUBJECTID, nc_researchgroup_uniqueid) ∧
  (nc_researchgroup_uniqueid IN [9612,4292]) ∧ (nc_experiment_uniqueid = 9610)

...

subject_dx("HID",SUBJECTID,
'Mental_Disorder>Psychotic_Disorder>Schizophrenia_Broad>Schizophrenia_Strict') <-
  HIDPSQLResource_nc_subjexperiment(uniqueid, tableid, owner, modtime, moduser,
       nc_experiment_uniqueid, SUBJECTID, nc_researchgroup_uniqueid) ∧
  (nc_researchgroup_uniqueid = 9611) ∧ (nc_experiment_uniqueid = 9610) ∧
  HIDPSQLResource_nc_assessmentinteger(tableid1, nc_assessmentdata_uniqueid1,
       scoreorder1, owner1, modtime1, moduser1, textvalue1, textnormvalue1,
       comments1, DATAVALUE1, datanormvalue1, storedassessmentid1,
       ASSESSMENTID1, SCORENAME1, scoretype1, ISVALIDATED1, isranked1,
       SUBJECTID, entryid1, keyerid1, raterid1, classification1, uniqueid1) ∧
  (ASSESSMENTID1 = 16415) ∧ (SCORENAME1 = "SCID_P47") ∧ (DATAVALUE1 = 3) ∧
  HIDPSQLResource_nc_assessmentinteger(tableid2, nc_assessmentdata_uniqueid2,
       scoreorder2, owner2, modtime2, moduser2, textvalue2, textnormvalue2,
       comments2, DATAVALUE2, datanormvalue2, storedassessmentid2,
       ASSESSMENTID2, SCORENAME2, scoretype2, ISVALIDATED2, isranked2,
       SUBJECTID, entryid2, keyerid2, raterid2, classification2, uniqueid2) ∧
  (ASSESSMENTID2 = 16415) ∧ (SCORENAME2 = "SCID_P53") ∧ (DATAVALUE2 = 1) ∧
  (ISVALIDATED1 = "TRUE") ∧ (ISVALIDATED2 = "TRUE")

imaging_protocol("HID", SUBJECTID, SZC_PROTOCOL_HIER, DATE, NOTES, DATAURI,
                MAKER, MODEL, FIELD_STRENGTH) <-
  HIDPSQLResource_nc_scannersbyscan (SUBJECTID, componentid, segmentid,
          SOURCE_PROTOCOL, DATE, nc_colequipment_uniqueid, SOURCE_MAKE,
          SOURCE_MODEL, DATAURI, NOTES) ∧
  MappingsMySQLResource_protocol_mappings(SZC_PROTOCOL_HIER, "HID",
                              SOURCE_PROTOCOL, ID1) ∧
  MappingsMySQLResource_scanner_mappings(MAKER, MODEL, FIELD_STRENGTH, "HID",
                              SOURCE_MAKE, SOURCE_MODEL, ID2)

imaging_protocol("XNAT", SUBJECTID, SZC_PROTOCOL_HIER, DATE, SCAN_ID,
                DATA_URI, "SIEMENS", "VISION 1.5T", 1.5) <-
  XnatMRSessionResource_xnat__mrSessionData(SUBJECTID, IMAGE_ID, SESSION_ID,
                     DATE, SCANNER, SCAN_ID, SCAN_TYPE, quarantine_status) ∧
  MappingsMySQLResource_protocol_mappings(SZC_PROTOCOL_HIER, "NUSDAST",
                              SCAN_TYPE, ID1) ∧
  Concat(IMAGE_ID, "/scans/", SCAN_ID, DATA_URI)

Fig. 5. SchizConnect schema mappings.

scanners values is achieved by joining with additional mapping tables (e.g., *MappingsMySQLResource_protocol_mappings*). The mediator also supports functional sources, such as concatenation (*Concat* in the last rule in Fig. 5). In general, the designer can define arbitrary Java functions and use them in the schema mappings to perform complex value transformations.

SchizConnect Harmonized Value	Source	Source Value
Imaging_Protocol>Functional> Task_Paradigm>Mismatch_Negativity	HID	cognitive task scan: MMN
Imaging_Protocol>Functional>Task_Paradigm> Sternberg_Item_Recognition_Paradigm	HID	cognitive task scan: SIRP
Imaging_Protocol>Functional>Task_Paradigm> Sternberg_Item_Recognition_Paradigm	HID	SIRP (ver121504)
Imaging_Protocol>Functional>Task_Paradigm> Sternberg_Item_Recognition_Paradigm	HID	sternberg_item_recognition
Imaging_Protocol>Functional>Task_Paradigm> Sternberg_Item_Recognition_Paradigm	COINS	Functional - Sternberg Item Recognition

Fig. 6. SchizConnect value mappings.

4.3 SchizConnect Value Mappings

In addition to mapping the schemas of the sources into the SchizConnect domain schema, we also harmonized the values for the attributes. This was achieved by developing mapping tables that relate values used in the sources with harmonized values in SchizConnect. These tables are stored in a separate relational database, which is treated as a regular data source for the mediator. For example, the source predicate *MappingsMySQLResource_protocol_mappings* stores the mappings for imaging protocols. Some sample mappings for this predicate appear in Fig. 6. Note that even within the same source, there are often several different values/codes for the same concept. For example, HID has several different codes for the Sternberg Item Recognition Paradigm protocol (since HID contains multiple substudies performed at different times, and no attempt at enforcing common values across substudies was made).

```
Imaging_Protocol
Structural
   Diffusion
   T1
        FLASH
        MPRAGE
   T2
Functional
   Resting_State
   Task_Paradigm
        Auditory_Oddball
        Breath_Hold
        Finger_Tapping
        Go_NoGo
        Mismatch_Negativity
        Sensory_Gating
        Sensory_Motor
        Sternberg_Item_
            Recognition_Paradigm
        Working_Memory
Field_Mapping
Perfusion
```

Fig. 7. Imaging protocol taxonomy

Many of the harmonized values in SchizConnect have a hierarchical structure. For example the current hierarchy for the imaging protocol appears in Fig. 7. Similar hierarchies for the diagnosis and cognitive assessments appear (partially) in Figs. 1(b) and 1(c). These hierarchies are easily extensible by updating the mapping tables.

The design of the harmonized values takes into account existing ontologies. A companion paper [16] describes in detail this design and the mapping of the SchizConnect value taxonomies to concepts in NeuroLex and other well-known ontologies.

4.4   Query Rewriting

Given a user query, the mediator uses the schema mappings defined for the application domain, to translate the query from the virtual domain schema into an executable query over the source schemas, a process called query rewriting. For GAV schema mappings, such as those in Fig. 5, query rewriting amounts to rule unfolding and simplification. We have also developed algorithms for query rewriting under LAV schema mappings [13] and GLAV rules, but they are not used in the current modeling of the Schiz-Connect domain.

We will describe the rewriting process by example. Consider a user query for all the available T1 scans: select * from imaging_protocol where szc_protocol like '%T1 %', and the schema mappings for **imaging_protocol** in Fig. 5. The rewritten query, expressed in SQL, appears in Fig. 8. This query is built by unfolding the definitions of imaging_protocol according to the schema mapping rules. In general, for GAV rewriting the system unifies each domain predicate with the corresponding consequent of the GAV rule (i.e., with the same predicate) and replaces it with the antecedent of the rule. After this unfolding process, the source-level queries are logically minimized to avoid probably redundant predicates (i.e., source invocations). For this simple example, the rewritten query is a union of conjunctive queries over the sources providing the data, including joins with the mapping sources to produce harmonized values, as we described in Sect. 4.3. The schema mapping for COINS and the corresponding portion of the rewriting is not shown for brevity.

4.5   Distributed Query Engine

Once the mediator has translated the user domain query into a source-level query (i.e., involving only source predicates), it must generate, optimize and execute a distributed query evaluation plan. Our current query engine is based on the Open Grid Services Architecture (OGSA) Distributed Access and Integration (DAI), and Distributed Query Processing (DQP) projects [14]. OGSA-DAI is a streaming dataflow workflow evaluation engine that includes a library of connectors to many types of common data sources such as databases and web services. Each data source is wrapped and presents a uniform interface as a Globus [15] grid web service. OGSA-DQP is a distributed query evaluation engine implemented on top of OGSA-DAI. In response to a SQL query, OGSA-DQP constructs a query evaluation plan to answer such query. The evaluation

```
(SELECT 'HID' as provenance, T6.subjectid as subjectid, T4.szc_protocol_hier as
    szc_protocol_hier, T6.date as img_date, T6.description as notes, T6.datauri as datauri,
    T2.maker as maker, T2.model as model, T2.field_strength as field_strength
FROM MappingsMySQLResource_scanner_mappings T2,
        MappingsMySQLResource_protocol_mappings T4,
        HIDPSQLResource_nc_scannersbyscan_mview T6
WHERE T2.source_make=T6.source_make AND T2.source_model=T6.source_model AND
    T2.source = 'HID' AND T4.source_protocol=T6.source_protocol AND T4.source = 'HID' AND
    T4.szc_protocol_hier LIKE '%T1%')
UNION
(SELECT 'XNAT' as provenance, T10.SUBJECT_ID as subjectid,
    T8.szc_protocol_hier as szc_protocol_hier, T10.SCAN_DATE as img_date,
    T10.SCAN_ID as notes, Concat(T10.IMAGE_ID,'/scans/',T10.SCAN_ID) as datauri,
    'SIEMENS' as maker, 'VISION 1.5T' as model, 1.5 as field_strength
FROM MappingsMySQLResource_protocol_mappings T8,
        XnatMRSessionResource_xnat_mrSessionData T10
WHERE T8.source_protocol=T10.SCAN_TYPE AND T8.source = 'NUSDAST' AND
        T8.szc_protocol_hier LIKE '%T1%')
```

Fig. 8. Executable query over the source schemas.

plan is implemented as an OGSA-DAI workflow, where the workflow activities correspond to relational algebra operations. The OGSA-DQP query optimizer partitions the workflow across multiple sources attempting to push as much of the evaluation of subqueries to remote sources. OGSA-DQP currently supports distributed SQL queries over tables in multiple sources. The OGSA-DAI/DQP architecture is modular and allows for the incorporation of new optimization algorithms, as well as mediator (query rewriting) modules, as plug-ins for new source types into the system.

We improved the OGSA-DAI/DQP query engine by adding a module to gather cost statistics from the sources, including table sizes and selectivity parameters, and by developing a cost-based query optimizer based on these statistics, as well as several other enhancements to specific optimization steps. The query plan optimizer proceeds in two phases. First, it applies a sequence of classical query plan transformations, such as pushing selection operations closer to their data sources, grouping operations on the same source and pushing subqueries to sources with query evaluation capabilities. Second, it searches how join operations can be ordered to minimize the cost of the overall plan. For complex queries, such as those described in Sect. 5 that involve conjunctive queries with 10–20 predicates, the enhanced cost-based optimizer produced plans that improved execution time by orders of magnitude.

4.6   Source Wrappers

The mediator can access sources of different types, including relational databases, such as HID, and web service APIs, such as XNAT. The actual data sources are wrapped as

OGSA-DAI resources. OGSA-DAI provides a common extensible framework to add new types of data sources.

For each non-relational source, we develop a *wrapper* that takes as input a SQL query (over predicates that encapsulate the data from the source), and translates this SQL query into the native query language of the source. Symmetrically, the wrapper takes data results from the source in their original format and converts them into relational tuples that can flow through the query engine.

For SchizConnect, we developed such a wrapper for XNAT. Consider the query:

select * from XnatMRSessionResource_xnat__mrSessionData where scan_type = 'T1'

This query invokes the wrapper for XNAT (see also the rewritten query in Fig. 8). This SQL query is translated to the native query language of the XNAT search service API, which is expressed as an XML document. The XNAT web service returns the results also as an XML document. The wrapper parses this document and translates it into relational tuples, following the schema of XnatMRSessionResource_xnat__mrSessionData. Now a uniform relational result, it is processed by the query engine as the data from any other source.

5 Experimental Results

The system is publicly deployed at SchizConnect.org. The web front-end is hosted at Northwestern University, the mediator is hosted at USC/ISI, and the sources are at UCI (the HID PostgreSQL DB), Washington University at Saint Louis (XNAT Central), and at USC/ISI (the MySQL database that hosts the replica COINS data).

Despite its nationwide distribution, the system performs well. We show some performance results for a representative set of queries in Fig. 9. The table of results is structured as follows. The first column is just the query id. The next two columns show the size of the tested domain query, and the specific predicates involved. All the tested domain queries are conjunctive. The following two columns show the structure and size of the resulting rewritten source-level query, which is generally much larger than the domain (user) query. The last two columns show the number of tuples in the answer to the user query and the total time in seconds to compute the answers (i.e., from sending the query to the mediator to returning the results to the user). For example, the fourth row shows the results for a domain query that asks for subjects with two assessments (of verbal episodic memory: HVLT-Delay and HVLT-Immediate), with two imaging protocols (T1, and sensory motor scans). The query involves the join of 7 domain predicates; namely, subject (s), in_project (ip), project (p), two instances of imaging_protocol (i), and two instances of cognitive_assessement (ca). The resulting rewritten query is a union of 5 conjunctive queries, each involving 16, 18, 17, 10, and 10 source predicates, respectively, for a total of 71 source predicates. The query returns 722 tuples and takes 12.1 s to complete.

The queries shown identify the subjects, imaging protocol, cognitive assessments, etc., satisfying the desired constraints, and return the desired data. However, the performance results in Fig. 9 do not include the transfer of the actual image files. For example, the seventh query asks for all the metadata about the 21447 imaging protocols currently accessible through SchizConnect from all the sources, which the mediator does return. However, the size of corresponding images is several hundred GBs ($\sim$173 GB compressed). So, when the user query identifies the subjects and scans of interest, SchizConnect schedules separate grid-ftp, ftp, and http connections to the original sources to obtain and package the images for the query subjects. In contrast, the cognitive and clinical assessment data are retrieved directly through the mediator, since these are smaller datasets. For example, the third query in Fig. 9, shows that asking for all the data on 13 cognitive assessments for all subjects produces a result set of 9318 tuples, which are returned in 8.9 s.

	Domain Query		Source-level Query		Result Size (#tuples)	Time (s)
	Size (#p)	Preds	Structure	Size (#p)		
1	6	ip, p, 4ca	U3CQ (10, 10,10)	30	189	7.8
2	1	s	U5CQ (4, 6, 2, 2)	14	1091	8.2
3	1	cad (13)	U2CQ (2, 3)	5	9318	8.9
4	7	s,ip,p,2i,2ca	U5CQ (16,18,17,10,10)	71	722	12.1
5	5	p,ca,i,s,ip	U5CQ (11, 13, 12,7,7)	50	1094	15.9
6	4	s,ip,p,i	U5CQ (9, 11, 10, 5, 5)	40	1462	17.3
7	1	i	U3CQ (3, 2, 1)	6	21447	18.7
8	4	s,ip,p,i	U5CQ (9,11,10,5,5)	40	19112	24.5

Fig. 9. Experimental results

The computation cost is a combination of the number final and intermediate results needed to compute the query, the number of sources involved, and the complexity of the rewritten queries, with large and more complex queries often taking more time, but not in a simple relationship.

6   Discussion

We have presented SchizConnect, a virtual data integration approach that provides semantically-consistent, harmonized access to several leading neuroimaging data sources. The mediation architecture is driven by declarative schema mappings that make the system easier to develop, maintain and extend. Our virtual approach allows the creation of large data resources at a fraction of the cost of competing approaches.

The system is publicly available at **SchizConnect.org**. Since its initial deployment in September 2014, the number of users, queries and image downloads has grown steadily (with over 50 registered users as of May 2015).

We are currently extending the coverage of different types data, specifically clinical assessments. We also plan to incorporate additional schizophrenia studies to Schiz-Connect. Finally, we plan to improve the underlying data integration architecture, specifically the performance of the query optimizer and adding a more expressive representational language for the domain schema, such as OWL2 QL.

Acknowledgements. SchizConnect is supported by a grant from the National Institutes of Health (NIH/NIMH), 5U01MH097435 to L. Wang, JL. Ambite, S.G. Potkin and J.A.Turner. The work on COINS is also supported by 5P20GM103472 (NIGMS) to V.D. Calhoun.

References

1. Turner, J.A.: The rise of large-scale imaging studies in psychiatry. GigaScience **3**, 29 (2014)
2. Glover, G.H., et al.: Function biomedical informatics research network recommendations for prospective multicenter functional MRI studies. J. Magn. Reson. Imaging JMRI **36**, 39–54 (2012)
3. King, M.D., Wood, D., Miller, B., Kelly, R., Landis, D., Courtney, W., Wang, R., Turner, J.A., Calhoun, V.D.: Automated collection of imaging and phenotypic data to centralized and distributed data repositories. Front. Neuroinform. **8**, 60 (2014)
4. Thompson, P.M., et al.: The ENIGMA consortium: large-scale collaborative analyses of neuroimaging and genetic data. Brain Imaging Behav. **8**, 153–182 (2014)
5. Keator, D.B., et al.: A national human neuroimaging collaboratory enabled by the biomedical informatics research network (BIRN). IEEE Trans. Inf. Technol. Biomed. **12**, 162–172 (2008)
6. Hall, D., Huerta, M.F., McAuliffe, M.J., Farber, G.K.: Sharing heterogeneous data: the national database for autism research. Neuroinformatics **10**, 331–339 (2012)
7. Wang, L., et al.: Northwestern University Schizophrenia Data and Software Tool (NUSDAST). Frontiers in Neuroinformatics **7**, 25 (2013)
8. Marcus, D.S., Olsen, T., Ramaratnam, M., Buckner, M.L.: The extensible neuroimaging archive toolkit (XNAT): An informatics platform for managing, exploring, and sharing neuroimaging data. Neuroinformatics **5**, 11–34 (2005)
9. Scott, A., Courtney, W., Wood, D., de la Garza, R., Lane, S., King, M., Wang, R., Roberts, J., Turner, J.A., Calhoun, V.D.: COINS: An innovative informatics and neuroimaging tool suite built for large heterogeneous datasets. Front. Neuroinform. **5**, 33 (2011)
10. Ashish, N., Ambite, J.L., Muslea, M., Turner, J.: Neuroscience Data Integration through Mediation: An (F)BIRN Case Study. Front. Neuroinform. **4**, 118 (2010)
11. Doan, A., Halevy, A., Ives, Z.: Principles of Data Integration. Morgan Kauffman, Waltham (2012)
12. Fagin, R., Kolaitis, P.G., Miller, R.J., Popa, L.: Data Exchange: Semantics and query answering. In: Calvanese, D., Lenzerini, M., Motwani, R. (eds.) ICDT 2003. LNCS, vol. 2572, pp. 207–224. Springer, Heidelberg (2002)
13. Konstantinidis, G., Ambite, J.: Scalable query rewriting: a graph-based approach. In: SIGMOD Conference, pp. 97–108. ACM (2011)
14. Grant, A., Antonioletti, M., Hume, A.C., Krause, A., Dobrzelecki, B., Jackson, M.J., Parsons, M., Atkinson, M.P., Theocharopoulos, E.: OGSA-DAI: Middleware for data integration: selected applications. In: Fourth IEEE International Conference on eScience (2008)
15. The Globus Project (1997). http://www.globus.org
16. Turner, et al.: Terminology development towards harmonizing multiple clinical neuroimaging research repositories. In: Proceedings of DILS 2015 (2015)

Ontology and Knowledge Engineering
for Data Integration

Annotating Medical Forms Using UMLS

Victor Christen[1]([⊠]), Anika Groß[1], Julian Varghese[2], Martin Dugas[2],
and Erhard Rahm[1]

[1] Department of Computer Science, Universität Leipzig, Leipzig, Germany
{christen,gross,rahm}@informatik.uni-leipzig.de
[2] Institute of Medical Informatics, Universität Münster, Münster, Germany
{Martin.Dugas,Julian.Varghese}@ukmuenster.de

Abstract. Medical forms are frequently used to document patient data or to collect relevant data for clinical trials. It is crucial to harmonize medical forms in order to improve interoperability and data integration between medical applications. Here we propose a (semi-) automatic annotation of medical forms with concepts of the Unified Medical Language System (UMLS). Our annotation workflow encompasses a novel semantic blocking, sophisticated match techniques and post-processing steps to select reasonable annotations. We evaluate our methods based on reference mappings between medical forms and UMLS, and further manually validate the recommended annotations.

Keywords: Semantic annotation · Medical forms · Clinical trials · UMLS

1 Introduction

Medical forms are frequently used to document patient data within electronic health records (EHRs) or to collect relevant data for clinical trials. For instance, case report forms (CRFs) ask for different eligibility criteria to include or exclude probands of a study or to document the medical history of patients. Currently, there are more than 180,000 studies registered on http://clinicaltrials.gov and every clinical trial requires numerous CRFs for data collection. Often these forms are created from scratch without considering existing CRFs from previous trials. Thus, there is a huge amount and diversity of existing medical forms until now, and this number will increase further. As a consequence, different forms can be highly heterogeneous impeding the interoperability and data exchange between different clinical trials and research applications.

To overcome such issues, it is important to annotate medical forms with concepts of standardized vocabularies such as ontologies [6]. In the biomedical domain, annotations are frequently used to semantically enrich real-world objects. For instance, the well-known Gene Ontology (GO) is used to describe molecular functions of genes and proteins [10], scientific publications in PubMed are annotated with concepts of the Medical Subject Headings (MeSH) [13], and concepts of SNOMED CT [5] are assigned to EHRs supporting clinical

© Springer International Publishing Switzerland 2015
N. Ashish and J.-L. Ambite (Eds.): DILS 2015, LNBI 9162, pp. 55–69, 2015.
DOI: 10.1007/978-3-319-21843-4_5

applications like diagnosis or treatment. These diverse use cases for annotations show that they can represent a variety of relationships between real-world objects improving semantic search and integration for comprehensive analysis tasks. In particular, ontology-based annotations of medical forms facilitate the identification of similar questions (items) and commonly used medical concepts. Well-annotated items can be re-used to design new forms avoiding an expensive re-definition in every clinical trial. Moreover, the integration of results from different trials will be improved due to better compatibility of annotated forms. Beside clinical trials, also other medical applications like routine documentation in hospitals can profit from form annotation. For instance, the fusion of two or more hospitals requires the integration of hospital data which will be less complex if data semantics are well-defined due to the use of ontology-based annotations.

The open-access platform *Medical Data Models* (MDM)[1] already aims at creating, analyzing, sharing and reusing medical forms in a central metadata repository [4]. Currently, MDM provides more than 9,000 medical form versions and over 300,000 items. Beside overcoming technical heterogeneities (e.g. different formats), MDM intends to semantically enrich the medical forms with concepts of the widely used Metathesaurus of the Unified Medical Language System (UMLS) [2], a huge integrated data source covering more than 100 different biomedical vocabularies. So far, medical experts could assign UMLS concepts to items of some medical forms in MDM, but many forms have no or only preliminary annotations. However, such a manual annotation process is a very time-consuming task considering the high number of available forms within and beyond MDM as well as the huge size of UMLS (> 2.8 Mio. concepts). Thus, it is a crucial aim to develop automatic annotation methods supporting human annotators with recommendations.

The automatic annotation of medical forms is challenging since questions are written in free text, use different synonyms for the same semantics and can cover several different medical concepts. Moreover, the huge size of UMLS makes it difficult to identify correct medical concepts. So far, there has been some research on processing and annotation of different kinds of medical texts (e.g. [9,12,19]). However, (semi-) automatic annotation of medical forms has only rarely been studied (see Related Work in Sect. 5). We propose an initial solution to semi-automatically annotate medical forms with UMLS concepts and make the following contributions:

- We first discuss the challenges to be addressed for automatically annotating items in medical forms (Sect. 2).
- We propose an annotation workflow to automatically assign UMLS concepts to items of medical forms. The workflow encompasses three phases: a novel semantic blocking to reduce the search space, a matching phase and a post-processing phase employing a novel grouping method to finally select the correct annotations (Sect. 3).
- We evaluate our approaches based on reference mappings between MDM forms and UMLS. Results reveal that we are able to annotate medical forms in a

---
[1] www.medical-data-models.org/?locale=en.

largely automatic way. We further manually verify recommended annotations and present results for this semi-automatic annotation (Sect. 4).

Finally, we discuss related work in Sect. 5 and conclude in Sect. 6.

Items			Associated UMLS concepts	
(a)	Patients with established **CRF (1)** as an indication for the **treatment (2)** of **anemia (3)**	○ yes ○ no	1 C0022661	Kidney Failure, Chronic
			2 C0039798	therapeutic aspects
			3 C0002871	Anemia
(b)	Patients who have had prior **recombinant erythropoietin (1)** treatment whose **anemia (2)** had **never responded (3)**	○ yes ○ no	1 C0376541	Recombinant Erythropoietin
			2 C0002871	Anemia
			3 C0438286	Absent response to treatment
(c)	**Ulcerating plaque (1)**	☐ yes	1 C0751634	Carotid Ulcer

Fig. 1. Example medical form items and associated annotations to UMLS concepts. (CRF = 'Chronic Renal Failure' = 'Chronic Kidney Failure').

2   Challenges

The automatic annotation of medical forms requires first of all the correct identification of medical concepts in form items. Figure 1 illustrates three annotated items: (a) and (b) ask for eligibility criteria for a study w.r.t. anemia, and item (c) asks for the abnormality 'ulcerating plaque' in the context of a quality assurance form. An item consists of the actual question and a response field or list of answer options. In our example, question (c) has one annotation, whereas (a) and (b) are annotated with three UMLS concepts. Thus, one form item can address several different aspects like diseases (e.g. CRF, anemia), treatments or a patient's response to a treatment. In the following we discuss general challenges that need to be addressed during the annotation process.

Natural Language Items: Typically, a form consists of a set of items. Questions can be short phrases like in item (c) or longer sentences written in free text (Fig. 1(a), (b)). It is a difficult task to correctly identify medical concepts in these natural language sentences. Moreover, the use of different synonyms complicate a correct annotation, e.g. in Fig. 1(a) 'CRF' (= Chronic Renal Failure) needs to be assigned to C0022661 ('Kidney Failure, Chronic'). Simple string matching methods are not sufficient to generate annotations of high quality for medical form items. We will thus apply NLP (natural language processing) techniques such as named entity recognition and document-based similarity measures like TF/IDF to identify meaningful medical concepts that can be mapped to UMLS.

Complex Mappings: Every question can contain several medical concepts and one UMLS concept might be mapped to more than one question. In our example in Fig. 1 three UMLS concepts need to be assigned to questions (a) and (b) and the concept 'anemia' occurs in both questions. By contrast, question (c) is only annotated with one concept. Thus, we might need to identify complex N:M mappings and do not know a priori how many medical concepts need to be tagged to one item. Conventional match techniques often focus on the identification of

1:1 mappings, but solely assigning one source concept to one target concept is a much simpler task. We thus need to develop sophisticated match techniques to correctly annotate items with several UMLS concepts.

Number and Size of Data Sources: There is high number of forms (e.g. 9000 only in MDM) that need be to annotated and every form can contain tens to hundreds of items. Moreover, UMLS Metathesaurus is a very large biomedical data source covering more than 2.8 million concepts. Matching 100 forms each comprising only 10 items to the whole UMLS would already require 2.8 billion comparisons. On the one hand this leads to serious issues w.r.t. memory consumption and execution time. On the other hand it is extremely hard to identify correct annotations in such a huge search space. It is thus essential to apply suitable blocking schemes to reduce the search space and restrict automatic annotation to the most relevant subset of UMLS.

Instances: Form items are not only characterized by medical concepts in the actual question but also by its possible instances or response options. Item answers have a data type (e.g. Boolean 'yes/no' in Fig. 1) and might be associated with value scales (e.g. between 1 and 5) or specific units (e.g. mg, ml). Often possible answers are restricted to a list of values (e.g. a list of symptoms). To improve the comparability of different forms, such instance information should be semantically annotated with concepts of standardized terminologies. In this paper, we focus on the annotation of item questions but see a correct annotation of answer options as an important future challenge.

In summary, the automatic identification of high-quality annotations for medical forms is a difficult task. However, studying automatic annotation is very useful to support human experts with recommendations. For a semi-automatic annotation process it is especially important to identify a high number of correct annotations without generating too many false positives. Thus, achieving high recall values is a major goal while precision should not be too low, since the number of presented recommendations should be manageable for human experts. Moreover, a fast computation of annotation candidates is desirable to support an interactive annotation process. To address these challenges, we present a workflow for semi-automatic annotation of medical forms in the following.

3   Annotation Workflow

Our annotation workflow semantically enriches a set of medical forms by assigning UMLS concepts to form questions. An annotation is an association between a question and an UMLS concept. UMLS concepts are identified by their *Concept Unique Identifiers* (CUI) and are further described by attributes like a preferred name or synonyms. To identify annotations for a given medical form F, we determine a mapping $\mathcal{M}$ between the set of form questions $F = \{q_1, q_2, ..., q_k\}$ and the set of UMLS concepts $UMLS = \{cui_1, cui_2, ..., cui_m\}$. The mapping covers a set of annotations and is defined as:

$$\mathcal{M}_{F,UMLS} = \{(q, cui, sim)|q \in F, cui \in UMLS, sim \in [0,1]\}.$$

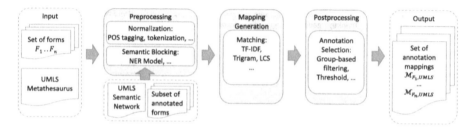

Fig. 2. Overview of the annotation workflow.

A question q in a form F is annotated with a concept *cui* from *UMLS*. Our automatic annotation method computes a similarity value *sim* indicating the strength of a connection. Greater *sim* values denote a higher similarity between the question and the annotated concept. Our annotation workflow (see Fig. 2) consists of three main phases that address the challenges discussed in Sect. 2. The input is a set of medical forms $F_1, \ldots, F_n$ each comprising a set of item questions as well as the UMLS Metathesaurus. During preprocessing we further use the UMLS Semantic Network and a subset of annotated forms. The output is a set of annotation mappings $\mathcal{M}_{F_1, UMLS}, \ldots, \mathcal{M}_{F_n, UMLS}$.

- In the *Preprocessing* phase we normalize input questions and UMLS concepts. Since a medical form is usually only associated to some domains covered by UMLS, we develop a novel semantic blocking technique to identify relevant concepts for the annotation generation. The approach is training-based and involves semantic types of UMLS concepts.
- In the *Mapping Generation* phase we identify annotations by matching the questions to names and synonyms of relevant UMLS concepts. We use a combination of a document retrieval method (*TF/IDF*) and classic match techniques (*Trigram, LCS (Longest Common Substring)*). By doing so we are able to identify complex annotation mappings for long natural language sentences as well as annotations to single concepts for shorter questions.
- During *Postprocessing* we remove probably wrong annotations to obtain a manageable set of relevant annotations for expert validation. Beside threshold selection we apply a novel group-based filtering to address the fact that questions might cover several medical concepts. For each question, we cluster similar concepts and keep only the best matching one per group.

Our workflow generates annotation recommendations which should be verified by domain experts since automatic approaches can not guarantee a correct annotation for all items. In the following, we discuss the methods in more detail.

3.1 Preprocessing

During preprocessing, we normalize the questions of a medical form as well as names and synonyms of UMLS concepts. In particular, we transform all string

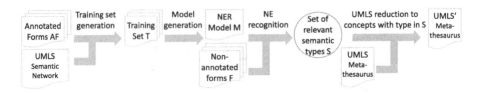

Fig. 3. Semantic blocking workflow. NER = Named Entity Recognition.

values to lower case and remove delimiters. We then remove potentially irrelevant parts of item questions. For instance, prepositions or verbs are typically part of natural language sentences, however they rarely cover information on medical concepts. We therefore apply a part-of-speech (POS) tagger[2] and keep only nouns, adjectives, adverbs and numbers/cardinals. We tokenize all strings into trigrams and word-tokens for the later annotation generation.

We further apply a semantic blocking to reduce the size of UMLS. UMLS Metathesaurus is a huge data source covering a lot of different subdomains. However, medical forms are usually only associated to a part of UMLS such that a comparison to the whole Metathesaurus should be avoided. We therefore aim at reducing UMLS by removing concepts that are probably not relevant for the annotation process. Our semantic blocking technique involves the UMLS Semantic Network. It covers 133 different semantic types and every UMLS concept is associated to at least one of the types. Our blocking technique follows a training-based approach and uses Named Entity Recognition (NER) to identify relevant semantic types for item questions. The general procedure is depicted in Fig. 3.

First, we build a training set T based on a subset of manually annotated forms AF. For each question in AF, we identify annotated named entities. Therefore, we compute the longest common part between a question and the names/synonyms of its annotated UMLS concepts. We then tag the identified question parts with the semantic types of the corresponding UMLS concept. Figure 4 illustrates an example for the training set generation. The given question is annotated with two UMLS concepts. The longest common part of the question and the concept *C0020517* is *Hypersensitivity*, while *C0015506* corresponds to the question part *Factor VIII*. Thus, *Hypersensitivity* is tagged with the semantic type of *C0020517* (*'Pathologic Function'*) and *Factor VIII* is labeled with *'Amino Acid, Peptide, or Protein'*. Based on the tagged training set T of forms AF we learn a NER-model M using the Open-NLP framework[3]. Our semantic blocking (see Fig. 3) then performs a named entity recognition using the model M to a non-annotated set of forms F. By doing so, we can recognize named entities for the questions in F and identify a set of relevant semantic types S. Finally, we reduce the UMLS Metathesaurus to those concepts that are associated to a semantic type in S and obtain the filtered $UMLS'$.

---

[2] http://nlp.stanford.edu/software/tagger.shtml.

[3] https://opennlp.apache.org/.

Question: Hypersensitivity to any recombinant Factor VIII product	Annotated concept	C0020517	C0015506
tagging ⬇	Names/ Synonyms	Hypersensitivity NOS, Allergy NOS, ...	FACTOR VIII, Antihemophilic factor
<Pathologic Function>Hypersensitivity </Pathologic Function> to any recombinant <Amino Acid, Peptide, or Protein> Factor VIII </Amino Acid, Peptide, or Protein> product	Semantic type	Pathologic Function	Amino Acid, Peptide, or Protein

Fig. 4. Training set generation: example for tagging a question with semantic types.

3.2   Matching Phase

We generate annotation mappings between a set of medical forms $F_1, \ldots, F_n$ and the reduced $UMLS'$ using a combination of a document retrieval method (TF/IDF) and classic match techniques ($ExactMatch$, $Trigram$, LCS). These methods can complement each other such that we are able to identify complex annotation mappings for long natural language sentences as well as shorter questions covering only one concept. To generate annotations for each considered form, we compute similarities between all questions of a form and every concept in $UMLS'$. Note that, we tokenized strings during preprocessing. To enable an efficient matching, we encode every token (word or trigram), and compare integer instead of string values. Furthermore, we separate UMLS into smaller chunks and distribute match computations among several threads.

We apply for each question the three match methods. $Trigram$ compares a question with concept names and synonyms, identifies overlapping trigram tokens, and computes similarities based on the Dice Metric. This is useful for shorter questions that slightly differ from the concept to be assigned. In our example in Fig. 1 the annotation for item (c) 'Ulcerating plaque' needs to be assigned to the concept C0751634 ('Carotid Ulcer'). This correspondence can be identified by the synonym 'Carotid Artery Ulcerating Plaque' of C0751634. Since there is only a partial overlap, it is feasible to identify the longest sequence of successive common word-tokens (LCS) between a question and a concept. LCS is also useful for complex matches when a question contains several medical concepts, e.g., 'recombinant erythropoietin' and 'anemia' in item (b) (Fig. 1).

Moreover, we use TF/IDF to especially reward common, but infrequent tokens between questions and UMLS concepts. For instance, in medical forms the token 'patient' occurs essentially more often then 'erythropoietin'. Thus, the computed similarity value should be higher for matches of rarely occurring, meaningful tokens compared to frequent tokens that appear in many questions and concepts. We compute tf-idf values for each token w.r.t. a question and an UMLS concept. The term frequency (tf) denotes the frequency of a token within the considered question or concept while the inverse document frequency (idf) characterizes the general meaning of a token compared to the total set of tokens. The tf-idf values are then used to compute the similarity between a token vector of the question and a token vector for names and synonyms of an UMLS concept. We choose a hamming-distance based measure to compare two token vectors. We compute distances between tf-idf values of two token vectors and normalize it based on the vector length. The normalized distance is converted

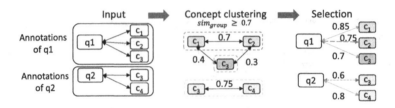

Fig. 5. Group-based filtering for two questions q_1 and q_2 and their annotations to concepts c_{1-4}. Uniformly colored concepts represent a group of similar concepts.

into a similarity value. We assign a smaller weight to the length of the longer vector to address cases, when one string consists of considerably more tokens than the other one, as this occurs for annotating long sentences. Thus, the measure does not penalize differences that are triggered by a differing vector length. High similarities between a shorter and a longer token vector can be achieved when a considerable number of meaningful tokens are contained in both vectors.

The generated annotation mappings are finally unified and similarities are aggregated by selecting the maximum *sim* value of a correspondence identified of several match methods to maximize the recall. Note that, we optimize the precision by performing the postprocessing phase. The match methods can identify overlapping results, but complement each other since they address different aspects of document and string similarity. We choose to adopt the three match methods in order to achieve a good recall by finding simple 1:1 as well as complex mappings for longer questions.

3.3   Postprocessing

Beside a simple threshold filtering, we apply a more sophisticated postprocessing step to filter the generated annotation mapping. Our aim is to identify all annotations to a question that are likely to be correct, i.e. to obtain high recall values. However, the result should not contain too many false positives in order to obtain a manageable set of recommendations to be presented to human experts. This is a complicated task when questions cover more than one medical concept, i.e. when we need to identify complex mappings. A simple approach would be to select the top k similar concepts for each question. However, it is possible that several annotations for the same medical concept in a question are among the top k. A top k selection could eliminate all annotations of medical concepts with lower *sim* values. We therefore apply a novel group-based filtering.

The group-based filtering first clusters concepts that are likely to belong to the same medical concept and then selects the most similar concept within a group. Figure 5 exemplarily describes the overall procedure for two questions q_1 and q_2 and their annotations to several concepts. Given a set of annotations for a question, we compute similarities between all UMLS concepts that are annotated to a question using trigram matching on concept names and synonyms. We than cluster concepts in one group if their similarity exceeds the required

sim_{group} threshold. In our example, we compare c_1, c_2 and c_3 for $q1$, and identify two groups $(\{c_1, c_2\}, \{c_3\})$. c_1 and c_2 are very similar $(sim_{group} \geq 0.7)$, while c_3 builds an own group. Finally, the best annotation per group is selected to be included in the final mapping based on the annotation similarities from the previous phase. For instance, we remove (q_1, c_2) due to the lower annotation similarity within its group. Applying a simple top 2 selection would have preserved (q_1, c_2) but removed (q_1, c_3), although (q_1, c_3) is likely to be the best match for a different medical concept covered by question q_1. Using the group-based filtering, we are able to keep one annotation for each medical concept in a question and thus allow for complex annotation mappings. In the following, we evaluate the proposed annotation methods for real-world medical forms.

4   Evaluation

To evaluate the proposed annotation workflow we consider three datasets covering medical forms from the MDM portal [4]. Figure 6 gives an overview on the number of considered forms, the average number of items per form, the average number of tokens per item question and the average number of annotations per item. The first set of medical forms considers *eligibility criteria* (EC) that are used for patient recruitment in clinical trials w.r.t. diseases like Diabetes Mellitus or Epilepsy. The dataset covers 25 medical forms each comprising about 20 items on average. To recruit trial participants, a precise definition of inclusion and exclusion criteria is required, such that most questions are long natural language sentences ($\sim$8 tokens on average) possibly covering several medical concepts. A correct identi-

Dataset	Eligibility criteria (EC)	Quality assur. (QA)	Top Items (TI)
#forms	25	23	1
avg (#items)	20.5	48.8	101
avg(#tokens)	8.3	3.3	2.4

Fig. 6. Overview of the used datasets.

fication of all annotations is very challenging for this dataset. Moreover, we consider medical forms for standardized *quality assurance* (*QA*) w.r.t. cardiovascular procedures. Since 2000 all German health service providers are obliged by law to apply these QA forms to prove the quality of their services [3]. The 23 QA forms contain about 49 items on average, but questions are shorter ($\sim$3 tokens on average). We further consider a set of top items (TI) from the MDM portal. In [20], these items have been manually reduced to the relevant semantic question parts resulting in a low token number per question. We handle the 101 top items as one medical form. For UMLS, we only consider concepts that possess a preferred name or term, which is the case for $\sim$1 Mio. UMLS concepts. We involve names and synonyms of these UMLS concepts.

   To evaluate the quality of automatically generated annotation mappings we use reference mappings between all considered MDM forms and UMLS. Our team consists of computer scientists as well as medical experts (two physicians), such that we could manually create the reference mappings based on expert knowledge. We compute precision, recall and F-measure for the annotation mappings of every medical form and show average values for the respective dataset (EC, QA or TI).

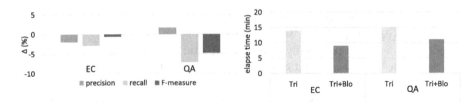

Fig. 7. Semantic blocking: quality differences (left) and execution time (right) for QA and EC, comparison of trigram without (*Tri*) and with semantic blocking (*Tri+Blo*).

Note, that the average of F-measures is not equal to a harmonic mean of average precision and average recall. Since a manual annotation is a difficult and time-consuming task, the initial reference mappings might not be complete. We therefore follow a semi-automatic annotation approach and manually validate the automatically generated annotations for the QA dataset to find further correct annotations (see Sect. 4.4). We first show evaluation results for EC and QA w.r.t. the methods of our annotation workflow (Sects. 4.1 and 4.2) and then give an overview on results for all datasets (Sect. 4.3).

4.1 Semantic Blocking

To evaluate our semantic blocking approach we measure the quality of the generated annotation mappings as well as matching execution times. We run experiments on an Intel i7–4770 3.4 GHz machine with 4 cores. Our aim is to reduce execution times without affecting the recall. The generation of training data is an important step for the semantic blocking. So far, we generated training data by randomly selecting half of the manually annotated datasets. Note, that the training sets have some bias since we consider a special type of medical forms, namely eligibility criteria and quality assurance forms. However, it is feasible to choose relevant semantic types in UMLS based on form annotations in the considered domain. It is an interesting point for future work to study the training set generation for the semantic blocking in more detail. We evaluate the impact of the semantic blocking using a basic trigram matching (*Tri*) without group-based filtering (threshold $t = 0.8$). Figure 7 shows quality differences and execution time results for QA and EC. The overall number of tokens was to small to apply the named entity recognition for TI. Applying the semantic blocking (*Blo*), UMLS could be reduced to ~600.000 concepts. This results in good execution time reductions of 26–36 % for both datasets. However, we observe for each dataset a reduction of the quality of −0.5 % for EC and −4.73 % for QA. In both cases, the semantic blocking might be too restrictive by filtering some relevant UMLS concepts. A reason might be that the selection of our training set is not representative for the unannotated set of forms. We plan to further study the NER model generation to improve the blocking of UMLS concepts. Overall, our semantic blocking leads to good execution time reductions by fairly preserving recall values.

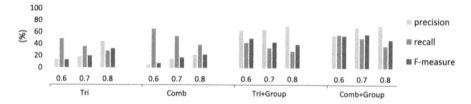

Fig. 8. Quality evaluation: comparison of trigram (*Tri*), combined matching (*Comb*) and group-based filtering (*Tri+Group* and *Comb+Group*) for QA forms.

4.2 Matching and Group-Based Filtering

We now generate annotation mappings by using a simple trigram matching (*Tri*), compare it to our combined match strategy based on TF/IDF, Trigram and LCS (*Comb*), and evaluate the impact of the group-based filtering (*Group*) for the QA dataset (see Fig. 8). We disable the blocking for this experiment and consider different threshold settings to evaluate the annotation quality. The combined match approach leads to higher recall values for all thresholds compared to trigram, since *Comb* detects a higher number of correct annotations compared to the single matcher. In particular, the combined matching achieves the best recall of ~66 % ($t = 0.6$) which is 17 % more than for trigram. Trigram is more restrictive and results in higher precision values, such that the overall F-measure is better for low thresholds. In general, increasing the threshold improves the overall annotation quality due to a higher precision, e.g. for $t = 0.8$ the F-measure is 15 % higher than for $t = 0.6$ (*Comb*). However, we want to find a high number of correct annotations (high recall) during the annotation generation phase. Therefore, we then filter wrong correspondences using our group-based selection strategy (Fig. 8 right). This leads to significantly improved precision values and preserves the high recall. Since the combined match strategy results in higher recall values than the trigram matching, the F-measure values of the combined match strategy with the group-based selection (*Comb+Group*) are better than the trigram matching with the group-based selection (*Tri+Group*). For $t = 0.7$, we achieve the best average F-measure of 57 % for the QA dataset. Thus, the group-based filtering is a valuable selection strategy to remove wrong but keep correct annotations.

4.3 Result Summary

To give a result overview w.r.t. the annotation quality, we show average F-measure values for all datasets (EC, QA, TI) in Fig. 9. Since the semantic blocking decrease the quality, we compare the trigram matching (*Tri*), trigram matching with group-based filtering (*Tri+Group*) and combined matching with group-based filtering (*Comb+Group*) Due to a different amount of free text within the datasets, a uniform threshold not results in the best quality for each dataset, e.g., the TI dataset consists of mostly two words per item compared to the QA and EC dataset which have mostly more than three words per item. Therefore, we calculate the average for the thresholds 0.6, 0.7 and 0.8. The vertical lines indicate the

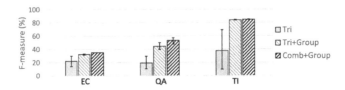

Fig. 9. Comparison of effectiveness of the combined matching strategy and group-based filtering approach for each dataset.

minimum and the maximum F-measure values for the underlying thresholds. We observe for each dataset an increasing of F-measure by applying group-based filtering compared to trigram matching. The precision increases heavily while most correct annotations are preserved. Since the combined matching strategy results in higher recall values than the trigram matching, the combination with group filtering leads to better F-measure values such that the difference of best F-measure values is ∼3 %(EC), ∼7 %(QA) and ∼0.5 %(TI). We achieve the best F-measure of ∼85 % for TI followed by ∼57 % for QA and ∼35 % for EC.

The automatic annotation of the EC dataset showed to be very difficult, since EC contains items with specifically long natural language sentences covering an unknown number of medical concepts. The annotation of QA forms leads to better results, but still needs improvement. For the annotation of the top items (TI) we achieve very good results. These items have been manually reduced to the relevant medical terms having a positive impact on the automatic assignment of UMLS concepts for this dataset. The semantic blocking was valuable to reduce executions times, and the combined match strategy together with the group-based filtering showed to produce very good results compared to a simple trigram matching. Overall, the automatic annotation of medical forms is a challenging task and requires future research, e.g. to further improve the recall.

4.4   Validation

We applied a semi-automatic annotation for the QA dataset by manually validating recommendations generated by our automatic annotation workflow. We computed mappings for all 23 QA forms using semantic blocking, combined matching and group-based filtering. For every form and question, we presented the expected correct annotations as well as our recommendations, and highlighted false negatives, false positives and true positives.

Medical experts could identify 213 new correct annotations out of the set of false positives. We further found 5 wrong annotations in the reference mappings based on our automatically generated recommendations. According to these findings we adapted the QA reference mappings leading to an average F-measure improvement of 9 % (for $t = 0.7$). Note, that we used these adapted QA reference mappings in the previous sections. Some of the recommendations were especially valuable. In particular, we found correct UMLS concepts for 38 so far not annotated questions, e.g.:

Question	Annotated concept
Heartbeat skipping (except for sleeping phases)	Dropped beats – heart (C0425591)
Ulcerating plaque	Carotid Ulcer (C0751634)
Malignant tumor (without curative treatment)	Malignant Neoplasms (C0006826)

The manual annotation of medical forms is difficult for curators. UMLS Metathesaurus is very huge, and even for medical experts it is hard to find a complete set of annotations. Sometimes it is difficult to decide for the correct concept, since UMLS contains similar concepts that might be suitable for the same medical concept in a question of a medical form [20]. Applying our automatic annotation workflow led to new correct annotations and could even indicate some false annotations. Our results point out the importance of semi-automatic annotation approaches. Combining manual and automatic annotation techniques (1) reduces the manual annotation effort and (2) leads to more complete and correct overall results. Semi-automatic annotation is especially relevant, since many medical forms are sparsely or not annotated. For instance, in MDM most items are only pre-annotated and need to be curated again. Part of the forms could not be annotated so far, and MDM is continuously extended by new non-annotated forms. Medical forms in MDM and can be semantically enriched by applying our annotation workflow in combination with expert validation.

5   Related Work

Our work on automatic annotation of medical forms is related to the areas of information retrieval [15] and ontology matching [8,17]. Both research fields have been studied intensively and provide useful methods to process free-text and match identified concepts to standardized vocabularies. Our system GOMMA [11] already allows for efficient and effective matching of especially large life science ontologies and can be a basis to align items with concepts of large ontologies. However, GOMMA does not provide methods to match free-text like form items.

In the medical domain, manual and automatic annotation methods have been studied to semantically enrich different kinds of documents. For instance, in [9] the authors clustered similar clinical trials by performing nearest neighbor search based on similarly annotated eligibility criteria. In [12] the application of a dictionary-based pre-annotation method could improve the speed of manual annotation for clinical trial announcements. The work in [19] focuses on the manual annotation process by presenting a semantic annotation schema and guidelines for clinical documents like radiology reports. The tool MetaMap [1] allows to retrieve UMLS concepts in medical texts based on information retrieval methods like tokenization and lexical lookup. In own initial tests by medical experts, MetaMap annotation results were not sufficient for our purposes. Moreover, there is evidence in the literature that MetaMap results are not fine-grained enough [14], contain too many spurious annotations [16] and do not cover mappings to longer medical terms [18]. In own previous work we already used manual annotations to compare and cluster different medical forms from the MDM platform [7]. We further identified most frequent eligibility criteria in clinical trial forms and performed a manual annotation for these top terms [20].

Previous research showed the usefulness of semantic annotations for different kinds of clinical documents. However, the problem remains that annotations, in particular, for medical forms are only sparsely available. So far, there is no automatic annotation tool to support the semantic annotation of large medical form sets as provided by MDM. In contrast to previous work on document annotation in the medical domain, we here focus on the development of automatic annotation methods for medical forms. In particular, we use a novel blocking technique to reduce the complexity of UMLS as well as a combined match approach to cope with shorter as well as free-text questions. A novel group-based filtering allows to select the most likely set of question annotations to be presented for further manual validation.

6   Conclusions and Future Work

We proposed a workflow to (semi-)automatically annotate items in medical forms with concepts of UMLS. The automatic annotation is challenging since form questions are often formulated in long natural language sentences and can cover several medical concepts. The huge size of UMLS further complicates the annotation generation. We used a combined match strategy and presented a novel semantic blocking as well as a group-based filtering of annotations. We applied our methods to annotate real-world medical forms from the MDM portal and performed a manual validation of the generated annotations. Our methods showed to be effective and we could generate valuable recommendations. Medical experts can benefit from automatic form annotation since it reduces the manual effort and can prevent from missing or incorrect annotations.

We see several directions for future work. We will extend our annotation workflow to enable an adaptive matching which automatically determines the thresholds and select a set of appropriate match approaches by considering useful dataset characteristics. We further plan to annotate the instance information of items, e.g. their response options or data types. To test whether recommendations computed by different annotation methods can complement each other, we will integrate results of other tools like MetaMap. Furthermore, we plan to develop a reuse repository to facilitate the annotation of existing and creation of new medical forms based on well-annotated items.

Acknowledgment. This work is funded by the German Research Foundation (DFG) (grant RA 497/22-1, "ELISA - Evolution of Semantic Annotations").

References

1. Aronson, A.R., Lang, F.M.: An overview of MetaMap: historical perspective and recent advances. J. Am. Med. Inform. Assoc. **17**(3), 229–236 (2010)

2. Bodenreider, O.: The Unified Medical Language System (UMLS): integrating bio-medical terminology. Nucleic Acids Res. **32**(suppl 1), D267–D270 (2004)
3. Bramesfeld, A., Willms, G.: Cross-Sectoral Quality Assurance. Â§137a Social Code Book V. Public Health Forum, pp. 14.e1–14.e3 (2014)
4. Breil, B., Kenneweg, J., Fritz, F., et al.: Multilingual medical data models in ODM format-a novel form-based approach to semantic interoperability between routine health-care and clinical research. Appl. Clin. Inf. **3**, 276–289 (2012)
5. Donnelly, K.: SNOMED-CT: The advanced terminology and coding system for eHealth. Stud. Health Technol. Inform. Med. Care Compunetics **3**(121), 279–290 (2006)
6. Dugas, M.: Missing semantic annotation in databases. The root cause for data integration and migration problems in information systems. Methods Inf. Med. **53**(6), 516–517 (2014)
7. Dugas, M., Fritz, F., Krumm, R., Breil, B.: Automated UMLS-based comparison of medical forms. PloS one **8**(7) (2013). doi:10.1371/journal.pone.0067883
8. Euzenat, J., Shvaiko, P.: Ontology Matching, vol. 18. Springer, Heidelberg (2007)
9. Hao, T., Rusanov, A., Boland, M.R., et al.: Clustering clinical trials with similar eligibility criteria features. J. Biomed. Inform. **52**, 112–120 (2014)
10. Huntley, R.P., Sawford, T., Mutowo-Meullenet, P., et al.: The GOA database: gene Ontology annotation updates for 2015. Nucleic Acids Res. **43**(D1), D1057–D1063 (2015)
11. Kirsten, T., Gross, A., Hartung, M., Rahm, E.: GOMMA: a component-based infrastructure for managing and analyzing life science ontologies and their evolution. J. Biomed. Semant. **2**(6), 1–24 (2011)
12. Lingren, T., Deleger, L., Molnar, K., et al.: Evaluating the impact of pre-annotation on annotation speed and potential bias: natural language processing gold standard development for clinical named entity recognition in clinical trial announcements. J. Am. Med. Inform. Assoc. **21**(3), 406–413 (2014)
13. Lowe, H.J., Barnett, G.O.: Understanding and using the medical subject headings (MeSH) vocabulary to perform literature searches. J. Am. Med. Assoc. (JAMA) **271**(14), 1103–1108 (1994)
14. Luo, Z., Duffy, R., Johnson, S., Weng, C.: Corpus-based approach to creating a semantic lexicon for clinical research eligibility criteria from umls. AMIA Summits Transl. Sci. Proc. **2010**, 26–30 (2010)
15. Manning, C.D., Raghavan, P., Schütze, H.: Introduction to Information Retrieval, vol. 1. Cambridge University Press, Cambridge (2008)
16. Ogren, P., Savova, G., Chute, C.: Constructing evaluation corpora for automated clinical named entity recognition. In: Proceedings of the Sixth International Conference on Language Resources and Evaluation (LREC), pp. 3143–3150 (2008)
17. Rahm, E.: Towards large-scale schema and ontology matching. In: Bellahsene, Z., Bonifati, A., Rahm, E. (eds.) Schema Matching and Mapping. Data-Centric Systems and Applications, pp. 3–27. Springer, Berlin (2011)
18. Ren, K., Lai, A.M., Mukhopadhyay, A., et al.: Effectively processing medical term queries on the UMLS Metathesaurus by layered dynamic programming. BMC Med. Genomics **7**(Suppl 1), 1–12 (2014)
19. Roberts, A., Gaizauskas, R., Hepple, M., et al.: Building a semantically annotated corpus of clinical texts. J. Biomed. Inform. **42**(5), 950–966 (2009)
20. Varghese, J., Dugas, M.: Frequency analysis of medical concepts in clinical trials and their coverage in MeSH and SNOMED-CT. Methods Inf. Med. **53**(6), 83–92 (2014)

OnSim: A Similarity Measure for Determining Relatedness Between Ontology Terms

Ignacio Traverso-Ribón[1](✉), Maria-Esther Vidal[2], and Guillermo Palma[2]

[1] FZI Research Center for Information Technology,
Karlsruhe Institute of Technology, Karlsruhe, Germany
`traverso@fzi.de`
[2] Universidad Simón Bolívar, Caracas, Venezuela
`{mvidal,gpalma}@ldc.usb.ve`

Abstract. Accurately measuring relatedness between ontology terms becomes a building block for determining similarity of ontology-based annotated entities, e.g., genes annotated with the Gene Ontology. However, existing measures that determine similarity between ontology terms mainly rely on *taxonomic* hierarchies of classes, and may not fully exploit the semantics encoded in the ontology, i.e., object properties and their axioms. This limitation may conduct to ignore the stated or inferred facts where an ontology term participate in the ontology, i.e., the term *neighborhood*. Thus, high values of similarity can be erroneously assigned to terms that are *taxonomically* similar, but whose neighborhoods are different. We present OnSim, a measure where semantics encoded in the ontology is considered as a *first-class* citizen and exploited to determine relatedness of ontology terms. OnSim considers the *neighborhoods* of two terms, as well as the object properties that are present in the neighborhood facts and the *justifications* that support the entailment of these facts. We have extended an existing annotation-based similarity measure with OnSim, and empirically studied the impact of producing accurate values of ontology term relatedness. Experiments were run on benchmarks published by the *Collaborative Evaluation of Semantic Similarity Measures (CESSM)* tool. The observed results suggest that OnSim increases the Pearson's correlation coefficient of the annotation-based similarity measure with respect to gold standard similarity measures, as well as its effectiveness is improved with respect to state-of-the-art semantic similarity measures.

1 Introduction

Semantic Web initiatives have fostered the development of large linked collections from different domains [11], as well as the collaborative definition of ontologies to semantically describe and annotate these data. Particularly, the biological and biomedical domain has been greatly benefited from these research movements, and a diversity of semantically annotated linked scientific datasets

© Springer International Publishing Switzerland 2015
N. Ashish and J.-L. Ambite (Eds.): DILS 2015, LNBI 9162, pp. 70–86, 2015.
DOI: 10.1007/978-3-319-21843-4_6

are publicly available, e.g., Chem2Bio2RDF[1], Bio2RDF[2], OpenPHACTS[3], and Linked Life Data[4]. Further, expressive ontologies have been defined, e.g., the Gene Ontology (GO)[5], and they have been extensively accepted by the scientific community as standards to describe the concepts and relations, and to replace textual descriptions by controlled vocabulary terms from the ontologies. For example, GO terms are extensively used for capturing functional information of proteins and genes as indicated in the Gene Ontology Annotation (UniProt-GOA) database[6], and there are international initiatives to collaboratively annotate organisms, e.g., the *Pseudomonas aeruginosa PAO1 genome*[7].

Ontology-based annotations provide the basis to uncover novel and interesting patterns, e.g., to predict gene functions across organisms, drug-target interactions, or to suggest families of drugs that interact in the effectiveness of other drugs. Annotations are also used to determine relatedness between annotated concepts that could not be observed only using structural properties of the entities. In this direction, several annotation-based similarity measures have been defined [4,12] and results of empirical evaluation studies suggest that considering ontology annotations can enhance the effectiveness of similarity measures [12,14]. Nevertheless, although the great effort conducted by the biomedical and Semantic Web communities, state-of-the-art annotation-based similarity measures may not fully explote all the semantics encoded in the annotations, and imprecisely assign high values of similarity to dissimilar entities [3,12].

Next, we illustrate the potential impact of semantics on the computation of relatedness. Figure 1 presents a taxonomy of relations (i.e., object properties) in the Gene Ontology (GO); *negatively regulates* (nr), *positively regulates* (pr), *regulates* (rg), *is-a* (sc), and *part of* (pf). These relations can refine a neighborhood-based similarity approach assuming that not only the neighbors of a concept influence in the similarity measure, but also the *justifications* that support the entailment of facts in the neighborhood. For example, even if the concepts A, B, C, and D have the same *taxonomic* properties, they should not be considered all equally identical, if they are related through the following relations or object properties: *(i)* A pf D; *(ii)* B nr D; and *(iii)* C pr D. Moreover, because nr and pr are more similar according to the object property hierarchy (See Fig. 1), both B and C must be more similar than A and B, or A and C. Additionally, existing annotation-based similarity measures do not take into account inferred facts or the *justifications* that support their entailment. However, considering the justifications of inferred facts may provide also insights of uncover properties required to accurately determine similarity of ontology-based annotated entities.

---

[1] http://chem2bio2rdf.org/.
[2] http://bio2rdf.org/.
[3] http://openphacts.org.
[4] http://linkedlifedata.com.
[5] http://geneontology.org/.
[6] http://www.ebi.ac.uk/GOA.
[7] http://www.pseudomonas.com/go_annotation_project_2014.jsp.

We propose OnSim, a novel semantic similarity measure for ontology
terms that is able to: *(i)* distinguish
the object properties that relate ontology terms with facts in their neighborhoods; and *(ii)* consider inferred
facts and the justifications that support their entailment.

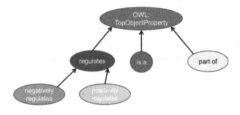

Fig. 1. GO taxonomy of object properties

We model OnSim as a 1-1 maximum weight bipartite matching of the
neighborhoods of two ontology terms, as well as of the justifications conducted to
infer facts in the neighborhoods. We extend the state-of-the-art annotation-based
similarity measure *AnnSim* [12] with OnSim to analyze the impact of considering the semantics of the annotations. *AnnSim* was selected as the baseline of our
evaluation because it has shown to effectively behave in a diversity of real-world
datasets of genes and their GO annotations, clinical trials, and human disease
benchmarks [12]. The *Collaborative Evaluation of Semantic Similarity Measures
(CESSM)*[8] tool was used to evaluate the correlation of *AnnSim*OnSim with
respect to domain-specific similarities considered as gold standards by the biomedical community: the *ECC* similarity [6], *Pfam* similarity [15], and Sequence
Similarity *SeqSim* [20]. The evaluation was conducted on two collections of pairs
of proteins published by the two available versions of the CESSM tool: the 2008
collection contains 13,430 pairs of proteins from UniProt-GOA[9], while the 2014
dataset comprises 22,302 pairs; annotations are from GO versions 2008 and 2014,
respectively. Reported plots are produced by the CESSM tool, and reveal that
*AnnSim*OnSim enhances the effectiveness of *AnnSim* by increasing the Pearson's
correlation coefficients with respect to the gold standard measures. Additionally,
*AnnSim*OnSim is compared to eleven state-of-the-art semantic similarity measures, and it is able to outperform all these measures with respect to Pfam, while
is competitive with the other two gold standard measures. Further improvements are observed in the CESSM 2014 collection, suggesting that high values
of *AnnSim*OnSim may provide evidences of high quality annotations.

*AnnSim*OnSim is also used to determining relatedness among patients annotated with the Human Phenotype Ontology (HPO)[10]. Patient data is produced
and managed to remotely monitoring patients in the FI-STAR project[11]. FI-
STAR detects anomalies in patient measurements and vital signs by exploiting
semantics and Complex Event Processing (CEP) technologies. FI-STAR man-
ages static and sensed data, as well as real-time predictions. Static data provide contextual information that improves the predictions of the system, and
are represented as ontology-based annotations of the patients. Pair-wise values of *AnnSim*OnSim computed from static data are exploited by FI-STAR

---

[8] http://xldb.di.fc.ul.pt/tools/cessm/about.php.
[9] http://www.uniprot.org/.
[10] http://www.human-phenotype-ontology.org/.
[11] https://www.fi-star.eu.

link prediction methods; the implemented hypothesis prediction establishes that patients with similar symptoms also suffer of similar diseases.

This paper is organized as follows: Sect. 2 provides a motivating example in the biomedical domain and Sect. 3 briefly describes preliminaries of our work. Section 4 presents the OnSim approach, and experimental results are reported in Sect. 5. Section 6 summarizes related research and Sect. 7 concludes.

2   Motivating Example

Figure 2 presents a portion of the neighborhoods of the GO terms *adaptation of rhodopsin mediated signaling* (GO:0016062), and *deactivation of rhodopsin mediated signaling* (GO:0016059). These terms are used to annotate entities from different collections. For example, in the UniProt-GOA dataset[12], they are used to annotate the proteins P10676 and P13217. These GO terms participate in different object properties; concretely, we observe in Fig. 2, that they occur in the object properties **rg** and **nr**, which are sub-properties of **rg** (Fig. 1). GO is described in OWL, which allows for representing logical axioms to describe the semantics of the object properties, e.g., include logical axioms to express transitivity or symmetry. Similarly to other biomedical ontologies, GO is continuously changing and therefore, these logical axioms may also change. In the GO version of 2008, **rg** is not associated with any logical axiom, while the GO 2014 version states that **rg** is transitive over **pf**. We focus on the 2008 version of GO in our motivating example, but we will see in our experimental results that more detailed definitions of logical axioms positively impact on the behavior of similarity measures. Figure 2 illustrates justifications of the inferred facts (GO:0016062 **rg** GO:0008150) and (GO:0016059 **rg** GO:0008150):

1. The first justification relies on: the *axiom of Instantiation of SubClassOf* (**sc**) over **nr** and the *axiom of Instantiation of SubPropertyOf* (**sp**) over **rg**. In Fig. 2, we observe that (GO:0016062 **sc** GO:0022401) and (GO:0022401 **nr** GO:0008150). Then, we can infer (GO:0016062 **nr** GO:0008150) by transitivity of the object property **nr** over **sc**. Finally, because **nr** is sub-property of **rg**, we can infer the fact (GO:0016062 **rg** GO:0008150).
2. This inference is justified by the *axiom of Instantiation of SubClassOf* (**sc**) over **rg**. In other way, every GO term inherits all the properties of its ancestors. The GO term GO:0050789 is an ancestor of GO:0016059, i.e., (GO:0016059 **sc** GO:0050789) and (GO:0050789 **rg** GO:0008150) hold; therefore, we infer the fact (GO:0016059 **rg** GO:0008150).

Existing ontology-based similarities mainly rely on *taxonomic* hierarchies of classes, and are not aware of these differences. For example, D_{tax} [1] and D_{ps} [13] are two taxonomic similarity measures that define similarity of two nodes in terms of the depth of the nodes to the root of class hierarchy, and the distance to their lowest common ancestor (LCA). D_{tax} and D_{ps} will assign relatively high values of similarities to GO:0016062 and GO:0016059, 0.625 and

---

[12] http://www.ebi.ac.uk/GOA.

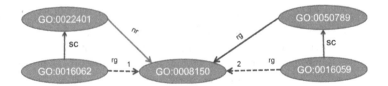

Fig. 2. Portion of the neighborhood from GO:0016062 and GO:0016059. Solid arrows represent stated object properties: *negatively regulates* (**ng**), *regulates* (**rg**), and *is-a* (**sc**). Dashed arrows represent inferred object properties.

0.55, respectively. Nevertheless, D_{tax} and D_{ps} ignore that both the neighborhoods of GO:0016062 and GO:0016059, and the justifications of their inferred facts are different. Therefore, D_{tax} and D_{ps} values may overestimate the real value of relatedness of these GO terms.

3   Preliminaries

AnnSim [12] and D_{tax} [1] have exhibited effective behavior on different domains, e.g., real-world datasets of genes and their GO annotations, clinical trials, and human disease benchmarks. Thus, we rely on these measures to evaluate the effectiveness of OnSim.

Consider two entities e_1 and e_2 annotated with the set of ontology terms A_1 and A_2. Let $BG = (A_1 \cup A_2, WE)$ be a weighted bipartite graph for set of terms A_1 and A_2, and $MWBG = (A_1 \cup A_2, WE_r)$ be 1-1 maximum weight bipartite matching for BG. Intersection of sets A_1 and A_2 is assumed empty, i.e., in case the same ontology term t occurs in A_1 and A_2, both occurrences of t are seen as different terms during the construction of BG and $MWBG$. The annotation-based similarity *AnnSim* is defined as follows:

$$AnnSim(e_1, e_2) = \frac{2 * \sum_{(a_1, a_2) \in WE_r} Sim(a_1, a_2)}{|A_1| + |A_2|}$$

A 1-1 *maximum weight bipartite matching* [17], $MWBG = (A_1 \cup A_2, WE_r)$ for a weighted bipartite graph $BG = (A_1 \cup A_2, WE)$, where edges are annotated with similarity *Sim* is as follows:

- $WE_r \subseteq WE$, i.e., *MWBG* is a sub-graph of BG.
- The sum of the weights of the edges in WE_r is maximized, i.e.,

$$max \sum_{(a_1, a_2) \in WE_r} Sim(a_1, a_2)$$

- for each node in $A_1 \cup A_2$ there is only one incident edge in WE_r, i.e.,
  - $\sum_{i=1}^{|A_1|}(a_i, a_j) = 1, \forall j = 1 \cdots |A_2|$
  - $\sum_{j=1}^{|A_2|}(a_i, a_j) = 1, \forall i = 1 \cdots |A_1|$

$Sim(a_1, a_2)$ is a generic similarity measure for ontology terms, but Palma et al. [12] reports on the benefits of using the taxonomic similarity D_{tax} [1]. D_{tax} computes taxonomic similarity values in terms of Lowest Common Ancestor. Given a directed graph G, the lowest common ancestor of two nodes x and y, is the node of greatest depth in G that is an ancestor of both x and y. Let $d(x, y)$ be the number of edges on the longest path between nodes x and y in a given ontology. Also let $lca(x, y)$ be the lowest common ancestor of nodes x and y, and $root$ is the root of the class hierarchy.

$$D_{tax}(x, y) = 1 - \frac{d(x, lca(x, y)) + d(y, lca(x, y))}{d(root, x) + d(root, y)}$$

4   OnSim: An Ontology Similarity Measure

OnSim is an ontology similarity measure that computes relatedness between ontology terms. OnSim not only relies on taxonomic hierarchies of the classes to decide relatedness, but also considers the neighborhoods of two terms, as well as the object properties that relate these terms with the facts in the neighborhoods and the justifications that support the entailment of these facts.

To illustrate the impact that considering additional knowledge may have on the computation of the similarity, consider the GO terms *adaptation of rhodopsin mediated signaling* (GO:0016062) and *deactivation of rhodopsin mediated signaling* (GO:0016059). As observed in Fig. 3(a) and 3(b), the neighborhoods of these terms are different, as well as the justifications that support the inference of these facts. Nevertheless, taxonomic similarity measures ignore this information and may assign relatively high values of similarity to these two terms. Contrary, OnSim detects that these two annotations are dissimilar in terms of the facts in the neighborhoods and their justifications, and assigns a lower similarity value, i.e., *OnSim(GO:0016062, GO:0016059)* is equal to *0.31*.

To represent neighborhoods and justifications, we define for each ontology term a_i, a set R_{a_i} that represent the neighborhood of a_i. Facts in the neighborhood are modeled as quadruples $t = (a_i, a_j, r_{ij}, E_{ij})$, where r_{ij} is an object property such that there is an out-going link from a_i to a_j in the ontology, and E_{ij} is a set of the instantiations of the *antecedents* of the axioms used to infer the fact $(a_i \; r_{ij} \; a_j)$[13]. Thus, $t_1 = (\text{GO:0016062}, \text{GO:0007165}, \text{rg}, \{(\text{nr sp rg}), (\text{GO:0016062 nr GO:0007165}), \text{Ax.4}\})$ is the quadruple that represents that the GO terms GO:0016062 and GO:0007165 are related through the object property rg (Fig. 3(b)). Further, t_1 states the justification of this inferred fact; in this case axiom Ax.4 is applied, and the instantiation of the antecedent of Ax.4 is (GO:0016062 nr GO:0007165). We define a quadruple t, based on the OWL2 axioms applied in a given justification.

Definition 1. *Given two ontology terms a_i and a_j, and an object property r_{ij}. A fact in the neighborhood of a_i establishing that a_i and a_j are related through*

---

[13] According to OWL2 semantics the inferred fact is a_i subClassOf r_{ij} some a_j.

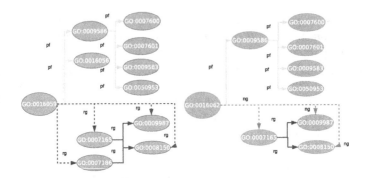

(a) Neighborhood of GO:0016059 (b) Neighborhood of GO:0016062

Fig. 3. Neighborhoods of GO terms. Object properties in inferred facts are represented with Dashed Arrows. Object properties are represented in arrows of different colors

r_{ij}, *i.e.,* $(a_i\ r_{ij}\ a_j)$, *is represented as a quadruple* $t = (a_i, a_j, r_{ij}, E_{ij})$, *where* E_{ij} *is a set of the instantiations of the antecedents of the axioms used to infer the fact* $(a_i\ r_{ij}\ a_j)$. *Depending of the axioms used to inferred the fact* $(a_i\ r_{ij}\ a_j)$, *the quadruple* t *is inductively defined as follows:*

1. *(Ax.1) Axiom of Symmetry Relation* r_{ij}:

$$\frac{(a_i\ r_{ij}\ a_j)}{(a_j\ r_{ij}\ a_i)} \implies t = (a_i, a_j, r_{ij}, \{(a_j\ r_{ij}\ a_i), Ax.1\})$$

2. *(Ax.2) Axiom of Instantiation of SubClassOf (sc) over* r_{ij}:

$$\frac{(a_i\ sc\ a_z) \wedge (a_z\ r_{ij}\ a_j)}{(a_i\ r_{ij}\ a_j)} \implies t = (a_i, a_j, r_{ij}, \{(a_i\ sc\ a_z), (a_z\ r_{ij}\ a_j), Ax.2\})$$

3. *(Ax.3) Axiom of Transitivity of SubClassOf (sc):*

$$\frac{(a_i\ sc\ a_z) \wedge (a_z\ sc\ a_j)}{(a_i\ sc\ a_j)} \implies t = (a_i, a_j, sc, \{(a_i\ sc\ a_z), (a_z\ sc\ a_j), Ax.3\})$$

4. *(Ax.4) Axiom of Instantiation of SubPropertyOf (sp) over* r_{ij}:

$$\frac{(r_z\ sp\ r_{ij}) \wedge (a_i\ r_z\ a_j)}{(a_i\ r_{ij}\ a_j)} \implies t = (a_i, a_j, r_{ij}, \{(r_z\ sp\ r_{ij}), (a_i\ r_z\ a_j), Ax.4\})$$

5. *(Ax.5) Axiom of Transitivity of SubPropertyOf (sp):*

$$\frac{(a_i\ sp\ a_z) \wedge (a_z\ sp\ a_j)}{(a_i\ sp\ a_j)} \implies t = (a_i, a_j, sp, \{(a_i\ sp\ a_z), (a_z\ sp\ a_j), Ax.5\})$$

6. *(Ax.6) Axiom of Transitivity Relation r_{ij}:*

$$\frac{(a_i\ r_{ij}\ a_z) \wedge (a_z\ r_{ij}\ a_j)}{(a_i\ r_{ij}\ a_j)} \implies t = (a_i, a_j, r_{ij}, \{(a_i\ r_{ij}\ a_z), (a_z\ r_{ij}\ a_j), Ax.6\})$$

7. *(Ax.7) Axiom of Transitivity of r_z over r_{ij}:*

$$\frac{(a_i\ r_z\ a_z) \wedge (a_z\ r_{ij}\ a_j)}{(a_i\ r_{ij}\ a_j)} \implies t = (a_i\ a_j, r_{ij}, \{(a_i\ r_z\ a_z), (a_z\ r_{ij}\ a_j), Ax.7\})$$

Inductive Case: *If $t_z = (a_z, a_k, r_{zk}, E_{zk})$ is part of the neighborhood of a_z, $t_i = (a_i, a_j, r_{ij}, E_{ij})$ is in the neighborhood of a_i, and $(a_z\ r_{zk}\ a_k) \in E_{ij}$, then eliminate t_i from the neighborhood of a_i and add the quadruple $t = (a_i, a_j, r_{ij}, \overline{E}_{ij})$ to the neighborhood of a_i, where $\overline{E}_{ij} = (E_{ij} - \{(a_z\ r_{zk}\ a_k)\}) \cup E_{zk}$.*

Let us consider the GO terms GO:0016062 and GO:0016059 in Fig. 4. The neighborhood of GO:0016062 represented by $R_{GO:0016062}$, comprises 12 quadruples associated with GO:0016062; the quadruples $t_{1.1}$ and $t_{1.2}$ describe the facts (GO:0016062 **rg** GO:0007165) and (GO:0016062 **rg** GO:0008150), respectively.

- $t_{1.1} = $(GO:0016062,GO:0007165,**rg**, {(**nr   sp   rg**), (GO:0016062 **nr** GO: 0007165), Ax.4}).
- $t_{1.2} = $(GO:0016062, GO:0008150,**rg**, {(**nr   sp   rg**), (GO:0016062 **sc** GO: 0022401), (GO:0022401 **nr** GO:0008150), Ax.2, Ax.4}.

Note that the quadruple $t_{1.2}$ represents the information of the justification of the fact (GO:0016062 **rg** GO:0008150), where more than one axiom support the inference, and the inductive definition of a quadruple (Definition 1) is applied to generate the quadruple, i.e., the justification is as follows:

$$(\text{GO:0016062 sc GO:0022401}) \wedge (\text{GO:0022401 nr GO:0008150})$$
$\Rightarrow \quad <\text{Ax.2}, (A\ \textbf{sc}\ B) \wedge (B\ \textbf{r}\ C) \Rightarrow (A\ \textbf{r}\ C) >$
$$(\textbf{nr sp rg}) \wedge (\text{GO:0016062 nr GO:0008150})$$
$\Rightarrow \quad <\text{Ax.4}, (r_i\ \textbf{sp}\ r_j) \wedge (B\ r_i\ C) \Rightarrow (B\ r_j\ C) >$
$$(\text{GO:0016062 rg GO:0008150})$$

Similarly, $R_{GO:0016059}$ describes the neighborhood of GO:0016059 and comprises 14 quadruples. The quadruple $t_{2.1}$ represents the fact (GO:0016059 **rg** GO:0008150):

- $t_{2.1} = $(GO:0016059,GO:0008150,**rg**, {(GO:0016059 **sc** GO:0050789), (GO: 0050789 **rg** GO:0008150), Ax.2}).

Given two quadruples, $t_{1i} = (a_1, a_i, r_{1i}, E_{1i})$ and $t_{2j} = (a_2, a_j, r_{2j}, E_{2j})$, the similarity of two quadruples $Sim(t_{1i}, t_{2j})$ is defined as the product triangular norm, TN, that combines the taxonomic similarity of t_{1i} and t_{2j} with the similarity of the sets E_{1i} and E_{2j} of justifications, $Sim_{justifications}(E_{1i}, E_{2j})$.

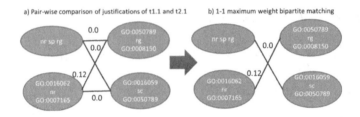

Fig. 4. Comparison of the justifications of quadruples $t_{1.1}$ and $t_{2.1}$; axiom identifiers are omitted for legibility: (a) Bi-partite graph from the pair-wise comparison of the justifications; (b) 1-1 maximum weight bipartite matching produced by the BlossomIV solver [2]

An item it_i in a justification can be an axiom identifier, or an RDF triple (b_i p_i c_i) that denotes the instantiation of one of the antecedents of the axiom. For example, the justification of the quadruple $t_{1.1} = $ (GO:0016062,GO:0007165,rg, {(nr sp rg), (GO:0016062 nr GO:0007165), Ax.4}) is a set that comprises three items; two items are RDF triples (nr sp rg) and (GO:0016062 nr GO:0007165), and the other item is the identifier of the applied axiom, i.e., Ax.4. The similarity of two justification items $it_i = (b_i$ p_i c_i) and $it_j = (b_j$ p_j c_j), named $Sim_{justification}(it_i, it_j)$, is defined as a product triangular norm that combines three taxonomic similarities: $D_{tax}(b_i, b_j)$, $D_{tax}(p_i, p_j)$, and $D_{tax}(c_i, c_j)$. Further, the similarity of the same axiom identifier is 1.0, while two different axioms are dissimilar, i.e., their similarity value is 0.0.

In our running example, if the taxonomic similarity is D_{tax} [1], the similarity of the justification items $it_1 = $ (GO:0016062 nr GO:0007165) and $it_2 = $ (GO:0050789 rg GO:0008150) is 0.12, where

- D_{tax}(GO:0016062,GO:0050789) is 0.55;
- D_{tax}(nr,rg) is 0.67;
- D_{tax}(GO:0007165,GO:0008150) is 0.33;
- $Sim_{justification}(e_1, e_2) = 0.55 \times 0.67 \times 0.33$.

Two justifications E_{1i} and E_{2j} are compared based on a similarity value. Formally, the similarity of two justifications is computed from a bipartite graph that corresponds to the 1-1 *maximum weight bipartite matching* of the edges in the Cartesian product of $E_{1i} \times E_{2j}$. Figure 4 presents the 1-1 maximum weight bipartite matching of the justification sets of $t_{1.1} = $ (GO:0016062,GO:0007165,rg, {(nr sp rg), (GO:0016062 nr GO:0007165), Ax.4}) and $t_{2.1} = $ (GO:0016059,GO:0008150,rg, {(GO:0050789 rg GO:0008150), (GO:0016059 sc GO:0050789), Ax.2}); axiom identifiers are omitted for legibility. We apply an exact solution to the problem of computing the *1-1 maximum weight bipartite matching* from a bipartite graph using the BlossomIV solver [2]. Values of justification similarity are used to compute the 1-1 maximum weight bipartite matching, and the sum of this similarity is maximized in the best matching. The time complexity of computing the 1-1 maximum weight bipartite matching is $O(m^4)$, where m is sum of the cardinalities of sets of justifications.

Once the 1-1 maximum weight bipartite matching $MWBM$ of $E_{1i} \times E_{2j}$ is computed, the similarity of these justifications is calculated as follows.

$$Sim_{justifications}(E_{1i}, E_{2j}) = \frac{\sum\limits_{(e_i, e_j) \in MWBM(E_{1i}, E_{2j})} Sim_{justifications}(e_i, e_j)}{Max(|E_{1i}|, |E_{2j}|)}$$

Particularly, the $Sim_{justifications}$ values for the 1-1 maximum weight bipartite matching of quadruples $t_{1.1}$ and $t_{2.1}$ in Fig. 4 is 0.06. Finally, we compute similarity $OnSim(a_1, a_2)$ based on the knowledge represented in quadruples t_{1i} and t_{2j} in the sets R_1 and R_2 associated with the ontology terms a_1 and a_2, respectively. First, a graph $GOS = (R_1 \cup R_2, EOS)$ is a labelled bi-partite graph comprised of the nodes in the sets R_1 and R_2, $EOS \subseteq R_1 \times R_2$, and edges are annotated with the similarity of the quadruples. EOS corresponds to the 1-1 maximum weight bipartite matching of the edges in the Cartesian product of $R_1 \times R_2$.

$$OnSim(a_1, a_2) = TN\left(D_{tax}(a_1, a_2), \frac{\sum\limits_{(t_{1i}, t_{2j}) \in EOS} Sim(t_{1i}, t_{2j})}{Max(|R_1|, |R_2|)}\right)$$

- TN is a product triangular norm;
- R_1 and R_2 are the sets associated with a_1 and a_2, respectively;
- EOS corresponds to the 1-1 maximum weight bipartite matching of the quadruples in the Cartesian product of R_1 and R_2 annotated with the similarity $Sim(t_{1i}, t_{2j})$;
- quadruples $t_{1i} = (a_1, a_i, r_{1i}, E_{1i})$ and $t_{2j} = (a_2, a_j, r_{2j}, E_{2j})$ belong to EOS; and

Dummy Quadruple	0.0	t2.2
Dummy Quadruple	0.0	t2.3
t1.2	0.75	t2.5
t1.1	0.45	t2.4
t1.3	0.27	t2.1
t1.4	0.52	t2.6
t1.5	0.0	t2.7
t1.6	0.94	t2.8
t1.7	1.0	t2.9
t1.8	0.0	t2.10
t1.9	0.91	t2.11
t1.10	0.93	t2.12
t1.11	0.11	t2.13
t1.12	0.95	t2.14

Fig. 5. Comparison of $R_{GO:0016062}$ and $R_{GO:0016059}$: 1-1 maximum weight bipartite matching produced by the BlossomIV solver [2]; Dummy Quadruples are added by the solver to find a matching that maximizes the sum of the similarity values

– $Sim(t_{1i}, t_{2j})$ is defined as a triangular norm TN^{14} that combines similarity values of the justifications of r_{1i}, r_{2j} with the taxonomic similarity of t_{1i} and t_{2j}.

Figure 5 presents the 1-1 maximum weight bipartite matching found by the BlossomIV solver [2] for the GO terms GO:0016062 and GO:0016059. We can observe that two dummy nodes are added to ensure that the sum of the similarity values is maximized. OnSim is computed on top of this 1-1 maximum weight bipartite matching and combined with the taxonomic similarity value of D_{tax}(GO:0016062,GO:0016059); thus, OnSim(GO:0016062,GO:0016059) corresponds to $0.488 \times 0.625 = 0.31$, which is lower than the values of D_{tax} and D_{ps} reported in Sect. 2.

5 Experimental Results

The goal of the study is to evaluate the impact of OnSim on existing annotation-based similarity measures. Our research hypothesis states that because OnSim considers the neighborhood of two ontology terms, the annotation-based similarity values of entities annotated with these terms are more accurate. We conducted an empirical study on the collections of proteins published at the Collaborative Evaluation of Semantic Similarity Measures (CESSM) portals of 2008^{15} and 2014^{16} using Hermit 1.3.8 as the OWL reasoner. The CESSM 2008 collection contains 13,430 pairs of proteins from UniProt with 1,039 distinct proteins, while the CESSM 2014 collection comprises 22,302 pairs with 1,559 distinct proteins. Both collections are annotated with 1,908 distinct terms from the August 2008 version of GO and 3,909 distinct terms from the December 2014 version, respectively. The class hierarchy of the 2008 GO version has a maximum depth of 15 levels, while the depth of the version of 2014 increases until 17 levels. Similarly, the number of axioms grows; the 2008 version has four object properties, and one of them is transitive (*Ax.6*); and the 2014 version has ten object properties, three are transitive (*Ax.6*), and five meet the Object-PropertyChain (*Ax.7*). Annotations are from UniProt-GOA, and are separated into the GO hierarchies of biological process (BP), molecular function (MF), and cellular component (CC). CESSM computes the Pearson's correlation coefficients with respect to three similarity gold standards: *ECC* similarity [6], *Pfam* similarity [15], and Sequence Similarity *SeqSim* [20]. The *ECC* similarity assigns values between 0 and 4 that measure the number of Enzyme Comparison (ECC) digits that are shared by two genes; high values of ECC indicate that both genes share several digits and are similar. The Pfam similarity (Pfam) of two genes corresponds to the Jaccard similarity as the ratio between the number of shared Pfam families and the total number of Pfam families of the two genes. Pfam similarity values are between 0.0 and 1.0. Finally, *SeqSim* produces normalized

---

[14] For this ontology we used the *Product TN* for Sim and Sim_D.

[15] http://xldb.di.fc.ul.pt/tools/cessm/.

[16] http://xldb.di.fc.ul.pt/biotools/cessm2014/.

values of the Sequence Similarity measure of BLAST that measures the sequence alignment of two genes or proteins; *SeqSim* is one of the gold standard measures for gene sequence alignment.

Eleven semantic similarity measures are compared; these similarity measures extend Resnik's(R) [16], Lin's(L) [9], and Jiang and Conrath's(J) [10] measures to consider GO annotations of the compared proteins, the information content (IC) of these annotations, and pairwise combinations of common ancestors. The average combination which is labeled A, considers the average of the ICs of pairs of common ancestors. Sevilla et al. [18] apply the corresponding measure, i.e., the Resnik's [16], Lin's [9], and Jiang and Conrath's [10] measures, to the maximum value of IC of pairs of common ancestors; these combined measures are distinguished with the labeled M. Measures labelled with B are combined with the best-match average of the ICs of pairs of disjunctive common ancestors (DCA) proposed by Couto et al. [4]. Finally, the set-based measures simUI (UI) and simGIC (GI) [14] apply the Jaccard index to sets of annotations together with domain-specific information. We evaluate two versions of *AnnSim* on the two CESSM collections: $AnnSimD_{tax}$ relies on D_{tax} to decide the relatedness of two annotations, while *AnnSim*OnSim uses OnSim.

Figure 6(a)–(d) report on the comparison of *SeqSim* with $AnnSimD_{tax}$, *AnnSim*OnSim, and the GO based extensions of the Resnik's [16], Lin's [9], and Jiang and Conrath's [10] measures. Annotations are restricted to GO Biological Process (BP) terms, the richer branch of GO in terms of axioms. Plots in Fig. 6(a) and 6(b) were generated on CESSM 2008, while Fig. 6(c) and 6(d) were returned by CESSM 2014. In almost all the cases, the studied similarity measures assign high similarity values to pairs of proteins that SeqSim also consider similar. Nevertheless, the problem is to precisely distinguish when two proteins are dissimilar. In the collections 2008 and 2014, simGIC (GI) [14] has the highest correlation with respect to SeqSim, *0.773* and *0.799*, respectively. In addition to GO annotations of the proteins, GI additionally exploits information content of the GO annotations in conjunction with the most informative ancestors of these annotations. Thus, a more precise estimate of the relatedness of two proteins is computed, i.e., both GI and SeqSim assign low similarity values to a large number of pairs of proteins. $AnnSimD_{tax}$ does not precisely distinguish dissimilar proteins in none of the collections, and the correlation with respect to SeqSim is *0.650* and *0.682*. Contrary, *AnnSim*OnSim considerably enhances *AnnSim*, and exhibits a performance more similar to GI in dissimilar pairs of proteins, i.e., pairs of proteins with low SeqSim values; thus, the correlation with respect to SeqSim is *0.732* and *0.772*. This improvement is the result of analyzing the neighborhoods of the GO terms that are compared during the computation of *AnnSim*OnSim, and corroborates our hypothesis that OnSim can positively impact on the effectiveness of annotation-based similarity measures. Another interesting issue to highlight is the impact that newer versions of GO and annotations may have on the behavior of semantic similarity measures. Although the CESSM 2014 tool only reports on eight similarities, clearly all of them behave better in the CESSM 2014 collection than in the CESSM 2008. This observation suggests an improvement in the quality of the GO taxonomy and axioms, as

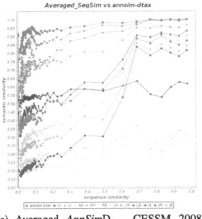

(a) Averaged $AnnSimD_{tax}$ CESSM 2008 Pearson's Correlation with SeqSim: 0.650

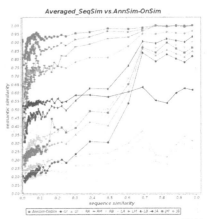

(b) Averaged $AnnSim$OnSim CESSM 2008 Pearson's Correlation with SeqSim: 0.732

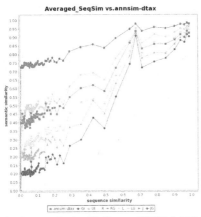

(c) Averaged $AnnSimD_{tax}$ CESSM 2014 Pearson's Correlation with SeqSim: 0.682

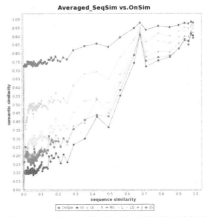

(d) Averaged $AnnSim$OnSim CESSM 2014 Pearson's Correlation with SeqSim: 0.772

Fig. 6. Results are produced by the CESSM tool for GO BP terms (versions 2008 and 2014). Average values for $AnnSimD_{tax}$ and $AnnSim$OnSim. The similarity measures are: simUI (UI), simGIC (GI), Resnik's Average (RA), Resnik's Maximum (RM), Resnik's Best-Match Average (RB), Lin's Average (LA), Lin's Maximum (LM), Lin's Best-Match Average (LB), Jiang&Conrath's Average (JA), Jiang&Conrath's Maximum (JM), Jiang&Conrath's Best-Match Average (JB)

well as on the annotations of the proteins provided by UniProt-GOA. Providing thus, this type of studies, not only the possibility of evaluating the effectiveness of existing measures, but also of analyzing the quality of existing ontologies and annotations.

Further, Table 1(a) and (b) report on the comparison of all the similarity measures with the gold standards: *ECC*, *Pfam*, and *SeqSim* on CESSM 2008 and 2014. Both tables report on Pearson's correlation coefficients, where the

Table 1. The Pearson's correlation coefficient between three gold standards and eleven similarity measures of CESSM. The top 5 correlations are highlighted in gray, and the highest correlation with respect to each gold standard is highlighted in *bold*.

(a) CESSM 2008				(b) CESSM 2014			
Similarity measure	*SeqSim*	*ECC*	*Pfam*	Similarity measure	*SeqSim*	*ECC*	*Pfam*
GI	**0.773**	0.398	0.454	GI	**0.799**	0.458	0.421
UI	0.730	0.402	0.450	UI	0.776	0.470	0.436
RA	0.406	0.302	0.323	R	0.794	0.513	0.424
RM	0.302	0.307	0.262	RG	0.794	0.513	0.424
RB	0.739	**0.444**	0.458	L	0.710	**0.511**	0.364
LA	0.340	0.304	0.286	LG	0.715	**0.511**	0.364
LM	0.254	0.313	0.206	J	0.715	0.451	0.355
LB	0.636	0.435	0.372	JG	0.715	0.451	0.355
JA	0.216	0.193	0.173	*AnnSim*D$_{tax}$	0.682	0.434	0.407
JM	0.234	0.251	0.164	*AnnSim*OnSim	0.772	0.439	**0.438**
JB	0.586	0.370	0.331				
*AnnSim*D$_{tax}$	0.650	0.388	0.459				
*AnnSim*OnSim	0.732	0.375	**0.514**				

top-5 values are highlighted in gray, and the highest correlation with respect to each of the baseline similarity measure is highlighted in bold. We can observe that both *AnnSim*D$_{tax}$ and *AnnSim*OnSim are among the top-5 more correlated measures to *SeqSim* and Pfam in CESSM 2008. However, in the version of 2014, only *AnnSim*OnSim is kept among the top-5 measures. While *AnnSim*D$_{tax}$ maintains its improvement in the correlation with SeqSim in the 2014 collection, it drops to the last position in terms of correlation. Similar to the results reported in Fig. 6(d), the enhanced effectiveness of *AnnSim*OnSim in this dataset suggests an improvement in the quality of the annotations and in the knowledge represented in GO. We hypothesize that most of changes in GO are related to axioms and object properties and not so much with the taxonomy. These characteristics of GO 2014 would explain the behavior of *AnnSim*D$_{tax}$ in this dataset. *AnnSim*OnSim is competitive because, unlike other top-5 similarity measures, it is a *generic* similarity measure and is not *tuned* for GO.

6   Related Work

A diversity of similarity measures have been proposed in the literature to compute relatedness between a pair of entities. Each measure exploits some knowledge including paths of relations with other entities, taxonomic hierarchies of the classes, and semantic knowledge. Path- or structure-based similarity measures compute the relatedness of two entities according to the properties of the paths that connect them (e.g., PathSim [21] or HeteSim [19]), or the structure of the graph that includes the two entities (e.g., SimRank [7]). High values of path- and structure-based similarity indicate that the entities are connected with a large number of paths that meet certain conditions, or the neighborhoods of these entities are highly connected. Taxonomic-based similarity measures, as D_{ps} [13] and D_{tax} [1], are a subset of structure-based similarity measures. They decide relatedness in terms of the class hierarchy of the ontology and usually consider only the *is-a* relation. High values of taxonomic similarities indicate that the entities share deep common ancestors in the ontology. In the context of Biomedicine, domain-specific similarity measures have been defined to measure relatedness between scientific entities. Smith and Waterman [20], BLAST[17] and FASTA[18] identify sequence alignment in sequences of nucleotides or amino-acids. Furthermore, domain-specific similarity measures rely on knowledge encoded in specific taxonomies to compute the similarity of two entities. For example, the GO semantic similarity measures assign values between GO terms according to the similarity measures proposed by Resnik et al. [16], Lin et al. [9], and Jiang&Conrath [8]. Finally, Couto et al. [3] propose a classification of similarity measures according to the semantics they exploit: Terminological measures compute relatedness between two entities by considering similarity between the names of the classes to which these entities belong; structural approaches decide similarity depending on the relations and attributes of the classes; extensional measures assign similarity values based on the cardinality of the intersection of the instantiations of the classes; and the semantic-based approaches take into account axioms that formalize properties of ontology classes to decide relatedness of two entities [5]. OnSim considers both, the ontology structure and logic axioms. Therefore, according to Couto et al., OnSim is classified as a structural and semantic-based similarity measure.

7   Conclusions and Future Work

We have defined OnSim, a similarity measure that exploits the semantics of ontology terms, i.e., object properties and axioms, to accurately determining relatedness. We extended the annotation-based similarity *AnnSim* with OnSim and conducted an extensive empirical study on collections available at the CESSM websites. Experimental results reveal that *AnnSim*OnSim is able to enhance *AnnSim* effectiveness with respect to biomedical gold standard similarity measures: *SeqSim*, *Pfam*, and *ECC*. Observed results also suggest that *AnnSim*OnSim and the other similarity measures are positively impacted by the evolution of the Gene Ontology and protein annotations; providing thus, a potential new application of these measures for suggesting quality issues.

In the future, we plan to study the impact of OnSim on other similarity measures, e.g., Cosine or GI. Further, we will formally analyze the effects of ontology and annotation evolution on the effectiveness of similarity measures; we hypothesize that these results will provide insights to define higher quality ontologies and annotations.

---

[17] http://blast.ncbi.nlm.nih.gov/.
[18] http://www.ebi.ac.uk/Tools/sss/fasta/.

Acknowledgments. This work was supported by the German Ministry of Economy and Energy within the TIGRESS project (Ref. KF2076928MS3) and the EU's 7th Framework Programme FI.ICT-2011.1.8 (FI-STAR, Grant 604691).

References

1. Benik, J., Chang, C., Raschid, L., Vidal, M.-E., Palma, G., Thor, A.: Finding cross genome patterns in annotation graphs. In: Bodenreider, O., Rance, B. (eds.) DILS 2012. LNCS, vol. 7348, pp. 21–36. Springer, Heidelberg (2012)
2. Cook, W., Rohe, A.: Blossom iv: code for minimum weight perfect matchings (2008). http://www2.isye.gatech.edu/wcook/software.html
3. Couto, F.M., Pinto, H.S.: The next generation of similarity measures that fully explore the semantics in biomedical ontologies. J. Bioinf. Comput. Biol. **11**(5), 1–12 (2013)
4. Couto, F.M., Silva, M.J., Coutinho, P.: Measuring semantic similarity between gene ontology terms. Data Knowl. Eng. **61**(1), 137–152 (2007)
5. d'Amato, C., Staab, S., Fanizzi, N.: On the influence of description logics ontologies on conceptual similarity. In: Gangemi, A., Euzenat, J. (eds.) EKAW 2008. LNCS (LNAI), vol. 5268, pp. 48–63. Springer, Heidelberg (2008)
6. Devos, D., Valencia, A.: Practical limits of function prediction. Proteins: Struct. Funct. Bioinf. **41**(1), 98–107 (2000)
7. Jeh, G., Widom, J.: Simrank: a measure of structural-context similarity. In: Proceedings of the Eighth ACM SIGKDD International Conference on Knowledge Discovery and Data Mining, pp. 538–543. ACM (2002)
8. Jiang, J.J., Conrath, D.W.: Semantic similarity based on corpus statistics and lexical taxonomy. CoRR, arXiv:cmp-lg/9709008 (1997)
9. Lin, D.: An information-theoretic definition of similarity. In: ICML, vol. 98 (1998)
10. Lord, P., Stevens, R., Brass, A., Goble, C.: Investigating semantic similarity measures across the gene ontology: the relationship between sequence and annotation. Bioinformatics **19**, 1275–1283 (2003)
11. Schmachtenberg, M., Bizer, C., Paulheim, H.: Adoption of the linked data best practices in different topical domains. In: Mika, P., Tudorache, T., Bernstein, A., Welty, C., Knoblock, C., Vrandečić, D., Groth, P., Noy, N., Janowicz, K., Goble, C. (eds.) ISWC 2014, Part I. LNCS, vol. 8796, pp. 245–260. Springer, Heidelberg (2014)
12. Palma, G., Vidal, M.-E., Haag, E., Raschid, L., Thor, A.: Measuring relatedness between scientific entities in annotation datasets. In: ACM-BCB 2013. ACM (2013)
13. Pekar, V., Staab, S.: Taxonomy learning: factoring the structure of a taxonomy into a semantic classification decision. In: Proceedings of the 19th ICCL, vol. 1, pp. 1–7. Association for Computational Linguistics (2002)
14. Pesquita, C., Faria, D., Bastos, H., Falcao, A., Couto, F.: Evaluating go-based semantic similarity measures. In: SMB/ECCB 2007 Bio-ontologies SIG (2007)
15. Pesquita, C., Pessoa, D., Faria, D., Couto, F.: Cessm: collaborative evaluation of semantic similarity measures. Challenges Bioinf. (JB2009) **157**, 190 (2009)
16. Resnik, P.: Semantic similarity in a taxonomy: an information-based measure and its application to problems of ambiguity in natural language. J. Artif. Intell. Res. **11**, 95–130 (1999)
17. Schwartz, J., Steger, A., Weißl, A.: Fast algorithms for weighted bipartite matching. In: Nikoletseas, S.E. (ed.) WEA 2005. LNCS, vol. 3503, pp. 476–487. Springer, Heidelberg (2005)

18. Sevilla, J.L., Segura, V., Podhorski, A., Guruceaga, E., Mato, J.M., Martínez-Cruz, L.A., Corrales, F.J., Rubio, A.: Correlation between gene expression and go semantic similarity. IEEE/ACM Trans. Comput. Biol. Bioinf. **2**(4), 330–338 (2005)

19. Shi, C., Kong, X., Huang, Y., Yu, P.S., Wu, B.: Hetesim: a general framework for relevance measure in heterogeneous networks. arXiv preprint arXiv:1309.7393 (2013)

20. Smith, T., Waterman, M.: Identification of common molecular subsequences. J. Mol. Biol. **147**(1), 195–197 (1981)

21. Sun, Y., Han, J., Yan, X., Yu, P.S., Wu, T.: Pathsim: meta path-based top-k similarity search in heterogeneous information networks. In: VLDB 2011 (2011)

AnnEvol: An Evolutionary Framework to Description Ontology-Based Annotations

Ignacio Traverso-Ribón[1]([⊠]), Maria-Esther Vidal[2], and Guillermo Palma[2]

[1] FZI Research Center for Information Technology, Karlsruhe Institute of Technolog,
Karlsruhe, Germany
traverso@fzi.de
[2] Universidad Simón Bolívar, Caracas, Venezuela
{mvidal,gpalma}@ldc.usb.ve

Abstract. Existing biomedical ontologies encode scientific knowledge that is exploited in ontology-based annotated entities, e.g., genes described using Gene Ontology (GO) annotations. Ontology-based annotations correspond to building blocks for computing relatedness between annotated entities, as well as for data mining techniques that attempt to discover domain patterns or suggest novel associations among annotated entities. However, effectiveness of these annotation-based approaches can be considerably impacted by the quality of the annotations, and models that allow for the description of the quality of the annotations are required to validate and explain the behavior of these approaches. We propose *AnnEvol*, a framework to describe datasets of ontology-based annotated entities in terms of evolutionary properties of the annotations of these entities over time. *AnnEvol* complements state-of-the-art approaches that perform an *annotation-wise* description of the datasets, and conducts an *annotation set-wise* description which characterizes the evolution of annotations into semantically similar annotations. We empirically evaluate the expressiveness power of *AnnEvol* in a set of proteins annotated with GO using UniProt-GOA and Swiss-Prot. Our experimental results suggest that *AnnEvol* captures evolutionary behavior of the studied GO annotations, and clearly differentiates patterns of annotations depending on both the annotation provider and on the model organism of the studied proteins.

1 Introduction

Semantic Web initiatives have fostered the collaborative definition of ontologies which have been used to semantically describe and annotate entities from different domains. Particularly, the biomedical science has greatly benefited from these research movements, and expressive ontologies have been defined, e.g., the Gene Ontology (GO)[1] and the Human Phenotype Ontology (HPO)[2]. Ontologies in the biomedical domain have been extensively accepted by the scientific community as standards to describe concepts and relations, and to replace

---

[1] http://geneontology.org/.
[2] http://www.human-phenotype-ontology.org/.

© Springer International Publishing Switzerland 2015
N. Ashish and J.-L. Ambite (Eds.): DILS 2015, LNBI 9162, pp. 87–103, 2015.
DOI: 10.1007/978-3-319-21843-4_7

textual descriptions by controlled vocabulary terms from the ontologies. For example, GO terms are extensively used for capturing functional information of proteins and genes as indicated in the Gene Ontology Annotation (UniProt-GOA) database[3], and there are international initiatives to collaboratively annotate organisms, e.g., the *Pseudomonas aeruginosa PAO1 genome*[4]. Furthermore, approaches have been defined for annotating clinical data with ontology terms from HPO to support phenotype analysis and discovery of genotype-phenotype relationships [4], as well as for predicting drug-target interactions [3,7] or determine relatedness of ontology-based annotated entities [6]. Accuracy and quality of all these approaches strongly depend on the quality of the ontology-based annotations, and several approaches have been defined to characterize GO annotations [5,10].

Annotation quality can be impacted by the evolution of the ontology, changes in the annotations and type of annotation. Ontology terms can be incorporated or eliminated from the ontologies, as well as annotations that describe scientific entities. Additionally, both ontology and annotation evolutions are not always monotonic, not all the annotated entities are equally studied and stability of their annotations is non-uniform. In order to describe the quality of the annotations, Gross et al. [5] propose an *evolution model* able to represent different types of changes in ontology-based annotated entities, quality of the changed annotations, and the impact of the ontology changes. In this direction, Skunca et al. [10] define three measures to compute the annotation quality of computationally predicted GO annotations: (*i*) *reliability*: proportion of electronic annotations confirmed by new experimental annotations; (*ii*) *coverage*: indicates the annotation predictive capability of existing annotation computational methods, and is computed as the power of electronic annotations to predict experimental annotations; and (*iii*) *specificity*: measures informativeness of an annotation. Both approaches are able to describe datasets of ontology-based annotated entities in terms of the evolution of the annotations over time, i.e., both approaches provide an *annotation-wise description* of ontology-based annotated entities. Conducting an *annotation-wise description* of the evolution of annotations allows for the discovery of relevant patterns, e.g., stability of the GO annotations of Swiss-Prot versus Ensembl annotations [5] or improvement of GO computationally inferred annotations. Nevertheless, changes of groups of annotations into similar annotations, elimination of groups of obsolete annotations, as well as the inclusion of recently annotations cannot be expressed, i.e., an *annotation set-wise description* of the ontology-based annotated entities is not performed.

We tackle this problem and propose *AnnEvol*, an evolutionary framework able to perform an *annotation set-wise description* of the evolution of an ontological annotated dataset. *AnnEvol* compares two versions of a dataset of entities d_i and d_{i+1} annotated with an ontology O in terms of the following parameters: (*i*) *group evolution* captures how groups of annotations in d_i evolve into groups of similar annotations in d_{i+1}, semantic similarity measures are used to

---

[3] http://www.ebi.ac.uk/GOA.
[4] http://www.pseudomonas.com/go_annotation_project_2014.jsp.

compute similarity of annotations; (ii) *unfit annotations* measures the number of annotations that are used in d_i but do not survive in d_{i+1}; (iii) *new annotations* measures the number of annotations that are used in d_{i+1} but are not in d_i; (iv) *obsolete annotations* measures the number of annotations that are used in d_i but did not survive in d_{i+1} because they became obsolete in O; and (v) *novel annotations* measures the number of annotations that are not used in d_i but are used in d_{i+1} after being included as part of O. We study the expressiveness power of *AnnEvol* on the four versions of the set of proteins available at the online tool Collaborative Evaluation of Semantic Similarity Measures (CESSM)[5]. GO Annotations of the studied set of proteins are from UniProt-GOA and Swiss-Prot, which is a subset of UniProt-GOA that only contains manually curated annotations. *AnnEvol* is able to capture different patterns in the evolutionary behavior of Swiss-Prot and UniProt-GOA annotations and different organisms. The reported results suggest that annotations gradually evolve into groups of similar annotations, as well as that evolution of the annotations not only depends on the type of organism of the protein (e.g., Homo Sapiens), but also to the type source of the annotation, i.e., Swiss-Prot and UniProt-GOA. These results although preliminary, reveal the power of an *annotation set-wise description* that relies on semantic similarity measures for computing the evolution of annotations.

   AnnEvol is also used to evaluate the quality of annotations of patient data in the FI-STAR project[6]. FI-STAR applies semantic and CEP (Complex Event Processing) technologies for remote patient monitoring. One of the goals is to support proactivity in detecting problems and alarm a patient ahead of time. To detect this problem, static, and sensed data and real-time predictions are considered. Static data provide contextual information that improves the predictions of the system; these data are represented as ontology-based annotations of the patient, e.g., a certain patient is diabetic. Some predictions may cause the addition of new static data, e.g., after detecting an epileptic seizure, a patient may be diagnosed with epilepsy; thus, the quality of the annotations (static data) impacts on the quality of the real-time predictions and vice versa.

   This paper is organized as follows: Sect. 2 provides a motivating example in the UniProt-GOA dataset and Sect. 3 briefly describes preliminaries of our work. Section 4 presents the *AnnEvol* evolutionary framework, and experimental results are reported in Sect. 5. Section 6 summarizes related approaches and Sect. 7 concludes.

2   Motivating Example

To motivative our work, we analyze the values of the semantic similarity measure $AnnSimD_{tax}$ [1] when is applied to dataset of 1,033 proteins from the online tool CESSM 2008. Different versions of annotations of these proteins are obtained

---

[5] http://xldb.di.fc.ul.pt/tools/cessm/about.php.

[6] https://www.fi-star.eu.

from the UniProt-GOA dataset[7] for February 2008, December 2010, November 2012, and November 2014. $AnnSimD_{tax}$ relies on the ontology-based annotations to assign values of similarity to two annotated entites. The hypothesis is that evolution of annotations enhances the knowledge about these proteins and increases the correlations of $AnnSimD_{tax}$ with domain gold standard similarity measures as ECC [2], $Pfam$ [9], and Sequence Similarity $SeqSim$ [11]. Table in Fig. 1 reports on the Pearson's coefficient between $AnnSimD_{tax}$, and ECC, $Pfam$ and $SeqSim$. Contrary to our hypothesis, the correlation values do not improve over time.

$AnnSimD_{tax}$ performs a 1-1 maximum weight bipartite match between the annotations of the compared proteins [6]. This kind of matching assigns low similarity values to pairs of proteins with very different number of annotations. We find a pair of proteins P48734 and P06493 that clearly justify the worsening of the $AnnSimD_{tax}$ values over this time period. SeqSim returns a high similarity value of 0.99 for P48734 and P06493.

	2008	2010	2012	2014
SeqSim	0.65	0.61	0.56	0.56
ECC	0.39	0.38	0.38	0.38
Pfam	0.46	0.45	0.43	0.43

Fig. 1. Pearson's coefficient between $AnnSimD_{tax}$, and ECC, $Pfam$ and $SeqSim$ for four annotation versions of UniProt-GOA proteins in CESSM 2008

However, AnnSimD_{tax} returns 0.81, 0.24, 0.23, and 0.21 in the datasets of 2008, 2010, 2012, and 2014, respectively. It is due to the non-uniform evolution of the annotation of these proteins. Annotations of P06493 increases from 7 annotations in 2008 to 55 in 2010, 70 in 2012, and 76 in 2014. Further, protein P48734 changes from having 6 annotations in 2008 to 8 in 2010, 9 in 2012, and 10 in 2014. We calculated the Gini's coefficient of the edit distance between the annotations of each protein in UniProt-GOA for generation changes 2008–2010, 2010–2012, and 2012–2014. The Gini's coefficient returns values between 0.0 and 1.0, where values close to 0.0 indicate, in this case, perfect equality in the evolution of the annotations, while values close to 1.0 indicate maximal inequality. The Gini's coefficient returns the values 0.65, 0.58, and 0.63 for the respective transitions. The number of annotation per protein is also non-uniform. Gini's coefficients for the annotation distribution for each dataset version are 0.40, 0.44, 0.45, and 0.45, respectively. The increase of the inequality of the distribution of annotations per protein and the inequality of the evolution of the proteins justify the worsening of $AnnSimD_{tax}$.

3   Preliminaries

We describe the ontology-based similarity measure D_{tax} [1] and the annotation-based semantic similarity measure $AnnSig$ [8]. D_{tax} is used to compute values of similarity of ontology terms based on the class hierarchy of O and the *lowest common ancestors*, e.g., the taxonomy induced by the *is-a* relationship between GO terms. Given a directed graph G, the *lowest common ancestor* of two ontology terms x and y, $lca(x, y)$, is the node of greatest depth in G that is an ancestor

---

[7] http://www.uniprot.org/.

of both x and y. Let $d(x,y)$ be the number of edges on the longest path between nodes x and y in an ontology O, and a *root* is a node root of the class hierarchy of the ontology O, $D_{tax}(x,y)$ is defined as follows:

$$D_{tax}(x,y) = 1 - \frac{d(x, lca(x,y)) + d(y, lca(x,y))}{d(root, x) + d(root, y)} \qquad (1)$$

Furthermore, given two ontology-based annotated entities e_i and e_j annotated with sets of ontology terms A_i and A_j, the semantic similarity measure $AnnSig(e_i,e_j)$ determines relatedness between e_i and e_j according to the minimal *many-to-many* matching between ontology terms of A_i and A_j; matching is computed in terms of $D_{tax}(x,y)$. A value of $AnnSig(e_i,e_j)$ close to 1.0 indicates that the majority of the terms of A_i are similar to at least one term in A_j and *vice versa*. Contrary, a value close to 0.0 indicates that there are a large number of terms in A_i (resp., A_j) that do not have at least one similar term in A_j (resp., A_i). $AnnSig(e_i,e_j)$ is defined in terms of a bipartite graph $BG = (A_i \cup A_j, WE)$ that represents the D_{tax} values of similarities of the terms in A_i and A_j, i.e., edges (x,y) in WE are annotated with $D_{tax}(x,y)$. Intersection of sets A_i and A_j is assumed empty, i.e., in case the same ontology term t occurs in A_i and A_j, both occurrences of t are seen as different terms during the construction of BG. The minimal *many-to-many* matching of terms in A_i and A_j corresponds to a (minimal) partition PA of WE such that the aggregate cluster density of PA is maximal, i.e., $\frac{\sum_{p \in PA} cDensity(p)}{|P|}$ is maximal, where $cDensity(p) = \frac{\sum_{(x,y) \in p} D_{tax}(x,y)}{|p|}$. The aggregate cluster density of PA corresponds to $AnnSig(e_i,e_j)$. Figure 2 illustrates a partitioning of bipartite

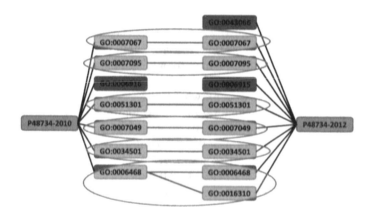

Fig. 2. Clusters (yellow ellipses) formed by *AnnSig* between annotations of protein P48734 in 2010 and 2012 (blue nodes). *AnnSig* similarity value is 0.95. BG is a bipartite graph between the set of GO annotations of protein P48734 in 2010 and 2012. Intersection between these two set of annotations is assumed empty, i.e., GO:0007067 in 2010 is considered different to GO:0007067 in 2012 in the bipartite graph BG (Color figure online)

graph of the sets of annotations of protein P48734 in 2010 and 2012 (blue nodes); parts or clusters of the partition are drawn as yellow ellipses. Note that even the same GO terms may appear in both set of annotations, they are considered as different terms, e.g., GO:0007067 in 2010 is considered different to GO:0007067 in 2012 during the construction of the bipartite graph. We can observe that except GO:0006916, GO:0016310, GO:0006915, and GO:00043066, the GO terms can be matched based on high values of D_{tax}, i.e., all these matchings have values of D_{tax} greater or equal to 0.5. $AnnSig$ is computed for this partitioning; the value is 0.95.

4   Our Approach

$AnnEvol$ is a framework to measure the evolution of the annotations of ontology-based annotated entities that comprise a given dataset. First, we will define the measures that allow for the description of the evolution of the annotations of a particular entity, and then, we will show the components of $AnnEvol$ that indicate the evolution of the annotations of a complete dataset of ontology-based annotated entities.

4.1   Evolution of Ontology-Based Annotated Entities

Annotations associated with entities may change over time, e.g., protein P48734 in Fig. 2 suffers several changes from 2010 to 2012: (i) GO:0006916 is removed, and (ii) GO:0016310, GO:0006915, and GO:00043066 are added. We define a generation of an entity e at time i, as a pair $g(e, i) = (A(e, i), O_i)$, where $A(e, i)$ is the annotation set of entity e at time i and O_i is the ontology version at time i. Then, to measure the evolution between two generations of the annotations of an ontology-based annotated entity e, we compare the set of annotations A_i and A_{i+1}, e.g., we compare the annotations of the protein P48734 at 2010 and 2012. We define the generation change of an ontology-based annotated entity between the generations $g(e, i) = (A(e, i), O_i)$ and $g(e, i + 1) = (A(e, i + 1), O_{i+1})$ as a quintuple $q(e|i, i + 1) = (s, n, w, o, v)$, where:

The *group evolution* of the annotations of e is represented by s in $q(e|i, i+1)$, and corresponds to the overall similarity of groups of annotations of e at time points i and $i + 1$. The *group evolution* is computed as the similarity value assigned by $AnnSig$ for the bipartite graph $BG = (A(e, i) \cup A(e, i+1), WE)$ and the ontology version O_{i+1}. Values close to 0.0 indicate that the annotations of e completely change during the two generations; while values close to 1.0 suggest that annotations either are maintained the same or are changed by similar terms. For example, Fig. 2 illustrates the bipartite graph between the annotations of protein P48734 at 2010 and 2012. To compute the similarity values of $AnnSig$, edges of this bipartite graph are partitioned into six clusters. Five out of these six clusters group the same GO term, e.g., GO:007067, and indicate that these five terms do not change in these generations. Further, the cluster that groups GO:0006468 and GO:00016310 indicates that the annotation GO:0006468 at 2010

changes into two terms GO:0006468 and GO:00016310 in 2012. Additionally, the
GO term GO:0006916 is not similar to any other GO term in the 2012 generation
of P48734, and similarly, GO terms GO:0006915 and GO:0043066 are dissimilar
to the GO terms in the generation 2010. Therefore, there is no cluster that
enclosed these GO terms. During the computation of *AnnSig*, values of similarity
of GO the terms in the same cluster are considered, as well as the number of
terms that cannot be included in a cluster; thus, the *group evolution* of P48734
at 2010 and 2012 is 0.95 indicating stability of the annotations of P48734 during
these generations.

Unfit annotations are represented by n in $q(e|i, i + 1) = (s, n, w, o, v)$, and
are modeled as the normalized number of annotations of the generation $g(e, i)$
which are not included in any cluster of the partition PA produced to compute
AnnSig. Formally, the number of *unfit annotations* is computed as $n = \frac{|a_n|}{|A(e,i)|}$,
where:

$$a_n = \{t | t \in A(e,i) \land t \in O_i \land t \in O_{i+1} \land \forall p \in PA, \forall x \in A(e, i+1) \Rightarrow \nexists (t, x) \in p\} \tag{2}$$

Values close to 1.0 indicate that $A(e, i + 1)$ does not contain most of terms in
$A(e, i)$ or terms similar with them. Values close to 0.0 indicate that $A(e, i + 1)$
contains either most of the terms in $A(e, i)$ or similar ones. To illustrate, although
the GO term GO:0006916 is not part of any cluster in the partition PA presented
in Fig. 2, also GO:0006916 is not in the GO version of 2012. Thus, GO:0006916
does not meet condition in Expression (2) and is not an *unfit annotation*; the
value of n is 0.0.

New annotations are represented by w in $q(e|i, i + 1) = (s, n, w, o, v)$, and
are modeled by the normalized number of terms contained in $A(e, i + 1)$ that
are in both ontology versions O_i and O_{i+1}, but are not part of $A(e, i)$ and
are not included in any cluster of *AnnSig*. The number of *new annotations* is
$w = \frac{|a_w|}{|A(e,i+1)|}$, where:

$$a_w = \{t | t \in A(e, i+1) \land t \in O_i \land t \in O_{i+1} \land \forall p \in PA, \forall x \in A(e, i) \Rightarrow \nexists (x, t) \in p\} \tag{3}$$

Values close to 1.0 indicate that most of the terms in $A(e, i + 1)$ are not in
$A(e, i)$ and are dissimilar to them. Values close to 0.0 indicate that most of
terms in $A(e, i + 1)$ that are not in $A(e, i)$ are present in clusters formed by
AnnSig and therefore their similarity is high. Although GO terms GO:0043066
and GO:0006915 are part of GO in 2010 and 2012, they are not annotations of
P48734 in the generation of 2010 and are not in any cluster of the partition PA
reported in Fig. 2. Thus, GO:0043066 and GO:0006915 meet Expression (3), and
both are *new annotations*; $w = \frac{2}{9} = 0.22$.

Obsolete annotations are represented by o in $q(e|i, i + 1) = (s, n, w, o, v)$, and
are measured as the normalized number of ontology terms used in $A(e, i)$ of the
annotation dataset that are not available in the version O_{i+1} of the ontology.
Formally, the number of *obsolete annotations* is computed as $o = \frac{|a_o|}{|A(e,i)|}$, where:

$$a_o = \{t | t \in A(e, i) \land t \in O_i \land t \notin O_{i+1}\} \tag{4}$$

Values close to 1.0 indicate that most of the terms in $A(e,i)$ are obsolete in O_{i+1}. For example, because GO:0006916 is not part of GO 2012, it is removed from the annotations of P48734 in the generation 2012. Thus, GO:0006916 does meet Expression (4) and is considered an obsolete term; $o = \frac{1}{7} = 0.14$.

Finally, *Novel annotations* are presented by v in $q(e|i, i + 1) = (s, n, w, o, v)$, and are measured as the normalized number of ontology terms used in $A(e, i+1)$ and that are not part of O_i; $v = \frac{|a_v|}{|A(e,i+1)|}$, where:

$$a_v = \{t | t \in A(e, i + 1) \land t \notin O_i \land t \in O_{i+1}\} \qquad (5)$$

Values close to 1.0 indicate that most of the terms in $A(e, i + 1)$ are novel. Note that GO:0043066 and GO:0006915 cannot be considered novel because even they do not belong to the annotations of P48734 in the generation of 2010, they are part of GO 2010, i.e., they do not meet Expression (5). Thus, there are no novel annotations, and $v = 0.0$.

Table 1 shows generation changes for proteins P48734 and P06493 between generations 2008–2010, 2010–2012, and 2012–2014, i.e., three quintuples are reported by both P48734 and P06493. Note that the *group evolution* is 1.0 for P48734 in the generations 2012–2014, and the rest of the components are 0.0. This indicates no changes of the annotations in these generations. On the other hand, annotations of P06493 in the generations 2010 and 2012 considerably change, i.e., two annotations in 2010 are removed in 2012 and two are included in 2012; one of the removed annotations is obsolete while one of the added annotations is novel.

We consider a sequence of generations of the same entity in a period $P = \{1, \ldots, n\}$ denoted as $g(e|P) = [g(e, 1), g(e, 2), \ldots, g(e, n)]$, e.g., to calculate

Table 1. AnnEvol descriptions for the proteins P48734 and P06493 between generations 2008–2010, 2010–2012, and 2012–2014. Rows describe the evolution of the annotations of an entity between two generations in terms of: *group evolution* (s), *unfit annotations* (n), *new annotations* (w), *obsolete annotations* (o), and *novel annotations* (v). Values of P48734 in the generations 2012–2014 indicate no changes of the annotations in these generations. Aggregated evolutionary behavior on the sequence of generations in terms of arithmetic mean.

Protein	Generations	s	n	w	o	v
P48734	2008–2010	0.95	0.0	0.14	0.0	0
	2010–2012	0.95	0.0	0.22	0.14	0.0
	2012–2014	1	0.0	0.0	0.0	0.0
	Aggregated	0.97	0.0	0.12	0.05	0.0
P06493	2008–2010	0.95	0.0	0.83	0.0	0.06
	2010–2012	0.91	0.02	0.13	0.04	0.01
	2012–2014	0.95	0.01	0.04	0.0	0.0
	Aggregated	0.94	0.01	0.33	0.01	0.02

aggregated values in Table 1 generations of the proteins P48734 and P06493 in the time period $P = \{2008, 2010, 2012, 2014\}$ are considered. In this case, we consider two-year separated generations, but a finer granularity may be computed. *Generation granularity* depends on the update frequency of the annotations of the dataset. Generations in $g(e|P)$ are ordered by date, so the oldest generation is the first in the list $g(e, 1)$ and the most current is the last $g(e, n)$. Sequences of generation changes on a time period $P = \{1, \ldots, n\}$ are represented as a quintuple list Q that contains one generation change for each pair of generations $Q(e|P) = [q(e|1, 2), q(e|2, 3), \ldots, q(e|n - 1, n)]$, where $q(e|i, i + 1)$ corresponds to the generation change of e between the generations $g(e, i) = (A(e, i), O_i)$ and $g(e, i+1) = (A(e, i+1), O_{i+1})$, e.g., generation changes of protein P48734 on the time period $P = \{2008, 2010, 2012, 2014\}$ are represented as $Q(P48734|P) = \{q(P48734|2008, 2010), q(P48734|2010, 2012), q(P48734|2012, 2014)\}$.

Measuring Evolution of the Annotations of an Entity in a Time Period.
Given an ontology-based annotated entity e and a *sequence of generation changes* of e in a time period $P = \{1, \ldots, n\}$, $Q(e|P) = [q(e|1, 2), q(e|2, 3), \ldots, \ldots q(e|n - 1, n)]$, the evolution of e given P is represented as a quintuple $\bar{Q}(e|P)$ that summarizes the evolution of the annotations of e over the time period P:

$$\bar{Q}(e|P) = < \bar{S}, \bar{N}, \bar{W}, \bar{O}, \bar{V} >$$

- $\bar{S}$ represents the aggregated value of *group evolution* of the annotations of e in the period P, i.e., $\bar{S} = F(\{s|(s, n, w, o, v) \in Q(e|P)\})$. Values close to 1.0 indicate that exist a stable group of annotations that survived all the generation changes. Values close to 0.0 indicate that does not exist such stable group and each generation change produce a total change in the annotation set. For example, consider the evolution of protein P06493 in the time period $P = \{2008, 2010, 2012, 2014\}$ (Table 1), and suppose $F(.)$ is the arithmetic mean function, then aggregated value of the *group evolution* is 0.94 and indicates that a high number of annotations either are maintained during the time period P, or are changed by similar GO terms.
- $\bar{N}$ represents the aggregated value of *unfit annotations* of e in the period P, i.e., $\bar{N} = F(\{n|(s, n, w, o, v) \in Q(e|P)\})$. A value close to 1.0 means that most of annotations do not survive more than one generation, while a value close to 0.0 means that most of them survive or evolve into similar annotations. For example, the evolution of protein P06493 in the time period $P = \{2008, 2010, 2012, 2014\}$ only few annotations are removed; thus, the arithmetic mean values of *unfit annotations* is low and corresponds to 0.01.
- $\bar{W}$ represents the aggregated value of *fit annotations* of e in the period P, i.e., $\bar{W} = F(\{w|(s, n, w, o, v) \in Q(e|P)\})$. A value close to 1.0 means that most of generations include a high proportion of new annotations that are not related with annotations in previous generation. A value close to 0.0 represents that most of generations contain a low proportion of new and different annotations. In our running example, new annotations are added to protein P06493 in all the generations (Table 1); thus, the aggregated value of *fit annotations* is 0.12.

- $\bar{O}$ represents the aggregated value of *obsolete annotations* of e in the period P, i.e., $\bar{O} = F(\{o|(s,n,w,o,v) \in Q(e|P)\})$. Values close to 1.0 indicate an inattention in the annotation of the entity since most of annotations remain obsolete in most of generation changes. Values close to 0.0 mean that most of generations have most of annotations up to date in relation to the ontology.
- $\bar{V}$ represents the aggregated value of *novel annotations* of e in the period P, i.e., $\bar{V} = F(\{v|(s,n,w,o,v) \in Q(e|P)\})$. Values close to 1.0 indicate that most of annotations of most of generations are terms that were added in the last ontology version. Values close to 0.0 indicate that few novel terms are introduced in most of generation changes.
- $F(.)$ is the average function but can be substituted by any other aggregation function, for example, the median.

Based on the results presented in Table 1 and setting $F(.)$ as the arithmetic mean function, the aggregated evolution of P06493 in the time period $P = \{2008, 2010, 2012, 2014\}$ is $\bar{Q}(P06493|P) = < 0.94, 0.01, 0.33, 0.01, 0.02 >$.

Interpretation of the Evolution of Annotations of an Entity: *AnnEvol* allows for the description of the following evolutionary properties of an ontology-based annotated entity e over a time period P.

Stable Evolution of Entity Annotations: Values of n and w of 0.0 suggest no significant changes in the annotation sets over a time period. Modified annotations are included in the clusters of *AnnSig* because they are similar to annotations in the next generation, e.g., in Fig. 2 GO terms GO:0006915, GO:0043066, and GO:0006915 are not part of any cluster because they are not similar enough to the other GO terms. Therefore, values of n and w are not 0.0 and suggest that the knowledge encoded in the annotations of protein P48734 is not completely stable during the generations 2010 and 2012. A value of s in the interval $(0.0, 1.0)$ may mean that: (i) the annotation set $A(e_{i+1})$ is extended with terms similar to the already existing in $A(e_i)$; (ii) the annotation set $A(e_i)$ is reduced but there are terms in $A(e_{i+1})$ which are similar to the removed; or (iii) some terms in $A(e_i)$ are substituted by similar terms in $A(e_{i+1})$.

Retraction of Significant Knowledge: A value of n higher than 0.0 means that some annotations are deleted, and there are no similar ontology terms in the current generation that represent this knowledge.

Addition of Significant Knowledge: A value of w higher than 0.0 means that new annotations are introduced in the annotation set, and that there are no similar annotations in the previous generation. For example, knowledge encoded in GO terms GO:0043066, and GO:0006915 is added in generation 2012 of protein P48734.

Elimination of Obsolete Knowledge: The component o of the quintuple allows us to identify how many ontology terms are obsolete in the more current version of the ontology. For example, because GO:0006916 is not part of GO 2012, the elimination of this annotation in the generation 2012 of protein P48734 corresponds to the elimination of *obsolete annotations*.

Improvements of Knowledge: Annotations can be improved in three ways: (*i*)Evolution of the ontology and the definition of new ontology terms, to afford a better description of the entity in terms of their annotations. The component v indicates that novel ontology terms are used in the more current version of the entity annotations. (*ii*) Annotations $A(e_i)$ can be extended in the version $A(e_{i+1})$ with new annotations related with those already present in $A(e_i)$. We measure the relatedness between two ontology terms with the ontology-based similarity measure D_{tax}. To discover this improvement, we consider the components s, n and w of a quintuple $q(e|i, i+1)$. The component s measure the similarity between the partitions formed by *AnnSig* in $A(e_i)$ and $A(e_{i+1})$. A value of s close to 1.0 and values of n and w of 0.0 indicate that all the terms in $A(e_i)$ and $A(e_{i+1})$ are included in clusters of *AnnSig*, i.e., these annotations are similar to other annotations. (*iii*) Annotations $A(e_i)$ can be extended in the version $A(e_{i+1})$ with new annotations not related to the annotations in $A(e_i)$. The component w indicates the number of annotations in $A(e_{i+1})$ that are not included in clusters of *AnnSig*, i.e., w indicates the terms in $A(e_{i+1})$ that are dissimilar to the terms in $A(e_i)$.

Annotation Stability: Given a sequence of generation changes of an entity e on a time period P, $Q(e|P)$, we measure the stability of its annotations as the proportion of quintuples in $Q(e|P)$ that indicates no change in the annotation sets. A quintuple $q(e|i, i+1)$ reflects stability if its components follow the expression $q(e|i, i+1) = (1.0, 0.0, 0.0, o, v)$. The value of the component s indicates that the same partitions are found in the two annotation sets $A(e_i)$ and $A(e_{i+1})$, while the values of n and w suggest that no term is deleted and no new term is added. The combination of these three values guarantee that $A(e_i) = A(e_{i+1})$. This property ensures that both o and v are equal to 0.0. We model the stability of the annotations of sequence of generation changes $Q(e|P)$ of an entity e on a time period P, as $stab(Q(e|P)) = \frac{|U|}{|Q(e|P)|}$, where:

$$U = \{(s, n, w, o, v) \in Q(e|P)|s = 1.0 \wedge n = 0.0 \wedge w = 0.0\} \tag{6}$$

Knowledge Monotonicity: Lower values of retraction of significant knowledge suggest higher evolution stability. We define the monotonicity of an annotated entity as the proportion of quintuples in $Q(e|P)$ that only reflects addition of knowledge. A quintuple $q(e|i, i+1)$ exhibits *monotonicity* if it meets the following condition:

$$q = (s, 0.0, w, o, v), \quad where \ s > 0 \tag{7}$$

Thus, entities do not lose meaningful annotations. Some annotations may be lost, but they are similar to other annotations present in the most current generation, and therefore, we do not consider this lost as a retraction of significant knowledge.

4.2   Measuring Evolution of the Annotations of Entities in a Dataset

Given a set of ontology-based annotated entities $E = \{e_1, e_2, ..., e_m\}$, we define
the generation changes at time i of the entities in E as $Dg(E|i) = \{g(e_i)|e \in E\}$,
e.g., a set generation of UniProt-GOA in 2010 contains one generation $g(p|2010)$
for each protein p in the dataset. Given two set generations $Dg(E|j)$ and
$Dg(E|k)$ and a period P from j to k, e.g., UniProt-GOA 2010 and 2012,
the dataset generation changes is defined as $DQ(E|P) = \{q(e|j,k)|g(e,j) \in$
$Dg(E|j) \wedge g(e,k) \in Dg(E|k) \wedge j \in P \wedge k \in P\}$ which contains generation
changes $q(e|j,k)$ for each entity e in E in the time period P. Considering
a dataset of two proteins $E = \{\text{P48734}, \text{P06493}\}$, two set generations, e.g.,
$Dg(E|2010)$ and $Dg(E|2012)$, and a time period P from 2010 to 2012, $DQ(E|P)$
contains all quintuples in each sequence of generation changes $Q(\text{P48734}|P) =$
$[q(\text{P06493}|2010, 2012)]$ and $Q(\text{P06493}|P) = [q(\text{P06493}|2010, 2012)]$, the dataset
generation changes corresponds to $DQ(E|P) = \{Q_{\text{P48734}} \cup Q_{\text{P06493}}\} =$
$\{q(\text{P48734}|2010, 2012), q(\text{P06493}|2010, 2012)\}$. Similar to when $AnnEvol$ is
applied to evaluate the evolution at the level of entities, $AnnEvol$ for a dataset E
allows for aggregating the evolutionary properties of the entities in E observed
over generations.

5   Related Work

Škunca et al. [10] define a methodology to measure the evolution of an annotated dataset in terms of electronic annotations. The methodology focuses on
the Gene Ontology and the UniProt dataset. Two *generations* of UniProt are the
input of the methodology which relies on three measures of annotations quality
for a GO term: (i) Reliability measures the proportion of electronic annotations
that were confirmed in the most current generation by an experimental annotation. (ii) Coverage measures the proportion of new experimental annotations
that were predicted by some electronic annotation in the previous generation.
(iii) Specificity measures how informative are the electronically predicted annotations. GO also evolves and GO terms are deleted and added over time. Reliability is the only measure that considers the removing of annotations but it
does not recognize if this removing is caused by a deletion of the term in GO
or the original term evolved into another more specific GO term. Coverage also
does not consider that some of the not predicted terms may not be available in
the corresponding ontology version and, therefore the prediction was impossible.
$AnnEvol$ solves this issues with the components s, v, and o of the quintuple.
The component s shows the evolution of ontology terms into similar ones. Components v and o show the evolution of the corresponding ontology, showing the
proportion of novel and obsolete terms, respectively.

Gross et al. [5] define a methodology to measure the quality of protein annotations. This methodology considers the annotation generation methods (provenance) and the evolution of the corresponding ontology. It is able to indicate
when the deletion of an annotation is due to a change in the ontology or not.
However it does not recognize if the addition of a new annotation is related to

the addition of a term in the ontology. They use three indicators to measure the quality of an annotation: (*i*) *type provenance* is represented by the Evidence Codes in the case of Ensembl and SwissProt; (*ii*) *stability* can take the values stable and not stable; and (*iii*) *age* can be *novel, middle,* and *old.* To represent *type provenance* and *age,* Gross et al. [5] also define numerical measures and thresholds for the different categories of annotations. Unlike *AnnEvol,* the methodology proposed by Gross et al. consider the *provenance* of a certain annotation, and defines the quality in terms of it. Provenance and quality are domain specific concepts; contrary, *AnnEvol* aims to be a generic methodology, and *AnnEvol* does focus in more domain-independent values. *AnnEvol* quintuples are *annotation-set oriented,* while the two presented methodologies are *annotation-oriented.* While these methodologies have finer granularity and report on information about each annotation of each resource, *AnnEvol* complements them providing information from a more general perspective, which also includes the relatedness between the annotations, measured in terms of D_{tax}.

6 Experimental Study

We conducted an empirical study on the collection of proteins published at the Collaborative Evaluation of Semantic Similarity Measures (CESSM) portals of 2008[8]. The CESSM 2008 collection contains 13,430 pairs of proteins from UniProt[9] with 1,033 distinct proteins present in both, UniProt-GOA and SwissProt. Annotations of these proteins are obtained from such datasets. We use *AnnEvol* to measure the evolution of both datasets. We consider three dataset generations with their corresponding ontology versions: 2010, 2012, and 2014. For each protein we have two quintuples per dataset, one per generation change: 2010–2012, and 2012–2014. Table in Fig. 3 reports on the number of annotations per protein for all the generations of each dataset. We observe that the average number of annotations for UniProt-GOA almost doubles the average of SwissProt. The explanation is that SwissProt contains only manually curated annotations, while UniProt-GOA additionally includes electronically predicted annotations.

Tendency of Changes in two Generations: The goal of this experiments is to study the tendency of the changes of the annotations in the datasets SwissProt and UniProt-GOA in the generation change 2010–2012. Figure 4(a) and (b) reflect the values of each generation change of each protein in the datasets. Different behaviors can be distinguished in these datasets. X-axis contains one quintuple per proteins. Quintuples are sorted on ascending values of the five components in

Dataset	2010	2012	2014
UniProt-GOA	12.21	14.69	16.13
SwissProt	5.39	8.11	8.66

Fig. 3. Average of annotations per protein

---

[8] http://xldb.di.fc.ul.pt/tools/cessm/.
[9] http://www.uniprot.org/.

order n, w, s, o, v. Y-axis represents the values of each component of the quintuple, whose values are in $[0.0, 1.0]$. Tendency of *group evolution* is reported with a blue line. We observe a larger amplitude of the blue line for values in SwissProt than in UniProt-GOA and a greater number of proteins whose group evolution value is 1.0. This indicates that fewer proteins change in SwissProt 2012. However, those proteins that change, undergoes major changes than in UniProt-GOA. Therefore, changes in SwissProt are less equally distributed than in UniProt-GOA. Tables 2 and 3 support this statement. Table 2 shows that the average value of *group evolution* in SwissProt is lower than in UniProt-GOA. Results on Table 3 suggest that SwissProt is more stable than for UniProt-GOA in 2010–2012. Tendency of *unfit annotations* is described with an orange line. As can be observed in Fig. 4(a) and (b), there are more proteins in SwissProt that experience removing of annotations (356 proteins in SwissProt versus 189 in UniProt-GOA). Moreover, area under the orange line in SwissProt is larger than in UniProt-GOA, i.e., the number of removed annotations is proportionally greater in SwissProt. This is confirmed by Table 2 where the normalized number of *unfit annotations* in SwissProt is almost the triple than in UniProt-GOA. Tendency of *new annotations* is reported with a yellow line. Figure 4(a) and (b) show that the number of proteins were annotations were added is slightly greater in SwissProt (566 vs. 549 proteins in UniProt-GOA). Table 2 indicates that the normalized number of *new annotations* for the generation change 2010–2012 is about the double in SwissProt, with a value of 0.249, while UniProt-GOA has a *new annotations* value of 0.129. The amplitude of the yellow line is also larger in SwissProt. This suggests that new annotations are more uniformly distributed in UniProt-GOA than in SwissProt. Tendency of *obsolete annotations* is described with a green line. There are more proteins in UniProt-GOA than in SwissProt 2010 that contain annotations that become obsolete in 2012 (171 versus 139 proteins). However, as the amplitude indicates, obsolete annotations are more equally distributed in UniProt-GOA and the proportional number of obsolete annotations per protein is lower in UniProt-GOA (0.026) than in SwissProt (0.033) (Table 2). Tendency of *novel annotations* is reported with a claret line. UniProt-GOA contains more proteins that include novel terms in their annotations (102 versus 69 proteins in SwissProt). The average of novel annotations per protein is also slightly higher in UniProt-GOA with a value of 0.009 versus 0.007 in SwissProt (Table 2). This suggests a tendency of using more novel terms in UniProt-GOA than in SwissProt. The combination of the results observed for *obsolete annotations* and *novel annotations* indicates that for the generation change 2010–2012 UniProt-GOA reacts quicker to the inclusion of new GO terms than SwissProt; however, UniProt-GOA seems to slower react to the deletion of terms in the ontology. Finally, Fig. 5(a)-(d) illustrate the evolutionary behavior of the annotations of the organisms Homo Sapiens and Mus Musculus in UniProt-GOA and SwissProt for the generation change 2010–2012. As observed, proteins of these two organisms follow a similar behavior to the rest of the proteins of the studied datasets.

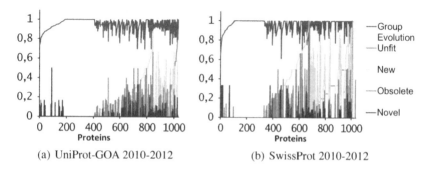

(a) UniProt-GOA 2010-2012   (b) SwissProt 2010-2012

Fig. 4. Generation changes of 2010–2012

Evolutionary Behavior. We report on aggregated values of *AnnEvol* for each dataset. We can generalize the behavior observed in the generation change 2010–2012 for *group evolution*. Table 2 contains group evolution values of 0.956 and 0.949 for UniProt-GOA and SwissProt, respectively. Stability values presented in Table 3 show an even higher stability of the SwissProt with respect to UniProt-GOA than the observed in generation change 2010–2012. Therefore we can conclude that, though fewer proteins change their annotations in SwissProt than

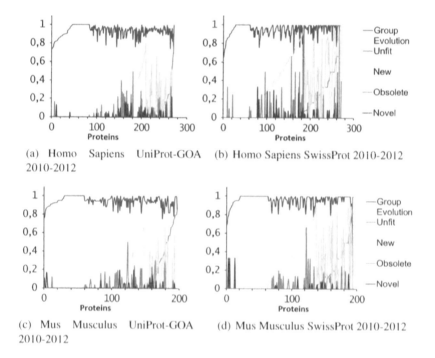

(a) Homo Sapiens UniProt-GOA 2010-2012   (b) Homo Sapiens SwissProt 2010-2012

(c) Mus Musculus UniProt-GOA 2010-2012   (d) Mus Musculus SwissProt 2010-2012

Fig. 5. Generation change 2010–2012 Homo Sapiens and Mus Musculus

Table 2. Aggregated behavior over generation changes 2010–2012 and 2012–2014 for UniProt-GOA and SwissProt

Dataset	Generations	Group evolution	Unfit annotations	New annotations	Obsolete annotations	Novel annotations
UniProt-GOA	**2010–2012**	0.946	**0.044**	**0.129**	0.026	0.009
	2012–2014	0.966	0.027	0.064	0.006	0.006
	Aggregated	0.956	0.036	0.097	0.016	0.008
SwissProt	**2010–2012**	0.930	**0.127**	**0.248**	0.033	0.007
	2012–2014	0.968	0.050	0.077	0.014	0.003
	Aggregated	0.949	0.089	0.163	0.024	0.005

in UniProt-GOA, changes in SwissProt are stronger than in UniProt-GOA. Monotonicity aggregated values in Table 3 also confirms that even the aggregated monotonicity value of SwissProt is higher than the observed in generation change 2010–2012, the monotonicity in UniProt-GOA is demonstrably higher than in SwissProt. Aggregated values contained in Table 2 confirm tendencies described for the generation change 2010–2012 with no remarkable changes.

Table 3. Stability and monotonicity values for each generation transition

Dataset	Generations	Stability	Monotonicity
UniProt-GOA	2010–2012	0.213	0.817
	2012–2014	0.418	0.816
	Aggregated	0.316	0.817
SwissProt	2010–2012	0.224	0.655
	2012–2014	0.518	0.790
	Aggregated	0.371	0.723

7   Conclusions and Future Work

We defined *AnnEvol*, a generic framework to measure the evolution of ontology-based annotated datasets. *AnnEvol* complements other evolution measures looking at the evolution from an annotation-set perspective. Experimental results reveal that *AnnEvol* is able to detect different behaviors in the annotation of the datasets and identify static and dynamic entities in terms of changes in their annotations. Results explain also that worsening of AnnSim is due to the unequal evolution of annotation proteins. In the future we plan to discover patterns in the evolution of the annotations for supporting users in the annotation task, e.g., to discover annotations that frequently appear together and common annotation substitutions.

Acknowledgments. This work was supported by the German Ministry of Economy and Energy within the TIGRESS project (Ref. KF2076928MS3) and the EU's 7th Framework Programme FI.ICT-2011.1.8 (FI-STAR, Grant 604691).

References

1. Benik, J., Chang, C., Raschid, L., Vidal, M.-E., Palma, G., Thor, A.: Finding cross genome patterns in annotation graphs. In: Bodenreider, O., Rance, B. (eds.) DILS 2012. LNCS, vol. 7348, pp. 21–36. Springer, Heidelberg (2012)
2. Devos, D., Valencia, A.: Practical limits of function prediction. Proteins: Struct. Funct. Bioinf. **41**(1), 98–107 (2000)
3. Ding, H., Takigawa, I., Mamitsuka, H., Zhu, S.: Similarity-based machine learning methods for predicting drug-target interactions: a brief review. Briefings Bioinform. **15**(5), 734–747 (2013)
4. Köhler, S., et al.: The human phenotype ontology project: linking molecular biology and disease through phenotype data. Nucl. Acids Res. **42**(D1), D966–D974 (2014)
5. Gross, A., Hartung, M., Kirsten, T., Rahm, E.: Estimating the quality of ontology-based annotations by considering evolutionary changes. In: Paton, N.W., Missier, P., Hedeler, C. (eds.) DILS 2009. LNCS, vol. 5647, pp. 71–87. Springer, Heidelberg (2009)
6. Palma, G., Vidal, M.-E., Haag, E., Raschid, L., Thor, A.: Determining similarity of scientific entities in annotation datasets. Database J. Biol. Databases Curation (2015). bau123. doi:10.1093/database/bau123
7. Palma, G., Vidal, M.-E., Raschid, L.: Drug-target interaction prediction using semantic similarity and edge partitioning. In: Mika, P., Tudorache, T., Bernstein, A., Welty, C., Knoblock, C., Vrandečić, D., Groth, P., Noy, N., Janowicz, K., Goble, C. (eds.) ISWC 2014, Part I. LNCS, vol. 8796, pp. 131–146. Springer, Heidelberg (2014)
8. Palma, G., Vidal, M.-E., Raschid, L., Thor, A.: Exploiting semantics from ontologies and shared annotations to find patterns in annotated linked open data. In: 3rd International Workshop on Linked Science 2013-Supporting Reproducibility, Scientific Investigations and Experiments, p. 15 (2013)
9. Pesquita, C., Pessoa, D., Faria, D., Couto, F.: Cessm: collaborative evaluation of semantic similarity measures. Challenges Bioinf. (JB2009) **157**, 190 (2009)
10. Škunca, N., Altenhoff, A., Dessimoz, C.: Quality of computationally inferred gene ontology annotations. PLoS Comput. Biol. **8**(5), e1002533 (2012)
11. Smith, T., Waterman, M.: Identification of common molecular subsequences. J. Mol. Biol. **147**(1), 195–197 (1981)

Terminology Development Towards Harmonizing Multiple Clinical Neuroimaging Research Repositories

Jessica A. Turner[1,2(✉)], Danielle Pasquerello[1], Matthew D. Turner[1],
David B. Keator[3], Kathryn Alpert[4], Margaret King[2], Drew Landis[2],
Vince D. Calhoun[2,5], Steven G. Potkin[3], Marcelo Tallis[6],
Jose Luis Ambite[6], and Lei Wang[4]

[1] Georgia State University, Atlanta, GA, USA
{jturner63,mturner46}@gsu.edu
[2] Mind Research Network, Albuquerque, NM, USA
{mking,dlandis,vcalhoun}@mrn.org
[3] University of California, Irvine, CA, USA
{dbkeator,sgpotkin}@uci.edu
[4] Northwestern University, Chicago, IL, USA
{k-alpert,leiwangl}@northwestern.edu
[5] University of New Mexico, Albuquerque, NM, USA
[6] University of Southern California, Los Angeles, CA, USA
{tallis,ambite}@isi.edu

Abstract. Data sharing and mediation across disparate neuroimaging repositories requires extensive effort to ensure that the different domains of data types
are referred to by commonly agreed upon terms. Within the SchizConnect
project, which enables querying across decentralized databases of neuroimaging,
clinical, and cognitive data from various studies of schizophrenia, we developed
a model for each data domain, identified common usable terms that could be
agreed upon across the repositories, and linked them to standard ontological
terms where possible. We had the goal of facilitating both the current user
experience in querying and future automated computations and reasoning
regarding the data. We found that existing terminologies are incomplete for
these purposes, even with the history of neuroimaging data sharing in the field;
and we provide a model for efforts focused on querying multiple clinical neuroimaging repositories.

Keywords: Neuroimaging · Data sharing · Clinical scales · Assessments ·
Mediation

1 Introduction

Using magnetic resonance imaging (MRI) in cognitive neuroscience and neuropsy-
chiatry has resulted in decades of study-specific datasets being stored at various
research institutions or in warehouses of archived data [1]. These data may or may not
have been used in a publication, or even analyzed; however, they can in many cases be

© Springer International Publishing Switzerland 2015
N. Ashish and J.-L. Ambite (Eds.): DILS 2015, LNBI 9162, pp. 104–117, 2015.
DOI: 10.1007/978-3-319-21843-4_8

combined in new analyses, or re-examined with new methods for new findings. They form an investment in brain images and information that needs to be capitalized upon.

As a result of the neuroimaging community's growing awareness that MRI datasets can and should be shared for accelerating scientific discovery, a large number of repositories have been developed and made available. Recent developments on data harmonization have led to the creation of national databases such as the National Database for Autism Research (NDAR) [2]. Within the imaging community studying schizophrenia, it was recognized that large scale datasharing would encourage reproducibility, generalizability, and special analyses of rare subjects [1, 3]. The data repositories developed by the Functional Imaging Biomedical Informatics Research Network (FBIRN; [3–5]), by the Mind Research Network (MRN) [6, 7], and the XNAT Central project [8–10], all included schizophrenia research imaging datasets, with the associated clinical and subject-specific information. These repositories were all developed with an eye toward solving the problem of data sharing: the FBIRN system, the Human Imaging Database, HID, is a federated system that allows the same database to be installed and queried across various collaborating institutions. It has a userbase of about 25, with several thousand downloads (D.B. Keator, 2015, personal communication). The database was carefully designed to be extensible and generalizable to archive clinical, imaging, and any other data type from any sort of study. The MRN system, the Collaborative Imaging and Neuroinformatics System or COINS, also includes a complex but extensible relational database to both archive data and manage ongoing projects, with additional tools for importing images and linking to imaging pipelines, anonymizing data on the fly for sharing, managing data sharing requests, etc. Including both data providers and data users, it has a userbase of over 1300 unique users in 38 states and 34 countries around the world (http://coins.mrn.org/index.php?page=userMap). The XNAT Central system is a lightweight data management system primarily for archiving and sharing imaging data from a variety of studies; it has a userbase in over 100 different institutions, each with approximately 50 users (D. Marcus, 2015, personal communication).

The SchizConnect project (www.schizconnect.org) [11] was developed to connect these and related imaging repositories so that a single query, e.g. for the data from all male subjects with schizophrenia and a DTI scan who have some measure of executive function, could return information from all the available schizophrenia imaging repositories. In these three example repositories noted above are data from several hundred patients and an equal number of control subjects from several different studies (for a total of 1091 subjects as of the time of writing). The data types per subject included the imaging data from structural and functional imaging, the subject specific demographics such as age, gender, diagnosis, and other measures, the subject's scores on clinical scales regarding various symptom profiles, and the subject's scores on cognitive test batteries. Each study in the various repositories had its own design, with its own choice of variables and scanning data for each subject. In some repositories, the imaging and clinical data are kept in separate databases with linking IDs; in others there are very stringent access rules to data, with complex layers of approval for any query that may vary with the study being queried. The details of SchizConnect's mediation system to solve this problem are presented in a companion paper. In this paper we describe the work we have done in harmonizing the terms used across the different sources and studies.

There are at least two usages of "harmonization" that come up in this project. The first is harmonizing data from different studies so that a data point from one study means the same thing as that data point in a different study from a different research team. We know, for example, that different MRI machines do not create identical pictures of the same brain [12–14]; different machines will provide unique regional contrast values across tissue types, and different imaging protocols will introduce specific distortions in the image. While cognitive neuropsychology tests are often harmonized, so that for example, an IQ of 100 is roughly comparable regardless of the specific standard IQ test, and clinical scales are standardized so that for a given scale neuropsychiatrists know what a score of 0,1,2, etc. should mean for the severity of the subject's symptoms, it turns out that without careful calibration of the observer or clinician, the same subject with the same clinical interaction may receive a different value from different raters. "Harmonizing" the data in this case means taking into account that both the people and the machinery used to collect the data introduce a bias or effect which is different from study to study, and harmonization methods remove that to make the data more directly comparable across sources. The best methods for taking this variation into account are not always known, and are outside the scope of SchizConnect.

The second meaning of "harmonization" is much simpler, on the one hand, but much more basic to the aims of datasharing, on the other. In building data repositories, many decisions are made that are specific to that particular repository or study, about what they will call different datatypes. The mediation efforts include implementing queries to each data source, so that the general user's query can be translated into a query that will retrieve the right data from each database regardless of differences in the database's structure. While the bulk of that work is in dealing with the structural differences in the database models, there are terminology differences which also need to be solved. In one study's data a structural MRI scan may be listed informatively as "T1-weighted scan", or something as complex as "5MPRAGE-AVG" or just "scan1", which assumes someone knows that to get the T1-weighted structural images they should look in "scan1". Harmonizing the data in this case means mapping the terms to standard terms that capture the semantics of what the data actually are, to help the user and eventually automated systems find the right data.

Lists of standard terms with definitions and uniform resource identifiers (URI) are often described as ontologies. Technically, a fully-developed ontology also includes logical definitions and relationships among the terms, rather than just a terminology list [15]. However, many ontologies or simpler lexicons have been published and shared for general use either with or without the more rigorous logical definitions, with the goal of providing standard terms that can be referred to by semantic web technologies. Ideally, within SchizConnect the terms being used for harmonization would also be standardized, with clear definitions and permanent URIs, so that there is less ambiguity both from the human user and from eventual automated systems when performing queries across resources.

Thus our goals in this part of the project were to develop three terminologies for the multiple data domains available across the resources: (1) imaging types, (2) cognitive measures, and (3) clinical variables, focused on the schizophrenia datasets. We first identified what the needed terms were, identified a basic data model for each domain, and examined the available ontologies and terminology resources for possible standardized terms. In many cases the existing terminologies were not adequate, which entails development and dissemination of new terms. This project builds on many previous efforts, and provides a research-oriented integration of several different facets in service of a single endeavor, as an example that can be leveraged in turn for other similar projects. We describe the needed steps and specific issues we faced; the specific terms and definitions are available for download from SchizConnect.org.

2   Methods

2.1   Identifying the Needed Terms from Sources

We extracted the database-specific terms from the different source repositories, and identified the different terms used for the same datatypes. Each data repository team provided a list of the variable names that could be queried, broken up into whether they referred to imaging data, or other variables. The terms were then compared, to identify which terms were actually referring to the same thing, or different things. This required extensive human interaction across teams, to identify when variable names were being used consistently both within and across repositories. The expertise needed for this effort included both the study-specific information from data collectors, database designers, and the domain expertise from neuroimagers and neuropsychologists.

A key issue in determining terms and definitions is to consider the granularity of the queries: Identifying that a subject has a particular standardized image type or clinical variable is one level, and that is the level that SchizConnect is focused on facilitating in this initial development. On the other hand, querying based on what the measure is about or what it is supposed to measure is a very different level of granularity. Many data points are actually composite, in that they are sums of measures on different questions about a subject's level of social function, for example; querying whether there is a measure of anxiety included on any test available in the repository requires a fine-grained semantic modeling which is not yet available through SchizConnect. Similarly, the functional MRI studies include cognitive behavioral tasks collected during the scan, measuring cognitive processes such as working memory or auditory processing; querying whether the fMRI data includes experimental conditions that entail specifically visual working memory, for example, requires an infrastructure that we want to be able eventually to include in our modeling.

2.2   Mapping the Source Terms to a Domain Model

Once the variables were identified and roughly defined, we then identified the domain model, or the hierarchy of terms for each of our three domains (imaging, clinical, or cognitive neuropsychological measures). In order to determine the hierarchy we compared our models with existing ontologies, and with the understanding of the relationships among the terms and models that the userbase for SchizConnect had.

For each term that we included in the domain model, we then identified the definitions of each term, mapping to other source ontologies when possible. We chose to use several established sources, namely UMLS (http://www.nlm.nih.gov/research/umls/), SNOMED (http://www.nlm.nih.gov/research/umls/Snomed/snomed_main.html), NIFSTD/Neurolex [4, 16, 17], and Cognitive Atlas/Cognitive Paradigm Ontology (CogPO; http://www.cognitiveatlas.org/ and http://cogpo.org/) [18, 19]. We also searched Bioportal.bioontologies.org [20] for potential matches, as that simultaneously searches several hundred biomedically relevant ontologies. However, we prioritized the ontologies listed previously as sources of terms, since not all ontologies that have been published are either complete or being actively maintained.

2.3   Build the Terms into the Mediator and Query Portal

The primary use of these terms in the current instantiation is for human users, to facilitate their understanding of how to query for what they might want. Thus these terms form the basic vocabulary for querying SchizConnect. As the hierarchies are developed, the querying interface develops to incorporate them, and the mediator system uses them and mappings to the terms in the sources to build the executable queries sent to the data sources. The details of how this is done are presented in a companion paper by Ambite et al. on the SchizConnect mediator.

3   Results

The spreadsheets of the different terms, their hierarchical structures and definitions are available for viewing and download at schizconnect.org. The terms are in the process of being submitted to Neurolex (www.neurolex.org) when Neurolex URIs do not already exist. The spreadsheets as current working drafts are available at http://schizconnect.org/documentation#data_models.

3.1   Imaging Hierarchy

Collecting all the specific variable names for the imaging sessions across the different repositories, we identified 632 idiosyncratic labels (e.g., "ep2d_words" for a particular task-based fMRI scan, "MR-010" for a structural scan). In order to find all the T1-weighted images that could be used to extract brain volumes from the COINS repository, for example, one needed to know that across all the available studies there were 29 different strings that labeled that kind of image. Our final, harmonized list currently consists of 22 unique terms, described generally below.

We modeled the original imaging labels as referring to several basic types of imaging data: *Structural, Functional, Fieldmapping* or *Perfusion*. Every imaging series that is collected can be in only one of these categories. *Structural* scans measure the anatomy of the brain, and under *Structural* scans we included *T1, T2,* and *Diffusion*. (See Fig. 1.) These are shorthand for, respectively "3D T1-weighted scan", or nlx_inv_20090243 from NeuroLex; "T2 weighted MRI 3D image", or nlx_156812; and "Diffusion weighted MRI 3D image", or nlx_156811. *Functional* scans are also referred to as functional MRI or fMRI, and measure the Blood Oxygenation Level

Dependent (BOLD) signal changes. This label is defined as "Functional MRI Assay" or nlx_inv_090914 from NeuroLex. Perfusion scans include Arterial Spin Labeling (ASL) scans, which measures the flow of blood through the brain, generally speaking. Fieldmapping are scans collected specifically to measure distortion in the magnetic field. Neither of these terms had matches in NeuroLex. The functional MRI scans were separated by "resting state" or "task-based", and if task-based, what the task was. The task could often be linked back to a pre-defined term in CogPO or Cognitive Atlas.

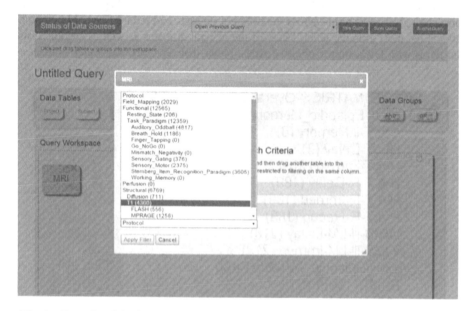

Fig. 1. Example of the imaging hierarchy being used in the query portal for SchizConnect.

This hierarchical structure specifically reflects the research community needs; it is very different, for example, from the hierarchical structure for RadLex [21, 22]. We decided on function or intent of the scanning protocol as the basis for categorization, rather than the imaging parameters per se. Radiologists and MRI physicists would organize the scanning types very differently, based on exactly what the scanning sequence parameters and details were. In our case, not all T2-weighted scans are structural; a T2-weighted scan that was used to measure some marker of brain function would be classified under "Functional." However, within the structural images, distinguishing a T1-weighted from a T2-weighted image is very important for analysis purposes and thus is modeled explicitly.

The choice of labels of "Structural" or "Functional" is shorthand for the benefit of the cognitive neuroscience or neuropsychiatric research community, who look for images that they can use to identify brain measures reflecting anatomy or physiology. This is very similar to the structure identified separately in the Quantitative Imaging Biomarker Ontology (http://purl.bioontology.org/ontology/QIBO) [23], which also explicitly breaks imaging measurements into "Anatomical" and "Functional" classes.

3.2   Neuropsychological Assessments Hierarchy

There were several standard cognitive batteries included with the various datasets, which overlapped in what they measured (attention, memory, verbal fluency) etc., but not in the particular test used. In consultation with neuropsychologists, we identified 11 subdomains, each of which had several specific tests or test modules which measured it. Examples are shown in Fig. 2 below. Specifically, under measures of "Verbal Episodic Memory", the available datasets included scores from several standardized tests of immediate or delayed recall and recognition. Overall, we began with 67 neuropsychological tasks terms across the different datasets and reduced it to 49 common tasks at the most granular level. Many of the general domains as well as specific tests had terms with URIs from Cognitive Atlas, rather than SNOMED or other sources.

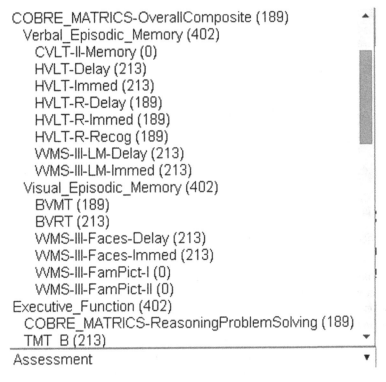

Fig. 2. Part of the neuropsychological assessment hierarchy for querying in SchizConnect. The number of subjects with data from each assessment are included in parentheses to help users identify the most common data types.

3.3   Clinical Hierarchy

Within the Clinical section we included the Subject Types and measures specific to aspects of disease. We started with approximately 70 idiosyncratic terms and reduced that to 55.

Given the datasets we were harmonizing worked primarily with studies of people with schizophrenia or healthy control subjects, the list of subject types was expected originally to include two terms: schizophrenia or control. That however did not fit the reality of the datasets. Some inclusion and exclusion criteria were different across datasets: Some included only subjects who strictly fit the definition of schizophrenia with no previous different diagnoses; other studies were more broad and allowed subjects with schizoaffective disorder. The "control" samples were even more heterogeneous, in that each had their own exclusion criteria and others were more lax, requiring only no history of clinical psychosis. The one aspect that could be agreed upon for the "control" subjects was that they had no known or listed diagnoses at the time of inclusion at the study. There is no guarantee across all studies that they were healthy from the point of view of their cardiovasculature, occasional illicit drug use, exercise or sleep habits, for example, since screening and exclusion criteria were study-specific.

Thus the hierarchy under "Diagnosis" included: either "Mental Disorder" or "No Known Disorder"; under Mental Disorder was included "Psychotic Disorder" (allowing for multiple diagnoses later perhaps including non-psychotic disorders); as subclasses of Psychotic Disorder, both "Bipolar Disorder", and "Schizophrenia (Broadly defined)"; then as subclasses of Schizophrenia (Broadly defined) were strict "Schizophrenia", and "Schizoaffective". See Fig. 3 below. This terminology is in principle expandable to include specific terminologies such as the ICD10 codes, or DSM-V codes, but that is not the researchers' data. Specific diagnostic codes were not available, only whether a person fell into one of two groups: cases or controls.

Symptom severity measures and other clinical measures draw largely from standardized, published scales that fall into specific classes based on what they measure. We identified 14 subdomains or aspects of disease measured in these studies, such as "Extrapyramidal symptoms", "Structured Interviews for Diagnosis", or "Mood," most of which had several scales used across the different studies. These classes do not have matches in any of the ontology sources we have examined to date; the standardized assessments largely can be pulled from SNOMED.

However, there were also idiosyncratic questionnaires to be included, such as specific post-imaging questionnaires assessing whether scanning exacerbated specific symptoms. That particular questionnaire may never be used again by another imaging study, but making it available through SchizConnect lets other researchers know it is there, leading them possibly to collect the same data, and more assessments may fall into that class in the future.

3.4   Evaluation

The SchizConnect portal has incorporated these terminologies in the querying capacity as shown above. Examples are shown in Figs. 4, 5, and 6. An example final query is below, showing a request for male subjects with broadly-defined schizophrenia and a DTI scan who have some measure of executive function. The numbers of subjects meeting each filter is given in the upper left of each square box. The interface is a drag and drop one, based on the current Data Exchange interface from COINS [24].

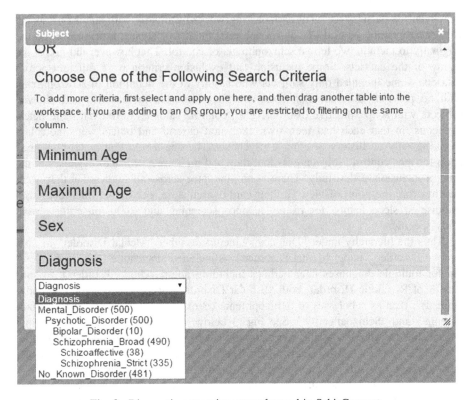

Fig. 3. Diagnostic categories currently used in SchizConnect.

The result in Fig. 5 is the number of imaging datasets from how many unique subjects available across the various repositories; in this case, 286 images from 140 subjects. The users can then proceed to request the data or go back and modify their query. After signing the appropriate data sharing agreements, the user can also obtain the individual-level data, an excerpt of which appears in Fig. 6.

Given the hierarchy we have included in the terms, investigators can query for subjects who have data at any level—requesting subjects who have any data on their executive function, for example, will return currently 402 subjects who have data from any of a number of cognitive tests. Or the query can drill down for only the subjects with data from the TrailMaking Test-B (TMT-B), to maximize comparability in the resulting dataset.

4   Discussion

Even with decades of work in the research community developing ontologies and terminologies to facilitate common communication across data repositories, we have identified several issues with the existing resources. It is simply not the case that we can identify the needed term for any given variable in any given clinical neuroimaging study from the work already done in UMLS or SNOMED or other sources. In this

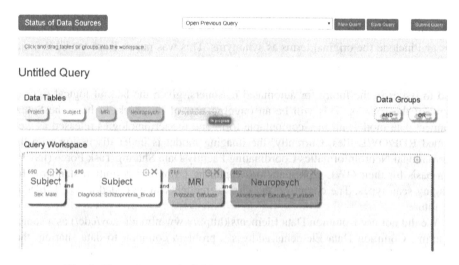

Fig. 4. Example query in Schizconnect, using the standardized terms.

Untitled Query Query Results

Your query returned 286 images and 6 assessments from 140 subjects. View My Query or Create New Query

• COBRE: 117 images and 3 assessments from 58 subjects
• MCICShare: 169 images and 3 assessments from 82 subjects

Note that some subjects have longidinal data, some visits contain multiple imaging sequences, and some scans have multiple formats

To review your query, please use the View My Query link (the back button will take you to a blank query creation page)

To download images and assessments and/or view summary data, please Sign in or Sign Up

Fig. 5. The results of the query from Fig. 4. The user can then proceed to request the data from the different repositories.

Provenance	Name	Budgecrtid	Age	Sex	Dx	Field strength	Img_date	Datauri	Maker	Model	Spc protocol_hier	Assessment	Assessment_description
COINS	COBRE	A00038624	45	male	Schizophrenia_Strict	3	2013-01-01 00:00:00.0	2294526	Siemens	MIND TRIO 3.01	Diffusion	WASI-Similarities	Wechsler Abbreviated Scale of Intelligence Similarities
COINS	MCICShare	A00038108	21	male	Schizophrenia_Broad	1.5	2008-01-01 00:00:00.0	1926323	Siemens	MIC SMS BON 1.5T	Diffusion	TMT_B	Trail Making Test B
COINS	MCICShare	A00038108	21	male	Schizophrenia_Broad	1.5	2008-01-01 00:00:00.0	1926323	Siemens	MIC SMS BON 1.5T	Diffusion	TowerLondon	Tower of London
COINS	MCICShare	A00038108	21	male	Schizophrenia_Broad	1.5	2008-01-01 00:00:00.0	1926323	Siemens	MIC SMS BON 1.5T	Diffusion	WAIS-III Similarities	Wechsler Adult Intelligence Scale-III Similarities

Fig. 6. An excerpt individual-level results of the query from Fig. 5. To obtain individual level results the user needs to sign the appropriate data sharing agreements.

work, out of almost 200 terms needed, fewer than 50 have already been defined and given URIs, and the rest need new terms. This work of harmonizing terms across repositories continues to be largely manual, although the goal eventually is to automatically map new terms to known terms as new repositories are integrated.

Given the close collaborations between NIF and other ontology developers, both Cognitive Atlas and CogPO terms have Neurolex IDs. We chose to use the Neurolex IDs and include the original terms as synonyms. This was not an issue for UMLS and SNOMed as the overlap between them and other sources was much less. This leads to the different terms used in SchizConnect having different source ontologies, which may lead to issues in the future for automated reasoners, given the lack of logical rigor in many of the sources. This will be an ongoing part of the work, to have the Schiz-Connect data models all in a computable form and the terminologies released as well formed RDF/OWL files. Currently, the imaging model is under discussion with the International Neuroinformatics Coordinating Facility Data Sharing Task Force (INCF), as a basis for their OWL representations capturing terms and definition standards for imaging scan types. The cognitive and clinical models can be coded as OWL files in the future.

We did not use Common Data Elements (http://www.nlm.nih.gov/cde/) as a source of terms. Common Data Elements address a problem common to data sharing, that different studies use different data collection questionnaires, scales, and assessments. The CDE effort for many biomedical research domains is attempting to identify a minimum common core of measures to collect, and tools with which to collect them. Thus CDEs are often just pdfs of questions, not compatible with semantic web needs. Rather than define what an existing dataset's assessments are, and represent the semantics in some way, they are proscriptive for future datasets. They reduce semantic uncertainty through providing a common set of measures, but not necessarily providing the semantic information regarding those measures. With the exception of the NINDS CDEs (http://www.commondataelements.ninds.nih.gov/CDE.aspx), there is a common lack of definitions and an overreliance on common usage, in the terms; URIs for individual terms are not always available; and they are often not available in an OWL/RDF format or other format which would allow extensions into computable representations of the terms, with automated reasoning available eventually. The NIH Toolbox, a set of cognitive assessments being recommended for use in clinical studies, was not used for any of the studies being modeled in the data repositories; if datasets which used the NIH Toolbox are accessed in SchizConnect in the future, we will assess the state of the relevant CDEs at that time. The CDEs are in ongoing development and will be integrated into the terminology usage whenever possible.

Common repositories of terminologies for clinical neuroimaging research are needed; UMLS is big, but not flexible enough for the day to day needs of modeling novel neuroimaging experiments where new variants of old concepts arise regularly. Bioportal [20] is useful as a repository of lexicons, for comparing across terminology sets to identify whether a term is already defined somewhere, and provides many tools for ontology-based data access; but in itself it doesn't solve the problem of semantically representing what a given dataset of values mean, and what conclusions they can be used to support. The Ontology of Biomedical Investigation (OBI) is incredibly thorough and logically rigorous for the domains that have worked on it (vaccines, for example), but it requires expert effort to extend into new areas [25, 26]. It is in many ways the standard to aspire to, for supporting logical reasoning. NeuroLex [17] as a repository of terms is flexible, extensible by the community, and well-structured, which is at least the first step in aggregating a common set of standardized terms.

Finding the neuroimaging and associated clinical data is one aspect of mining and re-using neuroimaging data; using it is another. SchizConnect has focused on identifying datasets which fit certain high-level characteristics (gender, age, diagnostic group, scan type etc.). Other collaborative groups include the INCF Neuroimaging Data Model (NI-DM), which focuses on models of individual subject neuroimaging data collection, processing methods, and individual or group statistical analysis [27, 28]. The terms for these more detailed concepts also need to be shared in ways that make their definitions clear, at the very least, for re-use in other projects like Schiz-Connect. Currently SchizConnect cannot answer more nuanced queries such as "Find cognitive and imaging datasets that show gray matter loss in the anterior cingulate in adult patients with childhood-onset schizophrenia", for example; one might be interested in the patterns of cognitive problems such patients have, and want to mine the available data to find out. With further development and interaction with the NI-DM development to represent gray matter loss analyses, and the Foundational Model of Anatomy (FMA) [29–31] to identify brain regions such as anterior cingulate cortex, such a query might be possible. This and other similar approaches being used in clinical research [32] would form the foundation for a truly innovative approach to large-scale, integrative biomedical science.

Acknowledgements. SchizConnect is supported by a grant from the National Institutes of Health (NIH/NIMH), 5U01MH097435 to L. Wang, JL. Ambite, S.G. Potkin and J.A.Turner. The work on COINS is also supported by 5P20GM103472 (NIGMS) to V.D. Calhoun. The authors would like to thank Derin Cobia, PhD, for help on constructing the SchizConnect neuropsychological assessment hierarchy.

References

1. Turner, J.A.: The rise of large-scale imaging studies in psychiatry. GigaScience **3**, 29 (2014)
2. Hall, D., Huerta, M.F., McAuliffe, M.J., Farber, G.K.: Sharing heterogeneous data: the national database for autism research. Neuroinformatics **10**, 331–339 (2012)
3. Keator, D.B., Helmer, K., Steffener, J., Turner, J.A., Van Erp, T.G., Gadde, S., Ashish, N., Burns, G.A., Nichols, B.N.: Towards structured sharing of raw and derived neuroimaging data across existing resources. NeuroImage **82**, 647–661 (2013)
4. Bug, W., Astahkov, V., Boline, J., Fennema-Notestine, C., Grethe, J.S., Gupta, A., Kennedy, D.N., Rubin, D.L., Sanders, B., Turner, J.A., Martone, M.E.: Data federation in the biomedical informatics research network: tools for semantic annotation and query of distributed multiscale brain data. AMIA Annu. Symp. Proc. 1220 6 November 2008
5. Ozyurt, I.B., Keator, D.B., Wei, D., Fennema-Notestine, C., Pease, K.R., Bockholt, J., Grethe, J.S.: Federated Web-accessible clinical data management within an extensible neuroimaging database. Neuroinformatics **8**, 231–249 (2010)
6. Scott, A., Courtney, W., Wood, D., de la Garza, R., Lane, S., King, M., Wang, R., Roberts, J., Turner, J.A., Calhoun, V.D.: COINS: an innovative informatics and neuroimaging tool suite built for large heterogeneous datasets. Front. Neuroinform. **5**, 33 (2011)
7. King, M.D., Wood, D., Miller, B., Kelly, R., Landis, D., Courtney, W., Wang, R., Turner, J. A., Calhoun, V.D.: Automated collection of imaging and phenotypic data to centralized and distributed data repositories. Front. Neuroinform. **8**, 60 (2014)

8. Marcus, D.S., Harwell, J., Olsen, T., Hodge, M., Glasser, M.F., Prior, F., Jenkinson, M., Laumann, T., Curtiss, S.W., Van Essen, D.C.: Informatics and data mining tools and strategies for the human connectome project. Front. Neuroinform. **5**, 4 (2011)

9. Marcus, D.S., Olsen, T.R., Ramaratnam, M., Buckner, R.L.: The extensible neuroimaging archive toolkit: an informatics platform for managing, exploring, and sharing neuroimaging data. Neuroinformatics **5**, 11–34 (2007)

10. Wang, L., Kogan, A., Cobia, D., Alpert, K., Kolasny, A., Miller, M.I., Marcus, D.: Northwestern university schizophrenia data and software tool (NUSDAST). Front. Neuroinform. **7**, 25 (2013)

11. Wang, L., Alpert, K., Calhoun, V.D., Keator, D.B., King, M.D., Kogan, A., Landis, D., Talllis, M., Potkin, S.G., Turner, J.A., Ambite, J.L.: SchizConnect: Mediating Schizophrenia Neuroimaging Databases for Large-Scale Integration. NeuroImage (Manuscript under review)

12. Jovicich, J., Czanner, S., Han, X., Salat, D., van der Kouwe, A., Quinn, B., Pacheco, J., Albert, M., Killiany, R., Blacker, D., Maguire, P., Rosas, D., Makris, N., Gollub, R., Dale, A., Dickerson, B.C., Fischl, B.: MRI-derived measurements of human subcortical, ventricular and intracranial brain volumes: reliability effects of scan sessions, acquisition sequences, data analyses, scanner upgrade, scanner vendors and field strengths. NeuroImage **46**, 177–192 (2009)

13. Jovicich, J., Czanner, S., Greve, D., Haley, E., van der Kouwe, A., Gollub, R., Kennedy, D., Schmitt, F., Brown, G., Macfall, J., Fischl, B., Dale, A.: Reliability in multi-site structural MRI studies: effects of gradient non-linearity correction on phantom and human data. NeuroImage **30**, 436–443 (2006)

14. Glover, G.H., Mueller, B.A., Turner, J.A., van Erp, T.G., Liu, T.T., Greve, D.N., Voyvodic, J.T., Rasmussen, J., Brown, G.G., Keator, D.B., Calhoun, V.D., Lee, H.J., Ford, J.M., Mathalon, D.H., Diaz, M., O'Leary, D.S., Gadde, S., Preda, A., Lim, K.O., Wible, C.G., Stern, H.S., Belger, A., McCarthy, G., Ozyurt, B., Potkin, S.G.: Function biomedical informatics research network recommendations for prospective multicenter functional MRI studies. J. Magn. Reson. Imag. JMRI **36**, 39–54 (2012)

15. Larson, S.D., Martone, M.E.: Ontologies for neuroscience: what are they and what are they good for? Front. Neurosci. **3**, 60–67 (2009)

16. Bug, W.J., Ascoli, G.A., Grethe, J.S., Gupta, A., Fennema-Notestine, C., Laird, A.R., Larson, S.D., Rubin, D., Shepherd, G.M., Turner, J.A., Martone, M.E.: The NIFSTD and BIRNLex vocabularies: building comprehensive ontologies for neuroscience. Neuroinformatics **6**, 175–194 (2008)

17. Larson, S.D., Martone, M.E.: NeuroLex.org: an online framework for neuroscience knowledge. Front. Neuroinform. **7**, 18 (2013)

18. Turner, J.A., Laird, A.R.: The cognitive paradigm ontology: design and application. Neuroinformatics **10**, 57–66 (2012)

19. Poldrack, R.A., Kittur, A., Kalar, D., Miller, E., Seppa, C., Gil, Y., Parker, D.S., Sabb, F.W., Bilder, R.M.: The cognitive atlas: toward a knowledge foundation for cognitive neuroscience. Front. Neuroinform. **5**, 17 (2011)

20. Whetzel, P.L., Team, N.: NCBO technology: powering semantically aware applications. J. Biomed. Semant. **4**(Suppl. 1), S8 (2013)

21. Mejino, J.L., Rubin, D.L., Brinkley, J.F.: FMA-RadLex: an application ontology of radiological anatomy derived from the foundational model of anatomy reference ontology. AMIA Annu. Symp. Proc. **2008**, 465–469 (2008)

22. Rubin, D.L.: Creating and curating a terminology for radiology: ontology modeling and analysis. J. Digit. Imag. **21**, 355–362 (2008)

23. Buckler, A.J., Liu, T.T., Savig, E., Suzek, B.E., Rubin, D.L., Paik, D.: Quantitative imaging biomarker ontology (QIBO) for knowledge representation of biomedical imaging biomarkers. J. Digit. Imag. **26**, 630–641 (2013)

24. Wood, D., King, M., Landis, D., Courtney, W., Wang, R., Kelly, R., Turner, J.A., Calhoun, V.D.: Harnessing modern Web application technology to create intuitive and efficient data visualization and sharing tools. Front. Neuroinform. **8**, 71 (2014)

25. Brinkman, R.R., Courtot, M., Derom, D., Fostel, J.M., He, Y., Lord, P., Malone, J., Parkinson, H., Peters, B., Rocca-Serra, P., Ruttenberg, A., Sansone, S.A., Soldatova, L.N., Stoeckert Jr., C.J., Turner, J.A., Zheng, J., Consortium, O.B.I.: Modeling biomedical experimental processes with OBI. J. Biomed. Semant. **1**(1), S7 (2010)

26. Kong, Y.M., Dahlke, C., Xiang, Q., Qian, Y., Karp, D., Scheuermann, R.H.: Toward an ontology-based framework for clinical research databases. J. Biomed. Inform. **44**, 48–58 (2011)

27. Poline, J.B., Breeze, J.L., Ghosh, S., Gorgolewski, K., Halchenko, Y.O., Hanke, M., Haselgrove, C., Helmer, K.G., Keator, D.B., Marcus, D.S., Poldrack, R.A., Schwartz, Y., Ashburner, J., Kennedy, D.N.: Data sharing in neuroimaging research. Front. Neuroinform. **6**, 9 (2012)

28. Breeze, J.L., Poline, J.B., Kennedy, D.N.: Data sharing and publishing in the field of neuroimaging. Gigascience **1**, 9 (2012)

29. Mejino Jr., J.V., Agoncillo, A.V., Rickard, K.L., Rosse, C.: Representing complexity in part-whole relationships within the foundational model of anatomy. AMIA Annu. Symp. Proc. 2003, 450–454 (2003)

30. Golbreich, C., Grosjean, J., Darmoni, S.J.: The foundational model of anatomy in OWL 2 and its use. Artif. Intell. Med. **57**, 119–132 (2013)

31. Nichols, B.N., Mejino, J.L., Detwiler, L.T., Nilsen, T.T., Martone, M.E., Turner, J.A., Rubin, D.L., Brinkley, J.F.: Neuroanatomical domain of the foundational model of anatomy ontology. J. Biomed. Semant. **5**, 1 (2014)

32. Sim, I., Carini, S., Tu, S.W., Detwiler, L.T., Brinkley, J., Mollah, S.A., Burke, K., Lehmann, H.P., Chakraborty, S., Wittkowski, K.M., Pollock, B.H., Johnson, T.M., Huser, V., Human Studies Database, Project: Ontology-based federated data access to human studies information. AMIA Annu. Symp. Proc. **2012**, 856–865 (2012)

Creating Biomedical Ontologies Using mOntage

Shima Dastgheib[1(✉)], Daniel Ian McSkimming[2], Natarajan Kannan[2], and Krys Kochut[1]

[1] Department of Computer Science, University of Georgia, Athens, GA 30602, USA
shida@uga.edu, kochut@cs.uga.edu
[2] Institute of Bioinformatics; Department of Biochemistry and Molecular Biology,
University of Georgia, Athens, GA 30602, USA
dim@uga.edu, kannan@bmb.uga.edu

Abstract. The growing volume of biomedical data available on the Web has contributed to numerous scientific advancements. At the same time, the complex, versatile and disparate nature of the data can overburden the knowledge discovery and data-driven hypothesis generation by scientists. Ontologies have been proposed to address the data integration challenge, however, creating useful domain-specific ontologies and populating them with high quality instances is tedious and time-consuming. In this paper, we present the mOntage framework to rapidly create ontologies representing data in a specific area of interest. We show how the mOntage framework can be used to create and populate biomedical ontologies from existing data sources. The classes and properties of the ontology being created are mapped to and instantiated from the existing data sources by executing suitable SPARQL queries. We illustrate our framework by creating a Phosphatase Ontology and show how it can serve as an important source of knowledge in the area of phosphatases.

1 Introduction

A vast amount of data related to life sciences is available and shared on the Web for the benefit of greater science [1]. However, because many of the data repositories have been developed independently, they tend to use different data schemas, incompatible terminology, and dissimilar data formats, such as spreadsheets, relational databases, XML, JSON, HTML, and many other, frequently non-standard formats [1]. In addition, Linked Open Data (LOD) [2] has recently emerged as "a set of best practices for publishing and connecting structured data on the Web" [2] in RDF format. Life sciences data providers have been publishing extensively on LOD, which, due to links established between data sources, could increase the potential of knowledge discovery and hypothesis generation. However, many of the highly curated biomedical data sources are provided only in their legacy formats, and even the LOD data sources are not highly integrated. Therefore, despite the vast amount of data available, data integration routinely overwhelms researchers who desire to find all data about an area of interest and to assemble it into a "useful block of knowledge" [1].

An ontological approach to the data integration challenge allows for creating a unified resource in a specific domain, which precisely represents the domain knowledge and enables hypotheses generation based on integrative analyses of the existing data in

© Springer International Publishing Switzerland 2015
N. Ashish and J.-L. Ambite (Eds.): DILS 2015, LNBI 9162, pp. 118–132, 2015.
DOI: 10.1007/978-3-319-21843-4_9

one place. An ontology is an "explicit specification of a conceptualization" [3], which represents concepts and concept taxonomies, as well as relationships existing among them. Ontologies not only conceptualize the knowledge of a domain, but also are designed to empower scientists to form and execute complex queries over data and associated relationships.

Domain-specific ontologies are ontologies that focus on concepts and relationships within a certain domain of knowledge. They serve an important purpose, not only as integral components of different semantics-driven applications, but also as important sources of knowledge in those domains. Numerous biomedical ontologies have been created so far which have had great impact on biomedical research. Many of these ontologies are included in well-known catalogues, such as the OBO Foundry [4] and BioPortal [5]. Ontologies, such as the Gene Ontology (GO) [6] and Protein Ontology (PO) [7], have been mainly developed for knowledge representation and organization, vocabulary standardization and data annotation purposes. However, these general-purpose ontologies do not capture information specific to a given domain. For example, information on human diseases is not conceptualized in GO, requiring domain-specific ontologies on human diseases such as Disease Ontology.[1]

In description logic, the *TBox* represents the schema (terminology) and the *ABox* defines individual assertions. The value of a domain-specific ontology is greatly amplified by the ABox, i.e. the actual data represented as instances of the concepts and relationships (TBox) in the ontology. On the other hand, creating a domain ontology populated with relevant and useful instances is a difficult and time-consuming task. Automatic population of domain ontologies by extracting data from text documents is difficult and error-prone. Similarly, writing specialized programs and scripts for extracting data from structured and semi-structured sources is time consuming. Yet, more and more domain ontologies will be required for a variety of specific applications. A high quality domain ontology should accurately define the domain knowledge in terms of classes and relationships, which are populated with instances obtained from well-curated data sources. Although the data sources containing the relevant data to fill these concepts and relationships are frequently available, the data of interest is often "buried" among large amounts of other less-relevant data. Further, the complex and disparate nature of the data sources overburdens the population process. Lastly, modifying the ontology to incorporate additional data sources or in response to updates of existing sources requires frequent changes to the underlying data models.

We believe that the massive biomedical data distributed among LOD and other data sources offers a great opportunity for domain experts to create high quality, well-populated domain ontologies. A new domain ontology can be created by defining its classes and properties, and then specifying how to obtain instance data in terms of the concepts and properties in the existing data sources [8, 9]. An ontology created in this way not only promotes the reuse of already existing concepts and properties, but also increases the interlinking of the new ontology to the existing data sources.

In [8, 9], we presented mOntage, a conceptual model and a framework for creating and populating domain-specific ontologies built from the existing data sources in the

---

[1] http://disease-ontology.org/.

LOD cloud. Classes and properties in a domain ontology being constructed are mapped onto parts of the available LOD data sets using our Protégé plugin and then automatically populated. However, many available data sources that could contribute to building new domain ontologies are not part of LOD and many of them have been developed using many dissimilar formats, such as RDB, XML, spreadsheets, and many others. For example, ProKinO [10–12], is a Protein Kinase Ontology created and populated from versatile data sources, such as COSMIC [13] (a TSV file), Reactome [14] (Rest Web Service), UniProt [15] (XML) and internally developed Sequence Alignment (a CSV file). A specialized population software has been developed to create and populate ProKinO from the underlying data sources. However, more and more domain ontologies will be expected for a variety of specific applications in the biomedical domain. In addition, existing domain ontologies, such as ProKinO, need to be expanded to cover more knowledge of their respective domains (e.g., drug data in the case of ProKinO). In this paper, we present an extended mOntage framework that can be used to create and populate domain ontologies not only from other already existing ontologies, but from structured data sources, as well. mOntage integrates data from other data sources considering both TBox and ABox. Hence, the resulting ontology not only represents the domain knowledge but also contains the actual data, which can be queried in an integrative way.

The rest of this paper is organized as follows. We begin by presenting motivating examples and discussing the related work. We then introduce a use-case driven conceptual model for our approach, followed by a case study implementation and evaluation of a phosphatase ontology. We end the paper with conclusions and future work.

1.1 Motivating Examples

The 518 proteins in the human kinome have been extensively studied for their role in multiple diseases, including a variety of cancers [16]. In [10–12], we reported on a special-purpose integrated framework for extracting data from heterogeneous sources to create ProKinO, an ontology for large-scale integrative analysis of protein kinase data used in cancer research. ProKinO is a valuable resource for mining and annotating the cancer kinome, allowing effective mining of cancer variants while facilitating hypothesis generation and testing. We have demonstrated the application of ProKinO in integrative data mining and systems analysis of protein kinase data [11].

While protein kinases are desirable drug targets and over two dozen kinase inhibitors have been developed thus far [16], protein phosphatases show promise as next-generation drug targets [17]. Phosphatases are enzymes, which remove a phosphate group from its substrate, in contrast to kinases, which modify substrates with the addition of a phosphate (phosphorylation). PTP1B, SHP2, LYB are examples of phosphatases with known associations with diseases, such as diabetes, obesity, leukemia, breast cancer and autoimmune disorders [16]. However, a more thorough exploration of phosphatase data could open new opportunities for innovative drug discovery targeting phosphatases [16, 18].

PhosphaBase [19] was published in 2005 as the first public resource of phosphatases, written in DAML+OIL [20], and populated with data from various biological sources (such as UniProt, InterPro [21], OMIM [22]) using Gene Ontology terms. The ontology is no longer available though. Moreover, since the supplying data sources such as UniProt release new versions frequently, the ontology update is crucial, which has not been done for PhosphaBase in the last ~6 years. Thus there is a need for automated methods to build and maintain biomedical ontologies.

Few phosphatase databases, such as the human DEPhOsphorylation Database (DEPOD) [23] cover some aspects of phosphates-related data, including the listing of identified phosphatases, their EC-Numbers, protein and non-protein substrates, etc. Large data sources, such as COSMIC, UniProt, and Reactome, encompass information about the variants, protein features, structures, and pathways of phosphatases, which are hidden among the other ~20,000 genes. As a consequence, in order to find phosphatase-specific information on cancer types mutated pathways and numerous other properties, one would have to query multiple datasets separately and then aggregate the results. Hence, performing a systems biology, hypothesis-driven analysis would be very time consuming and akin to looking for needles in a haystack.

This paper is focused on using mOntage to create biomedical ontologies such as phosphatase ontology from curated versatile data sources. The framework approaches the data integration challenge by *montaging* the subsets of relevant data from different data sources and creating a unified ontology in one place. While inspired by the methodology used in ProKinO and its specialized population software, mOntage does not require specialized programming for ontology creation, population and update.

Once the ontology is populated by mOntage, scientists would be able to create and execute integrative and hypothesis-driven queries, like the ones we used in ProKinO. For example, the mOntage-created Phosphatase Ontology will help identify phosphatase specific mutational patterns and effected pathways in a variety of disease states. This information, in turn, can be used to design treatment strategies based on the regulation of phosphatase activity, much like inhibitor use in kinases today.

Figure 1 shows an outline of the schema for such a Phosphatase Ontology along with the data sources supplying the required data.

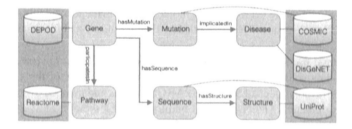

Fig. 1. An outline of the Phosphatase Ontology and the underlying data sources

2   Related Work

TopBraid Composer [24] and OntoStudio [25] provide tools for dynamic integration of other data sources, such as importing data from databases, XML files, spreadsheets, and others. Protégé [26] is an example of an open source ontology authoring software. It provides a plugin framework to extend the standard ontology editing functionality. However, not much work has been done towards using diverse and heterogeneous data sources in order to extract data relevant to a domain of interest and to create a domain ontology. LOGS[2] uses NLP techniques to construct lightweight ontologies from text. Cancer Biomedical Informatics Grid (caBIG) [27], which has been recently retired, was developed by the National Cancer Institute (NCI) to establish a common infrastructure to exchange cancer research data.

Karma [28] is an open source tool which models structured sources. It assigns the semantic types of a given ontology to the data source columns and enables users to create an integrative data model from other data sources including databases, spreadsheets, XML, JSON, Web APIs, etc. The system, then, learns to recognize the mapping of data to ontology classes and uses the ontology to propose a model that ties together these classes. Each data source should be separately imported and the user interface allows the domain expert to modify the mappings. Karma generates an integrative model of the data sources based on a given ontology, while mOntage populates a domain ontology using queries created by mapping the classes and properties of the ontology to the data sources. Also, in Karma, it is not possible to define the assignments in terms of SPARQL queries.

In [8, 9], we have reported on a framework to extract and integrate data from heterogeneous data sources to create ProKinO, an ontology for large-scale integrative analysis of protein kinase data. Sahoo, et al. described a system for creating a mash-up of gene and pathway resources and the creation of Entrez Knowledge Model which is then populated from publicly available gene and pathway resources [29].

As mentioned earlier, many ontologies and other sources have been available within the biomedical domain. Consequently, a significant part of the Linked Open Data is devoted to this area. Linking Open Drug Data (LODD) [30] links RDF data from Linked Clinical Trial (LinkedCT) [31] and various other sources of drug data in order to answer interesting scientific and business questions. Similarly, Linked Life Data (LLD)[3] is a project aiming to integrate heterogeneous biomedical knowledge available as LOD data sets into a common data model, extended with inference capabilities and semantic annotations.

The mOntage framework presented in this paper can be used to create ontologies from diverse data sources, spanning scores of domains. Subsets of the selected data sources are retrieved as needed through SPARQL queries and mapped to a new domain ontology being created. The constructed ontology can be thought of as a *montage* of existing data sources' fragments, integrated to form a cohesive domain ontology. An important feature of mOntage is that it automatically populates the ABox of the new ontology with instances obtained from the selected data sources.

---

[2] http://people.cis.ksu.edu/~rpr/TR/.

[3] http://linkedlifedata.com/.

3   Use Case-Based Conceptual Model

In [8, 9], we presented the mOntage framework, which allows for creating and populating domain ontologies from the data sources in the Linked Open Data cloud, which are all in the form of RDF, often available via SPARQL endpoints. In order to extend the framework to support structured data such as spreadsheets, XML, JSON and Relational Databases, we employ an RDF-Modeler, which, as its name suggests, models a variety of data formats as RDF. The RDF-Modeler has been implemented by taking advantage of available open source tools such as TARQL[4] and D2RQ.[5] As a result, the rest of the mOntage system did not have to be modified since the new data sources would be treated as the usual RDF data sources. The architecture of the mOntage system is shown in Fig. 2. Typically, the schema including the classes and relationships is defined by a domain expert and serialized as an OWL file, with the use of an ontology editing tool, such as Protégé. VoID+ [8, 9], our extension of VoID,[6] is a meta-data ontology describing the content of the available data sources, which is generated automatically by sending specialized queries to the data sources. Both the schema of the ontology being created and VoID+ are available to the Protégé plugin we have developed. They enable the domain expert to view the classes and properties of the schema along with the available classes and properties of each incorporated data source. Hence, the plugin can be used to easily create a set of human-readable maps of classes and properties onto the selected data sources. This effectively is a Global as View approach [32]. These maps are then imported to the Population Engine to be converted to SPARQL CONSTRUCT queries (e.g. Figure 3). The Population Engine also executes the queries included in the maps against the specified data sources and the ontology under construction and finally asserts the resulting triples in the new ontology. The details of the map formation are described in [8, 9]. As already discussed, most of the available data sources are not highly integrated and therefore we cannot treat them as well-aligned. As a consequence, we have to rely on the knowledge of domain experts in discovering, understanding and integrating fragments of domain-relevant data included in the existing resources. As mentioned in [8, 9], utilizing VoID+ can facilitate the discovery of the data sources.

Phosphatase Ontology (PhosphO). As discussed in Sect. 1.1, a number of data sources are available on the Web, which include information relevant to phosphatases. mOntage framework takes advantage of the existing data sources to create an ontology on phosphatases, which conceptually represents and integrates both the phosphatase domain knowledge and data in terms of mutations, diseases, pathways and structures, all in one place. Figure 1 shows an outline of the simplified schema of the Phosphatase Ontology (PhosphO), including its main classes and relationships. The Gene class is the focal class of this ontology, i.e. other classes and relationships are populated based upon and linked to the instances of this class. This class is populated with the instances of phosphatase. The Mutation class, on the other hand, is populated with the mutations found in phos-

---

[4] http://tarql.github.io/.

[5] http://d2rq.org/.

[6] http://void.rkbexplorer.com/.

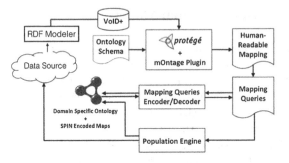

Fig. 2. mOntage architecture

```
CONSTRUCT {
            ?mut_ID rdf:type pho:Mutation.
            ?mut_ID pho:hasMutationAA ?mut_AA.
            ?Gene_name pho:hasMutation ?mut_ID
            }
FROM <PhosphO.owl>
{
  ?gene pho:Gene_name ?Gene_name.
    SERVICE <http://localhost:8890/COSMIC>
            {
               ?mut COSMIC:Mutation_ID ?mut_ID.
               ?mut COSMIC:Mutation_AA ?mut_AA.
               ?mut COSMIC:Gene_name    ?Gene_name
               }
}
```

Fig. 3. Fragment of a mapping query

phatases. Moreover, in order to be able to further bridge the PhosphO with ProKinO regarding the cancer data, the Disease class is only populated with cancer diseases. However, we retain Disease as the name of this class to maintain its extendibility to other disease types. Each phosphatase gene (an instance of Gene class) is related to its mutations, pathways that the gene participates in, sequences of the gene, its structure, and cancers associated with the gene. Note that a mutation of a gene may be implicated in some cancer type, which implies that the gene is associated with that cancer.

Figure 1 also shows (with dashed lines) the data sources used in populating the PhosPhO, based on the presented schema. DEPOD provides a database of phosphatases, their properties and classifications, substrate information and some pathway data in the form of CSV files. The sequence and structure data, as well as some supplementary information about the phosphatases is available from UniProt, in both RDF and XML formats. COSMIC provides a TSV file for mutation information of phosphatases. Pathways that phosphatases participate in can be retrieved from Reactome via its RESTful web service, which returns data in either XML or JSON format. DisGeNET [33], published as part of the LOD cloud, supplies disease-gene associations, to further populate the Disease class with cancer instances not affected by mutations. We also plan to include the phospahatse classifications using InterPro [21] in future.

The genes in DEPOD are identified by several identifier types, including UniProt and Ensemble identifiers. We use the former to get the relevant pathways from Reactome and the latter to get mutations from COSMIC, since the mentioned data sources use

UniProt and Ensemble identifiers, respectively, to identify the genes. Obviously, the UniProt identifiers are used to get the relevant data from UniProt.

3.1 Data Source Descriptions

In order to reuse the existing data sources for the construction of a domain specific ontology, one should have a clear understanding of the organization of information in these data sources. For example, once the domain expert notices that (1) DEPOD provides the Gene name, Ensemble id, UniProt id, etc. (2) COSMIC provides Gene id, Mutation id, Mutation AA, Mutation Description, etc., and (3) Reactome provides UniProt id, Pathway id and name, etc., she/he can decide to (a) populate Gene class in the new ontology with both UniProt ids and Ensemble ids, and the gene name from DEPOD, (b) use the Ensemble ids of the populated genes to get the relevant mutation data from COSMIC to populate Mutation class and its properties, such as Mutation AA, and (c) use the UniProt id of the populated genes to get the relevant pathway data from Reactome to populate Pathway class and its properties, such as the pathway name. We have collected the VoID+ information for the data sources chosen to populate the Phosphatase Ontology, including DEPOD, COSMIC, Reactome and DisGeNET. The populated VoID+ meta-data has been made available via a SPARQL endpoint and utilized in our mOntage framework.

It should be noted that the methodology used to populate our current VoID+ ontology can be used unchanged for any other data sources with similar data types, i.e. spreadsheets and CSV/TSV files, relational databases, XML, JSON, and RDF.

3.2 Defining Classes and Properties

After identifying the relevant data sources, the system populates VoID+ with the metadata of the data sources in order to display the structure and available contents of the data sources. Now, the domain expert can decide on (1) where to get the data to populate a class in the ontology based on the information available in a data source, e.g. how to obtain the gene instances from DEPOD to populate Gene class, (2) whether to retrieve all instances or only a subset of them that satisfy some conditions, e.g. retrieve all the genes available in DEPOD for the Gene class, but only cancer diseases from DisGeNET to populate the Disease class, and (3) how to establish URIs for the retrieved data to represent instances in the new ontology. For example, should the Gene class in the Phosphatase ontology use newly created URIs for its instances or reuse existing URIs from other sources? Similarly, the disease URIs can be newly created by concatenating the primary histology (cancer type) and histology subtype (cancer subtypes), generating a unique disease string.

The datatype and object properties are created based upon the expert knowledge. Frequently, these relationships can be established using the existing data and object properties, automatically retrieved from the relevant data sources and stored in VoID+. For example, the COSMIC meta-data in VoID+ reveals that this data source has *Mutation AA* (a combination of wild type, position and mutant type) as a property of mutation, which can be mapped to the same property in the Mutation class of the new ontology. In some cases, the properties in the selected data sources, especially object properties, are more complicated and require domain expert's knowledge. For example, in order to define the *implicatedIn* object property in the new ontology, based on the data available from COSMIC, the expert must decide how to map the domain and range of this property, since there is not an equivalent property directly retrievable from COSMIC. Hence, the Mutation class (domain) is mapped to Mutation id and the Disease class (range) is mapped to the concatenation of the primary histology and histology subtype (unique identifier for disease). In addition, the expert decides how the data from the two datasets should be integrated, if a link or the connecting variable is not explicitly available. For example, the genes in DEPOD are identified by several identifiers, including UniProt and Ensemble ids. We use the former to get the relevant pathways from Reactome and the latter to get mutations from COSMIC, since these data sources use UniProt id and Ensemble id, respectively.

3.3 Mapping Classes and Properties

Maps, which define the classes and properties of the new ontology in terms of the data available in the selected data sources, constitute the core of the mOntage system. The new domain-specific ontology with a defined schema is then incrementally populated, as each map is executed, based on an execution plan. Since the new ontology is stored locally while it is populated, we refer to it as the local ontology hereafter, as opposed to the underlying data sources, which we think of as remote. In [8, 9], we identified three general patterns that should be considered for designing the maps. We explain each pattern using the examples derived from the Phosphatase Ontology:

1. Instances for one or more mOntage classes and data properties are available from a single data source. For example, the instances of the Gene class are retrieved from DEPOD only. This pattern covers cases where a relationship (object property) between two instances exists in the data source at the time of the map execution, and can be executed without regard to the content of the local ontology.
2. A newly retrieved instance of a class must form a relationship with an already existing instance in the local ontology. In such case, we need to query the local ontology to retrieve the relevant instance. For example, only those instances of Pathways are retrieved from Reactome in which at least one already existing gene in the Gene class of the local ontology participates. Also, only those instances of the Mutation class are retrieved from COSMIC, which are found in at least one of the already existing genes in the Gene class of the local ontology.
3. Data type properties of a class exist when the instances of the class are being retrieved. For example, the instances of Mutation class are retrieved from COSMIC using the Mutation Id (e.g. Mutation-1000194); and at the same time, its Mutation_AA property (e.g. P642S) can be retrieved from the same data source.

Mappings are in the form of SPARQL CONSTRUCT queries designed to contain the instructions to (1) query the specified data source and retrieve the desired data, (2) check the local ontology for dependencies between the existing ontology instances and properties and the data retrieved from the data source, and (3) use the query results to populate the classes and properties of the ontology.

4   Creating the Phosphatase Ontology (PhosphO)

4.1   mOntage Protégé Plugin

We have developed the mOntage Protégé plugin to facilitate the definition of mapping between the classes and properties of a new ontology to the data in existing data sources. The schema of the new ontology can either be loaded into Protégé using an existing OWL file or be created in Protégé along with the mapping specification. The VoID+ ontology, which contains the meta-data of the available data sources, is accessible to the plugin from a SPARQL endpoint so that it can be queried to provide the data source organization to the user. The plugin provides a user-friendly interface that helps the expert to view all the information necessary for designing and creating the maps by selecting the suitable classes and properties. The output of the plugin is a set of human-readable maps that are later converted into CONSTRUCT queries in the format described in Sect. 3 and used to populate the new ontology.

A screenshot of the plugin is shown in Fig. 4. The domain ontology schema is created or loaded in Protégé first. The Data Source tree is populated by a query, which is automatically sent to VoID+ to get the list of all available data sources. Whenever a data source is selected, queries are submitted to VoID+ and the Class, Data Property and Object Property trees are populated accordingly. The bottom view of mOntage is the Protégé classic view of Class/Data and Object Property, which shows the new ontology schema. Providing the schema of the new ontology and the schema of the existing data sources makes the creation of the mapping definition more intuitive. For example, in PhosphO, to populate the Gene class, the user can select this class from the new ontology schema, select the DEPOD data source, view the list of its available classes and select the Gene class and finally press the "Map Class" button. This creates a map between the Gene class in PhosphO and genes in DEPOD, which are modeled as a class using the RDF Modeler. If the class has subclasses (e.g. once we add gene classification to PhosphO), user can map each subclass to the data in existing data sources. Using mOntage, it is also possible to add constraint expressions to filter the instances from an existing data source. For example, it is possible to populate the Mutation class in PhosphO using the Mutation ids in COSMIC, but only for the genes already acquired from DEPOD (i.e. phosphatases). Similarly, the user can map data and object properties. For example, *uniprotId*, one of the data properties of the Gene class, can be mapped to UniProtKB/Swiss-Prot AC available in DEPOD.

By default, when setting URIs for individuals in the new ontology, the plugin reuses the URIs obtained from the existing data sources. However, the user may decide to create new URIs to either make them meaningless to human (e.g. as required by OBO) or in case the new individual resource is composed from parts of multiple classes/data sources and hence does not directly correspond to an individual in any of the data sources used. For example, COSMIC provides Primary Histology and Histology subtype, but the domain expert may decide that neither of these alone can represent a disease in ontology. Consequently, the expert can select the Disease class in PhosphO and customize URI. In this case, the system uses an automatically incremented system variable to generate new URIs for the instances of the Disease class. The expert can map both diseaseType

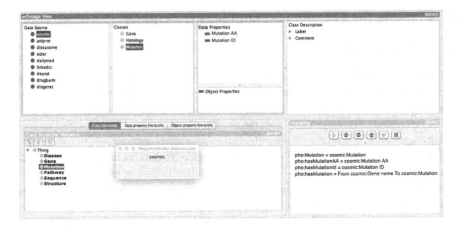

Fig. 4. A snapshot of mOntage Protégé plugin

and diseaseSubtype properties of the Disease class to Primary Histology and Histology Subtype in COSMIC (e.g., pho:mOntage0100018 represents a disease with *diseasetype* rhabdomyosarcoma and *diseaseSubtype* embryonal).

4.2 Ontology Population

Ontology population is the task of creating individuals (instances) in each class in the new ontology, adding data properties between the instances and the literal values and establishing object properties between instances in different classes. In mOntage, the ontology population is performed automatically and is accomplished by executing the class and property maps, as described in the previous section.

We based our population plan on the dependency between the population maps. The first class to be instantiated is the ontology focus class. A class is considered as the focus class depending on the theme of the domain ontology, i.e. the focus class is the concept that the entire ontology is created for. Every class in the domain ontology, directly or through other concepts, is related to the focus class. For example, in the Cancer Treatment ontology we created in [8, 9], Disease was used as the focus class and the drug instances asserted into the ontology were based on the cancer individuals already present in the ontology. In PhosphO, the Gene class is considered as the focus class and the mutations, pathways, diseases, etc. are populated based on the gene instances (i.e., phosphatases) created in the Gene class.

The remaining classes and properties should be populated according to their interdependency. For example, the Structure class in PhosphO should be populated after the Gene class and its certain data properties (e.g. UniProt id) are instantiated.

Once all of the maps have been executed, the new ontology is fully populated. This ontology represents a snapshot of the extracted data used to populate it. Due to the evolving nature of the underlying data sources, the new ontology should be versioned and periodically re-populated. We have explained the SPIN[7] encoding of the generated maps in [8] to enable the self-population of the ontology.

The prototype implementation of mOntage has been coded in Java and it uses Jena API for query processing, ontology storage and population.

5   Evaluation

While mOntage can be used to create large ontologies, PhosphO is an example ontology designed to show the utility of mOntage in biomedical domain, as required by a domain expert, a biologist in this case. The simplified schema (TBox) for PhosphO contained 6 classes, 5 object properties and 10 data properties (not shown in Fig. 1).

5.1   mOntage Evaluation

TBox Mapping. As described in Sect. 2, Karma is a tool that models the structured datasets and semi-automatically maps them to the schema of a user-selected ontology. However, there are some limitations that we address in mOntage: (1) The data sources should be explored a priori to see if the dataset really contains the data that the new ontology requires. mOntage uses VoID+ which retrieves and stores data source meta-data. (2) The ontology that the data source will be mapped to, should be created or if needed modified outside of the system. mOntage, as a Protégé plugin, allows for creating or modifying the domain ontology schema at the mapping time. (3) Each data source should be imported to and expressed in Karma separately. mOntage provides an easier access to the meta-data of the data sources and allows for alternating between the data source mappings.

ABox Assertions. Karma uses a base ontology to model the data sources by mapping the data sources to the ontology. On the other hand, mOntage creates the maps as SPARQL CONSRUCT queries, which are capable of querying the data source endpoints or local copies; and populates the designated classes/properties of the new ontology. Thus, both the TBox and ABox parts are included in the SPARQL query and further encoded in the ontology using SPIN, to create a self-populating ontology.

5.2   PhosphO Evaluation

The mOntage process of the selected data sources produced PhosphO with 8315 individuals, 38229 instantiated object properties and 136259 instantiated data properties. Using the established maps, new versions of PhosphO can be created whenever any of the data sources change. Creating new ontology versions is particularly needed for the biomedical ontologies, as new data is constantly released. Once a version of the ontology is populated, it can be queried using SPARQL to answer various scientific hypothesis-type

---

[7] http://spinrdf.org/.

questions (e.g. Fig. 5). For example, the Phosphatase ontology could provide answers to the following type of questions: (1) *Which biochemical pathways house mutated phosphatases in lymphomas?* (2) *Which phosphatases have modified residues that are mutated in with renal cell carcinoma?* (3) *Which phosphatases have mutations that occur in multiple disease types?*

```
SELECT ?pathway {
              ?gene rdf:type pho:Gene.
              ?gene pho:participatesIn ?pathway.
              ?gene pho:hasMutation ?mutation.
              ?mutation pho:implicatedIn ?disease.
              ?mutation pho:diseaseType "lymphomas"
          }
```

Fig. 5. SPARQL query for "pathways house mutated phosphatases in lymphomas" on PhosphO

The above queries would be difficult to answer without having this unified ontology. For example, the first query, formulated as shown in Fig. 5, requires mapping DEPOD, COSMIC and Reactome, while the second query requires mapping DEPOD, COSMIC and UniProt. The mappings would also be difficult since the data sources use different gene identifiers.

Comparing our automatically populated PhosphO with PhosphaBase was not possible since PhosphaBase is not publically available. Furthermore, search for specific genes in PhosphaBase resulted in an internal server error.

As a next step, we believe that linking the Gene classes of ProKinO and PhosphO will open new avenues for cancer and drug discovery research. Kinases and phosphatases regulate cellular activity through the respective addition or removal of a phosphate group from a target substrate. So, kinases in ProKinO can be linked to phosphatases in PhosphO through their shared molecular targets, offering a second set of proteins whose regulation can help stabilize intracellular signaling events [34, 35].

6   Conclusion and Future Work

mOntage, takes an ontology engineering approach towards data integration. Our protégé plugin allows a domain expert to map the ontology schema onto the available data in relevant data sources. The ontology will be populated as a montage of fragments of the data sources, by converting the maps to a set of SPARQL CONSTRUCT queries, which specify how the new ontology classes and properties will be automatically populated from the selected data sources. In this paper, we used mOntage to create and populate the first version of a Phosphatase Ontology, which integrates the data of phosphatases. mOntage allows for flexibly expanding the ontology schema and adding more data sources. For example, by incorporating sequence alignment ontology, which we are developing, we can relate mutations by their aligned position to increase the statistical power. Note that the created Phosphatase Ontology is our initial effort in creation and population of a more comprehensive ontology on phosphatases, akin to ProKinO for protein kinases. We would like to enhance this ontology and enrich it with more useful instances from a variety of well-curated data sources. We should note that mOntage accounts for verification, querying and update as well, which are beyond the scope of this paper. Once the mOntage system has been finished and fully tested, it will be available for download.

Acknowledgment. Funding for NK from the National Science Foundation (MCB-1149106) is acknowledged.

References

1. A prototype knowledge base for the life sciences. Available from: http://www.w3.org/TR/hcls-kb/
2. Bizer, C., Heath, T., Berners-Lee, T.: Linked data - the story so far. Int. J. Seman. Web Inf. Syst. **5**, 21 (2009)
3. Gruber, T.R.: Toward principles for the design of ontologies used for knowledge sharing. Int. J. Hum. Comput. Stud. **43**(4–5), 907–928 (1995)
4. Smith, B., et al.: The OBO foundry: coordinated evolution of ontologies to support biomedical data integration. Nat. BioTechnol. **25**(11), 1251–1255 (2007)
5. Noy, N.F., et al.: BioPortal: ontologies and integrated data resources at the click of a mouse. Nucl. Acids Res. **37**(suppl. 2), W170–W173 (2009)
6. Ashburner, M., et al.: Gene ontology: tool for the unification of biology. Gene Ontol. Consortium. Nat. Genet. **25**(1), 25–29 (2000)
7. Natale, D.A., et al.: The protein ontology: a structured representation of protein forms and complexes. Nucl. Acids Res. **39**(Database issue), D539–D545 (2011)
8. Dastgheib, S., Mesbah, A., Kochut, K.: Montage: creating self-populating domain ontologies from linked open data. Int. J. Seman. Comput. **7**(04), 427–453 (2013)
9. Dastgheib, S., Mesbah, A., Kochut, K.: mOntage: building domain ontologies from linked open data. In: International Conference on Semantic Computing (ICSC). IEEE, Irvine (2013)
10. Gosal, G., Kochut, K.J., Kannan, N.: ProKinO: an ontology for integrative analysis of protein kinases in cancer. PLoS ONE **6**(12), e28782 (2011)
11. McSkimming, D.I., et al.: ProKinO: a unified resource for mining the cancer kinome. Hum. Mutat. **36**(2), 175–186 (2015)
12. Gosal, G.P.S., Kannan, N., Kochut, K.J.: ProKinO: a framework for protein kinase ontology. In: 2011 IEEE International Conference on Bioinformatics and Biomedicine (BIBM). IEEE (2011)
13. Forbes, S.A., et al.: The catalogue of somatic mutations in cancer (COSMIC). Current Protoc. Hum. Genet. 10–11 (2008)
14. Croft, D., et al.: Reactome: a database of reactions, pathways and biological processes. Nucl. Acids Res. **39**(suppl. 1), D691–D697 (2011)
15. Bairoch, A., et al.: The universal protein resource (UniProt). Nucl. Acids Res. **33**(suppl. 1), D154–D159 (2005)
16. He, R.-J., et al.: Protein tyrosine phosphatases as potential therapeutic targets. Acta Pharmacologica Sinica **35**, 1227–1246 (2014)
17. McConnell, J.L., Wadzinski, B.E.: Targeting protein serine/threonine phosphatases for drug development. Mol. Pharmacol. **75**(6), 1249–1261 (2009)
18. Zhang, M., et al.: Viewing serine/threonine protein phosphatases through the eyes of drug designers. FEBS J. **280**(19), 4739–4760 (2013)

19. Wolstencroft, K., et al.: PhosphaBase: an ontology-driven database resource for protein phosphatases. Proteins: Struct. Funct. Bioinf. **58**(2), 290–294 (2005)
20. Horrocks, I.: DAML+OIL: a description logic for the semantic web. IEEE Data Eng. Bull. **25**(1), 4–9 (2002)
21. Apweiler, R., et al.: The InterPro database, an integrated documentation resource for protein families, domains and functional sites. Nucl. Acids Res. **29**(1), 37–40 (2001)
22. Hamosh, A., et al.: Online Mendelian Inheritance in Man (OMIM), a knowledgebase of human genes and genetic disorders. Nucl. Acids Res. **33**(suppl. 1), D514–D517 (2005)
23. Duan, G., Li, X., Köhn, M.: The human DEPhOsphorylation database DEPOD: a 2015 update. Nucl. Acids Res. **43**, D531–D535 (2014). doi:10.1093/nar/gku1009
24. Composer, T.: TopBraid Composer 2007 features and getting started guide version 1.0, created by TopQuadrant, US (2007)
25. Weiten, M.: OntoSTUDIO® as a ontology engineering environment. In: Davies, J., Grobelnik, M., Mladenić, D. (eds.) Semantic Knowledge Management, pp. 51–60. Springer, Heidelberg (2009)
26. http://protege.stanford.edu/
27. von Eschenbach, A.C., Buetow, K.: Cancer informatics vision: caBIG™. Cancer Inf. **2**, 22 (2006)
28. Knoblock, C.A., Szekely, P., Ambite, J.L., Goel, A., Gupta, S., Lerman, K., Muslea, M., Taheriyan, M., Mallick, P.: Semi-automatically mapping structured sources into the semantic web. In: Simperl, E., Cimiano, P., Polleres, A., Corcho, O., Presutti, V. (eds.) ESWC 2012. LNCS, vol. 7295, pp. 375–390. Springer, Heidelberg (2012)
29. Sahoo, S.S., et al.: An ontology-driven semantic mash-up of gene and biological pathway information: application to the domain of nicotine dependence. J. Biomed. Inf. **41**(5), 752 (2008)
30. Jentzsch, A., et al.: Linking open drug data. In: Triplification Challenge of the International Conference on Semantic Systems (2009)
31. Hassanzadeh, O., et al.: Linkedct: a linked data space for clinical trials (2009). arXiv preprint arXiv:0908.0567
32. Lenzerini, M.: Data integration: a theoretical perspective. In: Proceedings of the twenty-first ACM SIGMOD-SIGACT-SIGART Symposium on Principles of Database Systems. ACM (2002)
33. Queralt-Rosinach, N., Furlong, L.I.: DisGeNET RDF: a gene-disease association linked open data resource. In: SWAT4LS (2013)
34. Lin, Y.-C., et al.: SCP phosphatases suppress renal cell carcinoma by stabilizing PML and inhibiting mTOR/HIF signaling. Cancer Res. **74**(23), 6935–6946 (2014)
35. Humtsoe, J.O., et al.: Lipid phosphate phosphatase 3 stabilization of β-catenin induces endothelial cell migration and formation of branching point structures. Mol. Cell. Biol. **30**(7), 1593–1606 (2010)

Creation of Definitions for Ontologies: A Case Study in the Leukemia Domain

Amanda Damasceno de Souza[1](✉), Maurício Barcellos Almeida[2],
and Joaquim Caetano de Aguirre Neto[3]

[1] School of Information Science, Federal University of Minas Gerais, Belo Horizonte, Brazil
`amanda@ufmg.br`
[2] Department of Theory and Management of Information, Federal University of Minas Gerais,
Belo Horizonte, Brazil
`mba@ufmg.br`
[3] Centro de Qimioterapia Antiblastica e Imunoterapia, Belo Horizonte, Minas Gerais, Brazil
`caetanoaguirre@hotmail.com`

Abstract. The creation of the definitions it is an important stage of the activity of ontologies construction, insofar as the definitions provides the understanding of the meaning of classes. However, creating definitions is a complex and tiresome task. This study is part of an ongoing research that analyses some fundamental principles with the aim of formulating textual and formal definitions to be used in ontologies. The context of such analysis is a project of knowledge organization within the biomedical domain. The goal is to establish methodological guidelines for formulating the definitions in biomedical ontologies. In general, people building ontologies do not make use of consistent rules for the correct formulation of definitions, which, we believe, make our study a relevant initiative. As partial results, we present a list of topics that corresponds to the aforementioned methodological guidelines.

Keywords: Definitions · Biomedical ontologies · Leukemia

1 Introduction

In the context of the development of new information technologies, there are great potential for the use of ontologies for organizing medical information. Ontologies have been largely applied in the biomedical field, which demands semantic tools to better represent the large amount of medical entities and terms [1, 2]. Indeed, the use of ontologies is an alternative that has been receiving an increased amount of attention [3]. One step in building ontologies is the formulation of well-formulated definitions. Understanding how to create definitions is very important in order to organize concepts and terms for purposes of information representation and retrieval. This study aims to systematize the process of the creating definitions in the biomedical ontologies. In order to do this, we present a study case in the leukemia domain. Leukemia has having a strong impact in modern society due to the low rates of patients' survival. In addition, leukemia is a complex disease due of the phenotypic heterogeneity. The class called *Acute Myeloid*

© Springer International Publishing Switzerland 2015
N. Ashish and J.-L. Ambite (Eds.): DILS 2015, LNBI 9162, pp. 133–136, 2015.
DOI: 10.1007/978-3-319-21843-4_10

Leukemia (AML) corresponds to a set of heterogeneous diseases related to the clonality and chromosomal alterations [4].

Ontologies should provide clear and coherent definitions of the structures that are found in reality [5]. In order to make definitions understandable for computers, one has to create textual definitions and then translate them to some form of logic. An ontological hierarchy depends on the specification of properties that defines the essence of entities. This essence provides the basis on which such entities can be grouped together and distinguished one from another. The main role of definitions in ontologies is to emphasize those properties, as well as satisfying the need of transitive inheritance in hierarchies. The position of a class in a hierarchy can contribute to the understanding of its meaning [5].

In this paper, we discuss some ontological principles in the scope of construction of a large biomedical ontology (*Blood Ontology* – BLO [6]). We seek to formulate definitions for Leukemia within the cancer domain. One might claim that this effort does not present any research contribution or novelty. However, we believe in the relevance of our initiative, insofar as biomedical vocabularies and medical texts in general exhibit several sorts of mistakes in formulating definitions [14].

2   Methods

The terminological sample for our case study was taken from BLO. We aim to define a range of classes bellow AML, which contains 24 subclasses (Fig. 1). We also intend to define other hematological neoplasms, namely: (a) Myelodysplastic syndrome (containing 5 subclasses); (b) Myeloproliferative neoplasm (containing 11 subclasses).

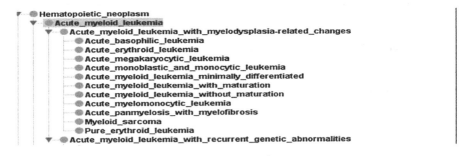

Fig. 1. - 24 classes of AML. Source: BLO in Protegé, Almeida *et al.* [6]

We have systematized criteria for the natural language and formal logic language definitions based on the best practices proposed in the literature [5, 7–12]. The steps of formulating textual definitions are part of our preliminaries results. In order to reach our preliminary findings we made use of a list of topics (from a to g):

(a) to understand the meaning of the term using more than one sources
(b) to establish the higher genus in the context of use of the term
(c) to establish the essential characteristic of the entity

(d) to formulate the definition in the form $S = Def.\ G\ which\ Ds$, where "G" stands for genus (the parent of S); and "S" stands for species

(e) to verify whether the definition is a statement of necessary and sufficient conditions

(f) to verify whether the definition is non-circular

(g) to verify the existence of multiple-inheritance and try to eliminate it.

The first class of our hierarchy, as well as its definition, came directly from BLO: "*An hematopoietic neoplasm is a hematologic malignancy which occurs in blood-forming tissues*". The second class was defined as acute myeloid leukemia (AML). Those definitions are the starting point of searching the essential feature of AML and its inheritance. Our next step in the context of the project is to formulate formal definitions using a logical language.

3   Preliminary Results

As we have mentioned before, some features of a class can be obtained by checking its inheritance. So, an AML received characteristics from the correspondent upper class, namely, hematopoietic neoplasm, which has characteristics in common with other classes in the hierarchy of BLO for blood cancers. The distinction between AML and other leukemia types is the myeloid cell lineage. Using the hierarchy of AML in BLO is possible to define the first relation of AML as a subsumption <is_a> relation, which connects a class to another one <class, class>. So, *acute myeloid leukemia is_a hematopoietic neoplasm*. Among other possible relations to define ALM, one can highlight the of the relation of derivation c <derives_from> $c1$, for example: *Acute Myeloid Leukemia derives-from hematopoietic stem cell*. Those relations are based on two material continuants [1], each one distinct of each other. Derivation is a relation between instances, where a simple continuant creates a plurality of other continuants. Some other examples of definitions based on class-class sort of relation are: <has_a> as in: *Acute Myeloid Leukemia has_a Clonal Disorder*; and *Acute Myeloid Leukemia has_a myeloid (monocytic) lineage*. Using the class-class relation <Located_in> relation, one can found: *Acute Myeloid Leukemia Located_in Blood* [13]. We used the definition of AML to illustrate the process of formulating textual definition on leukemia domain: Df = A leukemia that occurs when a hematopoietic stem cell undergoes malignant transformation into a primitive, differentiated cell with abnormal longevity and with abnormal proliferation of myeloid cells lineage. The main contribution of our approach is to emphasize the need of adopting some rules for creating definitions in ontologies. In general, people building ontologies don't follow any guidelines to create definitions.

4   Final Remarks

We present part of an ongoing project within Information Science field. We show our preliminary and partial results in defining a range of biomedical terms. This initial stage is presented with the aim of emphasizing the need of some guidelines or even a list of topics to formulate proper definitions. This will helps one, for example, to understand that the nature of things can be different (continuants and occurrents), as well as other required distinctions, for example, that relations among instances are different of relations among classes. So, we expect that in using our list of topics, one will be able to build better ontologies and provide advances in the development of expert medical systems. In reason of space limitations, we don't present any example here, but we intend to do this in future papers.

References

1. Spear A.D.: Ontology for the Twenty First Century: An Introduction with Recommendations. Institute for Formal Ontology and Medical Information Science (IFOMIS), Saarbrücken, Germany. University at Buffalo, New York. (2006). http://ifomis.buffalo.edu/bfo/documents/manual.pdf
2. Washington, N., Lewis, S.: Ontologies: Scientific Data Sharing Made Easy. Nat. Educ. 1(3), 5 (2008)
3. Almeida, M.B., Barbosa, R.R.: Ontologies in knowledge management support - a case study. J Am Soc. Inf. Sci. Technol. 60(10), 2032–2047 (2009)
4. Wernig, G., Gilliland, G.: Pathobiology of acute myeloid leukemia. In: Hoffman, R., et al. (eds.) Hematology: Basic Principle and Practice. 5th.ed. Churchill Livingstone, pp. 921–932. Elsevier, Philadelphia (2009)
5. Michael, J., Mejino Jr., J.L., Rosse, C.: The role of definitions in biomedical concept representation.In: Proceedings of the AMIA Symposium, pp. 463–467 (2001)
6. Almeida, M.B., et al. The Blood Ontology: an ontology in the domain of hematology. In: Proceedings of the International Conference of Biomedical Ontologies (2011). http://ceur-ws.org/Vol-833/
7. Köhler, J., et al.: Quality control for terms and definitions in ontologies and taxonomies. BMC Bioinf. 7, 212 (2006)
8. Smith, B., et al.: Relations in biomedical ontologies. Genome Biol. 6(5), R46 (2005)
9. Seppälä, S., Ruttenberg, R.: Survey on defining practices in ontologies: Report in the international workshop on definitions in ontologies. In: *ICBO 2013*, Montreal, Quebec, Canada (2013). http://definitionsinontologies.weebly.com/uploads/1/7/6/9/17696103/do2013_surveyreport_seppalaruttenberg.pdf
10. Petrova, A., et al.: Formalizing biomedical concepts from textual definitions. J. Biomed. Semant. 6, 22 (2015)
11. Seppälä, S., Schreiber, Y., Ruttenberg., A.: Textual and logical definitions in ontologies. In: Proceedings of DIKR 2014, IWOOD 2014, CEUR Workshop Proceedings, Houston, TX, USA, (1309), pp.35–41 (2014). https://seljaseppala.files.wordpress.com/2014/11/seppc3a4lc3a42014a.pdf
12. Tsatsaronis, G., et al.: Learning formal definitions for biomedical concepts.In: Srinivas, K, Jupp, S. (eds) Proceedings of the 10th OWL: Experiences and Directions Workshop (OWLED) (2013). https://ddll.inf.tu-dresden.de/web/LATPub509/en
13. Schulz, S., Kumar, A., Bittner, T.: Biomedical ontologies: what part-of is and isn't. J. Biomed. Inform. 39(3), 350–361 (2006)
14. Liss, P.E., et al.: Terms used to describe urinary tract infections–the importance of conceptual clarification. APMIS. 111(2), 291–299 (2003)

Biomedical Data Standards and Coding

Integration of Hematopoietic Cell Transplantation Outcomes Data

Data Standards Are Not Enough

Robinette Renner[1,2](✉), John Carlis[3], Martin Maiers[2], J. Douglas Rizzo[4],
Colleen O'Neill[1,2], Mary Horowitz[4], Katherine Gee[1,2], and Dennis Confer[1,2]

[1] Center for International Blood and Marrow Transplant Research, Minneapolis, MN, USA
r.renner@nmdp.org
[2] National Marrow Donor Program, Minneapolis, MN, USA
[3] University of Minnesota, Minneapolis, MN, USA
[4] Center for International Blood and Marrow Transplant Research, Milwaukee, WI, USA

Abstract. To complete large-scale clinical research, organizations must share data. Because institutional database schemas are inherently heterogeneous, they need a standard metadata representation in order to exchange and combine data for multi-center research. The AGNIS application (A Growable Network Information System) facilitates the exchange of hematopoietic cell transplantation outcomes data using data standards. However, adoption rates remain low due to a significant mapping burden. The AGNIS experience shows that developing a data standard is not enough. Tools and resources are needed to facilitate utilization of the standard.

Keywords: Data integration · Interoperability · Data standards · Hematopoietic cell transplant outcomes data

1 Introduction

Data standards are often viewed as the key to interoperability. If everyone speaks the same language, then data can flow freely among all interested parties. Unfortunately, the reality is not that simple. Multiple data standards and heterogeneous database systems preclude such a simplistic view. The reality often involves painstaking, labor-intensive manual mapping of a database system to a particular standard or standards only to find out later that the mappings must be updated because the standard has changed.

This reality is exemplified by the AGNIS application (A Growable Network Information System) developed by the Center for International Blood and Marrow Transplant Research (CIBMTR). The goal of the AGNIS project is to facilitate the integration of hematopoietic cell transplant (HCT) outcomes data. In this paper, we describe the AGNIS project, its current state, the challenges it has encountered, and potential strategies to address the challenges.

© Springer International Publishing Switzerland 2015
N. Ashish and J.-L. Ambite (Eds.): DILS 2015, LNBI 9162, pp. 139–146, 2015.
DOI: 10.1007/978-3-319-21843-4_11

2   Background

The CIBMTR is a research collaboration between the National Marrow Donor Program (NMDP)/Be The Match and the Medical College of Wisconsin. Its mission is to improve the outcomes of HCT and cellular therapies through observational and interventional research. The CIBMTR maintains a registry of outcomes data for more than 400,000 transplant recipients, with data submitted from 350 transplant centers worldwide [1]. This collaboration between the CIBMTR, transplant centers, data managers, clinicians, and researchers provides an invaluable resource for the medical community and the patients they serve.

The CIBMTR also maintains the Stem Cell Therapeutic Outcomes Database (SCTOD). The SCTOD is part of the C.W. Bill Young Cell Transplantation Program, known as the Program, established by the Stem Cell Therapeutic and Research Act of 2005. The Program collects a defined set of outcomes data, required when either the donor or the recipient is from the United States, to facilitate research that improves patient outcomes and increases the availability of adult volunteer donors and umbilical cord blood units [1]. Summaries of the outcomes data are publicly available via a Health Resources and Services Administration (HRSA) website [2].

To help transplant centers submit this federally required outcomes data, the CIBMTR developed FormsNet, a web-based application allowing real-time data entry and validation. While FormsNet collects high-quality data, for those centers with electronic medical records (EMRs) and/or local research databases, it requires double-data entry, an expense introducing the possibility of data transcription errors.

Eliminating double-data entry is crucial to cost-effective sharing of high-quality data. Indeed, Aljurf et al. say, "Many centers report data to a myriad of overlapping registries and databases. Integration, interfacing and interoperability are the key ingredients for optimum outcomes and use of these registries" [3]. To improve electronic data integration, the CIBMTR developed the AGNIS application, a web service based messaging system enabling the secure transmission of standardized data between disparate database systems [1]. Transplant centers can submit new or updated forms to the Java-based AGNIS server. The AGNIS server then submits those forms to the FormsNet system, which sends a response back to the center. Additionally, the FormsNet system periodically sends completed forms to the AGNIS server, which stores the forms in a MySQL database repository. Centers can retrieve the completed forms from the AGNIS repository [4]. AGNIS supports the transmission of all data required by the Program.

AGNIS serves strictly as a messaging system. In order for the messages to have meaning, both the transplant center's database and the FormsNet database must speak the same language. A standard language for the representation of the HCT outcomes data is critical to the implementation of AGNIS. The CIBMTR chose the cancer Data Standards Registry and Repository (caDSR), which is maintained by the National Cancer Institute (NCI) Center for Biomedical Informatics and Information Technology (CBIIT) [5], as that standard language because it uses an internationally-recognized metadata framework and provides metadata management tools.

The semantics of a data point in the caDSR are expressed using an internationally recognized framework, ISO/IEC 11179. Its high-level construct is a Common Data

Element (CDE), which is comprised of two parts: a Data Element Concept (DEC) and a Value Domain (VD). The DEC is a contextual representation of the data element – roughly equivalent to the form question. The VD is a physical representation of the data element which describes how the answer to the question gets stored in the database (data type, maximum length, and list of allowed values if applicable) [6].

The caDSR provides a wealth of web-based metadata development, deployment, and maintenance tools. These tools include the Curation Tool, the CDE Browser, Form Builder, and the Sentinel Tool. The Curation Tool walks the end-user through all steps needed to create well-defined CDEs linked to a common terminology maintained by the NCI Enterprise Vocabulary Services. The CDE Browser allows searching the caDSR CDEs, viewing results via a graphical user interface, and downloading the CDEs in Excel or Extensible Markup Language (XML) format. The Form Builder website is CIBMTR's primary means of organizing the CDEs for mapping by the transplant centers. The CDEs are arranged in a manner that mimics the CIBMTR's data collection forms. The CDEs are presented in the order in which they appear on a form along with form headers and instructions. Finally, the caDSR's Sentinel Tool supports monitoring changes to either CDEs or Form Builder reports via email alerts. This monitoring helps maintain the overall metadata quality by showing changes that may negatively impact content [5, 7].

To supplement caDSR tools, the CIBMTR has developed a custom reporting tool that supports its robust, multi-step review process. It automatically verifies that each CDE complies with established caDSR best practices and does not violate the CIBMTR's metadata business rules. A metadata analyst then generates detailed reports to facilitate a comprehensive CDE review that verifies that each CDE accurately captures the data element semantics and is constructed according to proper ISO/IEC 11179 guidelines. A more general report facilitates the review of each CDE for correct semantics by a clinician. This detailed review process ensures CDE quality.

These CDEs serve as the standard language for data transmission via AGNIS. To use AGNIS, each transplant center or software vendor must map their data elements to the AGNIS CDEs.

3 Current State of AGNIS Data Transmission

To date, 26 HCT recipient outcomes forms and their associated 6,795 FormsNet database fields have been released in the caDSR. 1,515 CDEs are used to represent the database fields on those forms. These forms represent 71.5 % of all completed recipient forms in the FormsNet database.

Four vendors, four domestic transplant centers, and one international registry are using AGNIS to submit data to the CIBMTR. The vendor applications are being used by twenty-six centers. The number of centers utilizing AGNIS represents 13 % of all domestic transplant centers. The transplant centers support an average of seven forms; the vendors support an average of 18 forms.

Unfortunately, use of AGNIS has yet to reach its full potential. In 2014, AGNIS was used by US transplant centers to submit 7,700 forms which represents just 4 % of all recipient forms and 6 % of AGNIS-supported forms collected by the CIBMTR. While the utilization of AGNIS has increased since its initial release in 2009, this valuable resource is still underutilized.

In the remainder of the paper, we explore some of the possible reasons for this underutilization and potential strategies for increasing it.

4   Challenges in Integrating Data

Mapping the transplant center's database to the CDEs is by far the largest barrier to the utilization of AGNIS. As Warzel et al. say, "Complex metadata requirements, overlapping and competing medical terminology standards, and inconsistent information models presented challenges and obstacles to CDE standardization" [8]. Their challenges are similar to those in the AGNIS project, which we group into three broad categories: complexities of the mapping process; changes to clinical practice; and inconsistencies and evolution of the data standard.

Complex Mappings. Mapping from heterogeneous database systems to a data standard is complex. It requires an in-depth knowledge of the database system, the clinical domain, and the business process. The transplant center's EMR may consist of separate databases for information about laboratory results, accounting information, HCT - related information, and others. Consequently, the human mapper may be required to search through several systems to obtain an accurate mapping. Additionally, the mapping to one CDE may require applying complex business rules and calculations to several database fields. Involving clinicians and business process subject matter experts helps ensure that these complex mappings are semantically accurate.

Changes to the Clinical Domain. The nature of the clinical domain necessitates change. As clinical practice changes, new CDEs are created, and old CDEs are removed in order to maintain data that is timely and useful. Therefore, the CIBMTR periodically reviews and revises forms to ensure that they are consistent with current medical practice. The latest round of form revisions was released in the FormsNet application in 2013. During this revision cycle, 26 recipient forms were revised. Of these, seven were supported by AGNIS. In the AGNIS supported forms alone, 801 questions were added, and 580 questions were deleted. These essential changes burden the transplant centers with the task of updating their mappings.

Inconsistencies in and Evolution of the Standard. Inconsistencies commonly exist within a data standard [9–14]. The CIBMTR has not been immune to this universal challenge. For example, the CIBMTR employs a form-based data management approach. Historically, each form question was defined independently from other forms. Therefore, semantically identical data points were defined multiple times, resulting in inconsistencies across forms. The CIBMTR has addressed these inconsistencies by linking the questions to a robust data dictionary. In November, 2013, the CIBMTR released forms revised using the new data dictionary structure. They had 62 % data dictionary instance reuse versus a previous 4 %. The new forms' questions were more consistent, facilitating the transplant center's mapping effort.

In addition, best practices for CDE development have evolved. In AGNIS version 1.0, the XML message structure allowed a particular CDE to be used only once per form. This created a conflict between clinical practice and functional capability. For example, forms commonly collect data for the same data element at multiple time points. Due to XML messaging structure limits, two or more CDEs would be created for this data element. In AGNIS version 2.0, the XML messaging structure allowed for the repetition of a CDE within a form. Thus, more generic CDEs facilitating CDE reuse are possible. In the long-term, this change eases the transplant center's mapping effort. In the short-term, the change complicates overall mapping efforts because the centers must update their mappings to reflect the usage of the new CDEs. To minimize the impact of these changes, new CDEs are incorporated only when the CIBMTR releases new revisions of the forms, and comprehensive change notes that map the old CDEs to the new, semantically equivalent CDEs are provided.

5   Strategies to Resolve Data Integration Problems

While the adoption rate of AGNIS among transplant centers is low now, this is a very exciting time for the AGNIS project. The CIBMTR has created a solid foundation for the integration of HCT outcomes data, and there are several innovative strategies that can facilitate the increased utilization of AGNIS. Since each transplant center is different, there is not a one-size-fits-all approach, as center size, patient volume, and available information technology resources will vary. Some strategies to facilitate AGNIS adoption are: the BRIDG project; mapping aids; annotation with other standards; and marketing AGNIS and its potential return on investment.

BRIDG. The Biomedical Research Integrated Domain Group (BRIDG) Model represents collaboration between the NCI, the Clinical Data Interchange Standards Consortium, Health Level Seven International, and the Food and Drug Administration. Its goal is "to produce a shared view of the dynamic and static semantics for the domain of protocol-driven research and its associated regulatory artifacts" [15]. The model is an implementation agnostic representation of the semantics of clinical research that does not provide a physical database model. The CIBMTR, in collaboration with a team of subject matter experts from BRIDG and MD Anderson Cancer Center, along with Computer Science graduate students from the University of Minnesota and NMDP summer interns, mapped the HCT CDEs to the BRIDG Model. This mapping served as the foundation for the development of a BRIDG-compliant physical database for the HCT domain. The broader HCT community is now reviewing the first version of the physical database.

The next step of the project is to develop an integration engine that will allow for bi-directional transmission of data between the BRIDG-compliant physical database and the FormsNet database. The integration engine will contain all of the mappings and business rules needed for data transmission. This strategy is helpful for primarily those transplant centers that either do not have a database system or are looking to replace their existing one. For them, the combination of the integration engine and the physical database can facilitate the development of electronic data submission to the CIBMTR by significantly reducing their mapping efforts. In addition, they can extend the database model to capture information specific to their needs.

For those transplant centers who already have an integrated database system, the BRIDG-compliant physical database will not significantly reduce their mapping efforts. To utilize the integration engine, they will still need to map their database to the BRIDG-compliant database. While there may be fewer attributes to which to map, the mapping effort will not be eliminated entirely.

Mapping Aids. Since the mapping of database fields to either the CDEs or the BRIDG-compliant physical database will never be eliminated completely, innovative solutions are needed to reduce the mapping burden. Interesting research is being conducted into ways to do so. For example, Lin et al. have developed a process that combines CDEs, ontologies, and natural language processing to develop a query tool that matches form question texts to a list of potential CDEs. While the tool is still a prototype, initial tests yielded a 90 % accuracy rate along with favorable feedback [16].

The work of Lin et al. is not the only work being done is this field. As another example, the MAPONTO tool uses the web ontology language (OWL) and SQL DDL declarations to map an existing database to an ontology [17]. An evaluation of this tool found that it was "able to infer the semantics of many relational tables occurring in practice in terms of an independently developed ontology" which resulted in "significant saving in terms of human labors" [18].

Also, the Karma system, as described by Knoblock et al., provides a semi-automated way to match structured data such as databases to ontologies. Karma not only determines the most likely mapping, but it also provides an interface so that the user can modify the mapping. The goal is to facilitate the work of the subject matter expert while shielding them from the complexities of the mapping process [19]. Karma has been used to meet the needs of several projects such as a mapping project conducted by the Smithsonian American Art Museum [20].

This is just a small sampling of the work that is being done in the field of ontology mapping, and it indicates that there is significant work upon which a mapping aid for AGNIS can be built.

Annotation of Other Standards. EMRs use a wealth of standards, including controlled vocabularies such as LOINC, SNOMED CT, and ICD, which liberate one from the curse of free text. Ideally, there would be one standard used for the capture of all clinical information. Until that time, annotating the CDEs used by AGNIS with the appropriate code from the most commonly used standards may help facilitate the mapping of a transplant center's database to the CDEs. Annotation of multiple standards would serve as a type of Rosetta Stone. The transplant center may not understand all of the standards, but knowing part may help them understand the whole. The effort needed to annotate the CDEs with other standards would be significant. Prior to beginning the annotation project, it would be critical to survey the AGNIS end-users so that work could begin on the highest-impact standards first.

Communicating and Marketing the Standard. To date there has not been a strong effort to market the AGNIS application. The primary means of marketing employed the

CIBMTR websites, AGNIS user groups, presentations at transplant conferences, 27 visits to transplant centers, and word of mouth. Despite these efforts, some centers are not aware of either AGNIS or the data elements defined in the caDSR.

In addition, clearly communicating the return on investment that might be realized with an AGNIS implementation can help facilitate its adoption. The CIBMTR has produced documentation about the estimated costs associated with the mapping process. Unfortunately, the documentation does not consider the potential long-term cost savings of the mapping effort [18]. Surveying current AGNIS users to better estimate those cost savings would provide potential users with a clearer understanding of the benefits of AGNIS and help them advocate for an AGNIS implementation project.

6   Conclusion

The AGNIS project is an excellent case study of the universal challenges in data stand-ards adoption. The complexities of the mapping process, the changing nature of the clinical domain, and inconsistencies within the standard itself hinders the widespread adoption of data standards. While progress has been made since the 2008 update on the NIH Roadmap for Reengineering Clinical Research [21], of which AGNIS is a part, additional work remains.

The move from an underlying form-based model to the BRIDG model, with its focus on a structure common to all protocol-driven research, has potential to lower the barrier to adoption. Transplantation is an area of biomedical research where data sharing has been essential and productive. It stands to reason that the value of a shared domain model and semantics for protocol-driven research will be realized in due time in other fields, whether the motivation is financial, regulatory or scientific. Clear, quantitative commu-nication of the benefits of standards adoption along with tools and resources to facilitate its adoption will go a long way towards bridging the gaps in data standard utilization. After all, a standard is worthless unless it is being used.

Acknowledgements. Support for this project was partially provided by contract ADB. No. N01-HC-45215 / HHSN268200425215C from the National Heart, Lung, and Blood Institute and the NMDP. Thanks are extended to all who reviewed the document and provided their thoughtful feedback. In addition, Kirt Schaper, Bridget Wakaruk, and Tony Wirth helped calculate the metrics gathered here.

References

1. CIBMTR Progress Report 2014. http://www.cibmtr.org/About/ProceduresProgress/Pages/index.aspx
2. HRSA Blood Cell Transplant. http://bloodcell.transplant.hrsa.gov
3. Aljurf, M., Rizzo, J., Mohty, M., Hussain, F., Madrigal, A., Pasquini, M., Passweg, J., Chaudhri, N., Ghavamzadeh, A., Solh, H., Atsuta, Y., Szer, J., Kodera, Y., Niederweiser, D., Gratwohl, A., Horowitz, M.: Challenges and opportunities for HSCT outcome registries: perspective from international HSCT registries experts. Bone Marrow Transplant. **49**, 1016–1021 (2014)

4. AGNIS Service - Technical Description. http://www.agnis.net/uploadedFiles/Documentation/docs/AGNISService.pdf

5. caDSR. https://cbiit.nci.nih.gov/ncip/biomedical-informatics-resources/interoperability-and-semantics/metadata-and-models

6. ISO/IEC 11179 Information Technology. http://metadata-standards.org/11179/

7. Komatsoulis, G., Warzel, D., Hartel, F., Shanbhag, K., Chilukuri, R., Fragoso, G., Coronado, S., Reeves, D., Hadfield, J., Ludet, C., Covitz, P.: caCORE version 3: implementation of a model driven, service-oriented architecture for semantic interoperability. J. Biomed. Inform. **41**, 106–123 (2008)

8. Warzel, D.B., Andonyadis, C., McCurry, B., Chilukuri, R., Ishmukhamedov, S., Covitz, P.: Common data element (CDE) management and deployment in clinical trials. In: AMIA Annual Symposium Proceedings, p. 1048 (2003)

9. de Coronado, S., Wright, L., Fragoso, G., Haber, M., Hahn-Dantona, E., Hartel, F., Quan, S., Safran, T., Thomas, N., Whiteman, L.: The NCI thesaurus quality assurance life cycle. J. Biomed. Inform. **42**, 530–539 (2009)

10. Jiang, G., Solbrig, H., Chute, C.: Quality evaluation of cancer study common data elements using the UMLS semantic network. J. Biomed. Inform. **44**, S78–S85 (2011)

11. Adamusiak,T., Bodenreider, O.: Quality assurance in LOINC using description logic. In: AMIA Annual Symposium Proceedings, p. 1099 (2012)

12. Elhanan, G., Perl, Y., Geller, J.: A survey of SNOMED CT direct users, 2010: impressions and preferences regarding content and quality. J. Am. Med. Inform. Assoc. **18**, i36–i44 (2011)

13. Jiang, G., Solbrig, H., Chute, C.: Quality evaluation of value sets from cancer study common data elements using the UMLS semantic groups. J. Am. Med. Inform. Assoc. **19**, e129–e136 (2012)

14. Mougin, F., Bodenreider, O.: Auditing the NCI thesaurus with semantic web technologies. In: AMIA Annual Symposium Proceedings, pp. 500–504 (2008)

15. BRIDG. http://www.bridgmodel.org

16. Lin, C., Wu, N., Liou, D.: A multi-technique approach to bridge electronic case report form design and data standard adoption. J. Biomed. Inform. **53**, 49–57 (2015)

17. An, Y., Borgida, A., Mylopoulos, J.: Refining semantic mappings from relational tables to ontologies. In: Bussler, C., Tannen, V., Fundulaki, I. (eds.) SWDB 2004. LNCS, vol. 3372, pp. 84–90. Springer, Heidelberg (2005)

18. An, Y., Mylopoulos, J., Borgida, A.: Building semantic mappings from databases to ontologies. In: Proceedings of the National Conference on Artificial Intelligence, p. 1557. AAAI Press, MIT Press (2006)

19. Knoblock, C.A., et al.: Semi-automatically mapping structured sources into the semantic web. In: Simperl, E., Cimiano, P., Polleres, A., Corcho, O., Presutti, V. (eds.) ESWC 2012. LNCS, vol. 7295, pp. 375–390. Springer, Heidelberg (2012)

20. Szekely, P., Knoblock, C., Yang, F., Fink, E., Gupta, S., Allen, R., Goodlander, G.: Publishing the data of the Smithsonian American Art Museum to the linked data cloud. Int. J. Humanit. Comput. **8**, 152–166 (2014)

21. Williams, R.L., Johnson, S., Greene, S., Larson, E., Green, L., Morris, A., Confer, D., Reaman, G., Madigan, R., Kahn, J.: Signposts along the NIH roadmap for reengineering clinical research: lessons from the Clinical Research Networks initiative. Arch. Intern. Med. **168**, 1919–1925 (2008)

ICD Code Retrieval: Novel Approach for Assisted Disease Classification

Stefano Giovanni Rizzo[1]([✉]), Danilo Montesi[1], Andrea Fabbri[2], and Giulio Marchesini[3]

[1] Department of Computer Science and Engineering, University of Bologna, Mura Anteo Zamboni 7, 40127 Bologna, Italy
stefano.rizzo8@unibo.it
[2] Local Public Health Unit of Forlì, Emergency Department, Hospital Morgagni-Pierantoni, via Forlanini 34, 40121 Forlì, Italy
[3] Department of Medicine, University of Bologna, via Massarenti 9, 40138 Bologna, Italy

Abstract. The task of assigning classification codes to short medical text is a hard text classification problem, especially when the set of possible codes is as big as the ICD-9-CM set. The problem, which has been only partially tamed for a subset of ICD-9-CM, becomes even harder in real world applications, where the labeled data are scarce and noisy. In this paper we first show the ineffectivenesss of current Text Classification algorithms on large datasets, then we present a novel incremental approach to clinical Text Classification, which overcomes the low accuracy problem through the top-K retrieval, exploits Transfer Learning techniques in order to expand a skewed dataset and improves the overall accuracy over time, learning from user selection.

Keywords: ICD-9-CM · Text classification · Transfer learning · Learning to rank · Document expansion · Icd coding task

1 Introduction

The International Classification of Diseases (ICD) is a standard, broadly used classification system, that codes a large number of specific diseases, symptoms, injuries and medical procedures into numerical classes. Assigning a code to a clinical case means classifying that case into one or more particular discrete class, hence allowing further statistics studies and automated calculations. The possibility to have a discrete code instead of a text in natural language is intuitively a great advantage for data processing systems. The use of such classification is becoming increasingly important for, but not limited to, epidemiological, economic and policy-making purposes.

The presentation of this work has been partly funded by FIRB project Information monitoring, propagation analysis and community detection in Social Network Sites.

© Springer International Publishing Switzerland 2015
N. Ashish and J.-L. Ambite (Eds.): DILS 2015, LNBI 9162, pp. 147–161, 2015.
DOI: 10.1007/978-3-319-21843-4_12

While the ICD Classification is clearly useful on many aspects, physicians and clinical personnel think and write in natural language and, after that, assign the right code to their text description aided by manuals, guidelines, or their own memory.

The ICD-9-CM contains more than 14 thousand classification codes for diseases, meaning that manual methods are inadequate to locate the right classes in a real-world scenario, even for expert clinical coders. In some medical departments the codes used are just a tiny subset of the ICD classification set, hence the problem is reduced, but in many other and in generic departments like the Emergency, this subset covers a big portion of the classification codes. An accurate system that assist the medical personnel in the task of coding is needed to reduce costs and to provide better standardization of the medical data (Table 1).

Table 1. Samples of medical text with the associated ICD-9-CM codes

Clinical short text	ICD-9-CM labels
5-year-old male with cough, normal slightly hypoventilatory chest x-ray, no pneumonia	786.2
Urinary tract infections. Normal sonographic appearance of the kidney bilaterally. Trace amount of nonspecific free fluid in the pelvis	599.0, 780.31, 780.39
Vesicoureteral reflux followup. Normal renal ultrasound. Mild intermittent left hydroureter proximally at the renal pelvis	593.70, V13.09, 593.5

Among the many attempts to simplify or automate the coding task of medical text we can distinguish between two approaches: the **Information Retrieval** (IR) of codes from a dictionary and the machine learning or rule-based **Text Classification** (TC).

In the first approach a typical boolean IR model allows the personnel to search the dictionary for a set of one or more terms. Often these systems allow also to search for disjunction and conjunction of terms (boolean queries), exact text matching (full-text search) and the use of jolly characters, to expand the queries (regular expressions). Nevertheless these methods represent the most used techniques in real world applications, due to their simplicity of implementation and their ability to cover seamlessly an entire set with thousands entries.

Over the last years, TC has received attention as a valuable solution to medical text coding [3,8]. The described problem fall into a TC problem with some properties:

1. Multi-class Classification: the number of output classes (ICD codes) can be very high, contrary to the simplest binary classification.
2. Multi-label Classification: a text instance can be associated with more than one label. This is true for two reasons: because a text can include different diseases (e.g. injuries to different arms) and because there might need more than one code to describe a clinical condition (primary and secondary).

The TC approach to the problem is the most promising one, since it aims at providing automatic code assignment, without any user interaction. Unfortunately, even getting a clean and balanced training set of labeled medical text, TC achieved great results on small datasets, but almost fails in classifying large-scale taxonomies, like the ICD, in both classification accuracy and performance. The effectivenesss of cutting-edge classification algorithms is heavily reduced when applied to very large taxonomies. We will conduct a short survey on classification accuracy in Sect. 3.1, showing the accuracy degradation over increasing number of classes.

The code retrieval approach that we propose is a mixed approach, as it shares features and ideas of both IR and TC. The proposed approach is based on learning from labeled samples and auxiliary sources, retrieving the K most relevant classes based on term-frequency similarities and improving the ranking by learning from the users feedback. The impossibility to achieve a reasonable accuracy on a large class space, together with the online assisted coding approach, leads to prefer a top-K retrieval model over a strict text classifier. Instead of precisely selecting the right number of labels for a medical text, we are interested in showing the most relevant codes, and then let the user to choose the appropriate ones. Moreover this ensures associations with the right codes, allowing a running system to further learn and improve itself, using the users' selection as a continue flow of training data.

In order to address the lack of high-quality annotated examples we took some ideas from Transfer Learning, that is a set of methods to extract useful knowledge from different but related auxiliary domains [16]. Using the ICD code as an attribute to match related contents, we augmented our training set with knowledge from auxiliary sources (e.g. Wikipedia, ICD Manuals, etc.), thus obtaining a model with a greater accuracy.

In Sect. 2 we present the related work. In Sect. 3 we outline the addressed problem and we lay the foundations for the proposed approach. In Sect. 4 we present the approach in further details showing our implementation. In Sect. 5 we evaluate the accuracy of the system in different settings on medical datasets. In Sect. 6 we summarize the contributions of the paper and propose further experiments.

2   Related Work

The goal of fully automating the ICD-9-CM assignment of codes to medical text is unrealistic for many practical reasons we will outline hereafter. Nevertheless some attempts and studies have been made by researchers in the last two decades, most of which have been conducted on a small subset of the coding classes. Larkey and Croft [10] trained three statistical classifiers for the automatic assignment of ICD-9 codes, and then combined their results to obtain a better classification. Their work is based on discharge summaries, for which the number of labels per document is from 1 to 15. This combined classifier produces a ranked list of the top-K most relevant codes, which makes it very similar to our approach, but the instances domain is different, as discharge summaries have different terms distribution than short diagnosis. Lussier et al. [13] studied the feasibility of automating the ICD-9-CM coding task, concluding that more external knowledge bases and manual revisions where needed to improve accuracy.

The lack of a shared, publicly available training and testing dataset with labeled medical text discouraged further reasearches, until the CMC Challenge in 2007 [17]. The challenge consisted in building a classifier that could automatically encode medical text in ICD-9-CM classification. For the challenge purposes, data were collected from the Cincinnati Childrens Hospital Medical Centers (CCHMC) Department of Radiology. Since code annotation is a difficult task, each document in the corpus was evaluated by three expert annotators. A gold annotation was created by taking the majority of the annotators. With only 45 ICD codes, this corpus is still really far from the ideal. A group of 50 teams and individuals submitted their results for the challenge. The best results for classification accuracy have been scored by rules-based systems [7], which dominated the challenge. These systems were based entirely or partly on hand-crafted expert rules. In the challenge context this was a feasible approach and has been proved to be the best model in terms of prediction accuracy. However it would be very time-consuming, if not impossible, to hand-craft expert rules for all ICD codes. Another approach is the machine learning one [20], in which the classifier is automatically built from the training data, without the need for human intervention. We will show in Sect. 3.1 that the accuracy tends to drop dramatically as the number of classes increases [12].

3   ICD Code Retrieval

Our work is focused on the practical problem that medical personnel face on a daily basis. Medical personnel manually assign ICD codes while or after examinations and procedures. The code assignment task has become part of the procedure and is not an a posterieri practice, therefore a coding system should help the personnel during the coding. This significant property of the problem should be exploited with a new approach to overcome the low accuracy of automated solutions.

3.1   Text Classification Accuracy Decay

In the task of Multi-label TC we have a set of text instances such that each instance must be associated with a subset of all possible classes $\mathcal{Y} = \{c_1, ..., c_n\}$.

TC on large taxonomies, like ICD-9-CM codes set, is a major challenge for state-of-the-art machine learning algorithms, including Support Vector Machines (SVM). Machine learning algorithms, like SVM, have achieved great results in classifying small text collections [4], but proved to be less and less accurate when the number of classes starts growing [4,12].

As discussed in [11,18], current machine learning methods need significant improvement when applied to very large-scale datasets. Effectiveness of state-of-the-art models is unacceptable on large-scale applications, partially due to the data sparseness in rare classes.

In order to show the relation between number of classes and classification accuracy, we conducted a short survey on classification performance, summarized in Fig. 1. Accuracy values are measured as F1 score, a popular measure of accuracy in classification problems. Given the number of true positive results (TP), false positives (FP) and false negatives (FN), the F1 score is calculated as:

$$F1 = \frac{2TP}{2TP + FP + FN} \tag{1}$$

The Macro-averaged F1 is the average of the F1 scores of each instance in the specific test collection.

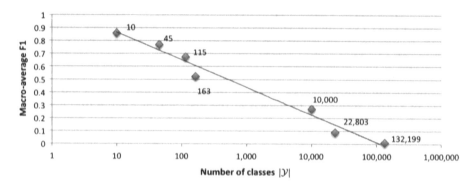

Fig. 1. Values of accuracy (Macro-averaged F1) using SVM on datasets with different $|\mathcal{Y}|$ value (classes space size). Trend and class space scale are logarithmic.

Results from various multi-label classification experiments on small, medium and large popular datasets are shown. In particular, we selected results of Support Vector Machines (SVM) algorithms on collections with different size $|\mathcal{Y}|$ of the target class space $\mathcal{Y}$: $|\mathcal{Y}| = 10$ and $|\mathcal{Y}| = 115$ are from *Reuters 21578* [4], $|\mathcal{Y}| = 45$ is the best result for the CMC Challenge [20], $|\mathcal{Y}| = 163$ is from the *LookSmart* web directory [2], $|\mathcal{Y}| = 22,803$ is from the *MERG* subset of *Yahoo! Directory* [12], $|\mathcal{Y}| = 132,199$ is from *Yahoo! Directory* [11]. All the results are obtained using SVM algorithms except for the CMC Challenge ($|\mathcal{Y}| = 45$), which derives from a rule-based system. Those results come from different works on text categorization, therefore the SVM implementation may vary slightly, but the overall degradation of accuracy on larger datasets is evident in Fig. 1.

3.2   Top-K Code Retrieval

As pointed out in [15,21], there is no obvious winner in multi-class classification techniques. For practical problems, the choice of approach will have to be made depending on the constraints, e.g. the desired accuracy level, the time available, and the nature of the problem.

In the hard version of the classification problem, a particular set of labels is explicitly assigned to the instance, whereas in the soft version of the classification problem, a score is assigned to the each label. The approach for interactive TC that we refer to as the code retrieval approach solve a soft version of the TC problem. It has been applied on the ICD-9-CM classification problem by Larkley and Croft [10] in 1995. A similar approach is found more recently in [14] in which a semi-automatic approach is proposed to automatically classifying the easiest associations while hardest instances are left to the user judgement.

In a top-K IR model, results are displayed in a ranked order to the user. Similarly, in code retrieval, most probable ICD codes for a medical text are retrieved and displayed in ranked order. In most multi-label TC algorithms, a ranked set of the best scoring classes is also produced, however a thresholding strategy exists to select how many codes, from the best scoring ranked set, should be assigned to the text instance.

In multi-label TC, different choices of the threshold strategy lead to different accuracy results [6], while in our approach results are presented in ranked order, without a thresholding strategy. Since no specific set of codes is assigned in code retrieval, accuracy measures are evaluated over the first K ranked results returned, for different values of K. Each value of K can be considered as the number of ranked results to be shown in the first Search Engine Results Page (SERP). It is important to note that the total lack of the right code in the retrieved results is unacceptable: the end-user must be able to get more than K results whenever he asks to. However, it is desirable to obtain the right codes in the first SERP: from a user point of view, earlier researches have shown that only 30 % of users view results past the first SERP in search engines [9], which in the average case counts 10 results.

3.3 Transfer Learning

Dealing with a collection of real labeled data provided by partner hospitals, we came across different issues regarding its use as a training set:

1. **Data Sparseness**: uncommon or specific clinical conditions are never or rarely present in the data.
2. **Unreliable Labels Association**: due to the coding task complexity, the chosen labels (ICD codes) are not always objectively accurate. The construction of a reliable ground truth would involve several experts to individually vote for every association, as in the CMC Challenge for radiology department [17].
3. **Unbalanced Distribution of Labels**: while less common diseases or very specific codes are missing or scarce, generic codes and codes related to common clinical conditions are used very often resulting in over abundance of positive samples for a small subset of the labels space.

When a valid training set is not available, one strategy to improve the learning is to expand the training set with text-code associations from auxiliary sources, a practice that falls under the Transfer Learning category. Transfer Learning refers to the framework of methods for machine learning where training data or classification model are extracted from an auxiliary source to augment the original learning model. In a Transfer Learning setting a *transfer* of knowledge occurs from a source domain (the auxiliary source) to the target domain (the domain of the model you want to learn). Apart from this common meaning, many different settings and definitions of the Transfer Learning model exist and found application in different contexts of classification [16]. Our scenario fits in an *inductive* Transfer Learning setting, in which labeled data from the source domain are used to induce a predictive model for the target domain. Since a lot of labeled data are available in the source domain, the *inductive* Transfer Learning setting aims at improving the learning task in the source domain by transferring knowledge from the source task.

4   Implementation

The overall architecture of the implementation is shown in Fig. 2. The main processes of the implementation are:

1. **Training Set Learning**: labeled samples, consisting of diagnoses labeled with codes from the ICD standard, compose the training set of the original domain.
2. **Trasfer Learning**: external sources, like dictionary entries and encyclopedia articles, are extracted along with the related ICD codes. Generic codes are mapped onto a subset of the labels set $\mathcal{Y}$.
3. **Text Preprocessing**: a set of filters is applied on the text data from both the training set and the auxiliary domains, in order to improve the final accuracy and reduce the index size.
4. **TF/IDF Indexing**: the preprocessed text data, with the associated labels, is indexed in a vector space using standard term weighting based on terms frequency.
5. **Top-K Retrieval**: when a user issue a set of words describing a disease (query), the K best scoring labels are selected using a textual similarity model, and provided to the user for manual picking. We evaluated three different similarities: Vector Space Model, Language Model and Okapi BM25, in the implementations provided by the *Apache Lucene*[TM]framework[1]. We found the BM25 similarity to be the most effective similarity model for this task.
6. **Learning to Rank Cycle**: from the set of K relevant codes, the user select the right ones. The user selection feedback allows further improvement of future scoring: the issued query text is used as a positive training sample for the hand-picked labels.

---

[1] http://lucene.apache.org.

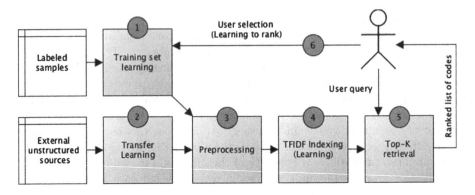

Fig. 2. The architecture of the ICD code retrieval implementation, showing the data flow involved in the main processes.

4.1   Preprocessing and Indexing

In order to improve efficiency and effectivenesss of the classification and reduce the index size, some pre-processing actions must be taken. The pre-processing filters are applied in sequence to the textual data. Apart from the HTML filter, which is applied only to the auxiliary domain instances coming from web sources, the rest of the pipeline is applied on all the text involved: labeled samples, auxiliary instances, test instances (user queries).

All the modules in the pre-processing pipeline are:

1. HTML Code Removal: this filter applies only on auxiliary instances coming from web sources. If the text data is in unformatted form, the filter is ignored.
2. Keep Word Filter: this module ensures that the words on a list are not discarded or altered by the pre-processing. The keep list is populated with abbreviations and expressions from the medical jargon.
3. Stop Word Removal: common words (e.g. "the", "that", "a", "an") are discarded in order to reduce index size and improve effectivenesss.
4. Lowercase Filter: transforms the letters in each term to lowercase only letters, in order to reduce the number of tokens.
5. Porter Stemmer: Porter's stemming algorithm is applied to remove the commoner morphological and inflexional endings of the terms, improving recall and reducing the index size.
6. Shingle Filter: combine together adjacent terms to form n-grams of terms, producing a new token for every combination, therefore improving precision without affecting the recall of single terms.

The last two filters significantly improved accuracy on both general and medical TC.

4.2   Cross-Domain Transfer Learning

For each auxiliary domain a specific *crawler* is required to retrieve all the documents associated with ICD codes. Each document is then processed with a *scraper*, built on a set of hand-crafted regular expression, which extract different fields of a semi-structured document, along with the attribute related to the ICD-9-CM code (see Fig. 3).

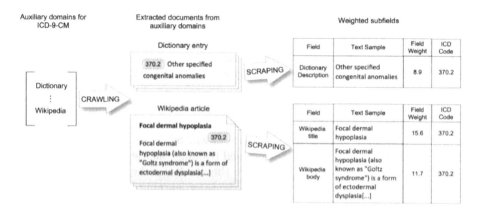

Fig. 3. Cross-domain data extraction and mapping for Transfer Learning. New features from different domains are extracted and decomposed into fields with specific weights.

Transfer learning is a valuable solution when the training set is small relatively to the number of classes and the labels distribution is unbalanced. It improves the recall of the system, expanding the terms in the training set with synonyms and related words. However this augmentation may associates terms which are not strictly related to a disease, whose relationship makes sense only in the context of the source domain.

A strategy to address the degradation of precision is to weight differently the domains and the fields involved in the training, as in Fig. 3. Given the set of all fields $T = \{t_1, ..., t_r\}$ from all domains, a weight vector $W = \{w_1, ..., w_r\}$ is computed, denoting the relative significance of every field. At retrieval time, the probability of a code c with respect to a text is computed as the linear combination of the probabilities of each single field t_i associated with c, with w_i the coefficient for t_i. The Apache DisMax query parser allows to alter the similarity model by specifying different weights for different fields of a structured document, therefore implementing the linear combination described.

The optimal weight vector W depends on the involved auxiliary domains and can be determined empirically, selecting the vector that maximize the overall accuracy. While this exhaustive search can be viable for the small CMC Corpus, it becomes extremely time-consuming for larger datasets. In this case the weight w_i of each field t_i can be approximated as the accuracy produced by the system trained with t_i only. This means training the system r times with a different binary permutation of the vector W.

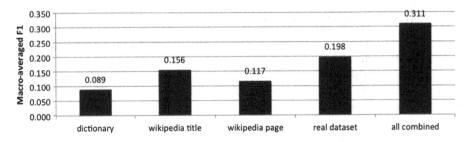

Fig. 4. Accuracies (macro-averaged F1 scores) obtained training with each single field only. The first field is the description of official italian dictionary of all ICD-9-CM codes. From italian wikipedia pages of diseases are extracted the title and the whole article. The real dataset are text medical reports from the *ITA50*.

We conducted the experiment on the *ITA50* corpus [5] using the known minimum K for every instance of the testing set. The resulting accuracies are shown in Fig. 4 for 4 different domain fields, of which 3 fields comes from transfer learning. The first 4 accuracies are obtained training the sistem with each single field alone. The rightmost accuracy show the results of the linear combination of all the fields, proving the advantage of transfer learning.

4.3   Incremental Learning to Rank

The learning to rank paradigm allows a running system to improve the ranking relying on past user selections. Based on this idea, the proposed code retrieval approach increase its capabilities over time, using additional knowledge and users interaction.

In the typical scenario, when a coding assistant software is not yet deployed, there are no labeled instances for training yet, or the ones available are not reliable. With no other supplementary knowledge, the best and only help a non-expert code can get is a search engine on the dictionary.

Our approach permits, within a single framework, to first relying solely on a simple search engine and a provided dictionary. Then to increase the system capability providing other knowledge bases, like encyclopedia and manuals, assuming these are properly structured. Finally, every medical text issued in the system, along with the selected codes, will contribute at improving the system.

The user query text, together with the subset of codes in the ranked list selected by the user, is regarded as a labeled sample, in the same domain of the training set, therefore weighted accordingly.

5   Experimental Results

Since it has not been possible to test the implementation with medical personnel, we conducted several experiments on labeled corpuses to assess the benefits of the proposed approach. The indexing, preprocessing and scoring tasks have been carried out using the *Apache Lucene*^{TM} framework.

5.1 Dataset

Popular TC datasets, such as *Reuters 21578* and *20 Newsgroups* have been first used to evaluate the model as a classic text categorization algorithm, obtaining average results. The CMC corpus [17] and a set of 50 thousand text-label associations for short clinical reports from italian hospitals (*ITA50* [5]) have been used for accuracy testing on medical text data.

Since there is no publicly available English dataset for medical classification with a label space $\mathcal{Y}$ larger than 45 codes, the *ITA50* corpus represented the most reliable dataset to validate our approach in a realistic scenario. The *ITA50* corpus is a set of human labeled samples from real hospital clinical reports, edited in italian language and coded accordingly to the ICD-9-CM guidelines. Albeit the learning sources involved in training and Transfer Learning are obviously language dependent, the proposed approach abstracts from any specific language. The *ITA50* corpus is composed of 14,304 different medical records and 50,078 text-label associations, meaning an average of 3.5 labels per text record. The distribution of classes among the records is strongly unbalanced: 3,259 different classes of which 1,061 associated with only 1 record instance, while the 4 most frequent classes alone counts 5,187 records. The average number of words per text record is 18.

5.2 Evaluation

The commonly used performance evaluation criteria for multi-label classification is the F1 accuracy score. Since our approach is strongly related to Information Retrieval, significant measures considered in our tests comprise also precision and recall measures at specific K values. In fact, since a fixed K of results will be returned, it is crucial to investigate recall and precision over K.

The precision score denotes the fraction of TP in the returned results:

$$Precision = \frac{TP}{TP + FP} \tag{2}$$

The recall score denotes the fraction of TP in the set of right codes:

$$Recall = \frac{TP}{TP + FN} \tag{3}$$

In the evaluation on the *ITA50* corpus we considered the total set of ICD-9-CM classes (14,170 in the italian dictionary), despite the *ITA50* comprises only 3,259 labels, of which 1,061 labels are either in the training or in the testing set. Given the imbalance in the number of samples per class, we splitted the corpus with a ratio 10/90 between testing and training set.

Using values of K from 1 to 100 we evaluated the overall system accuracy under precision, recall and macro-averaged F1, as shown in Fig. 5.

With only 3.5 right labels per test instance on average, accuracy measures taking into account false positives (i.e. precision and F1) are clearly disadvantaged for larger values of K. We are instead mostly interested in the recall of the

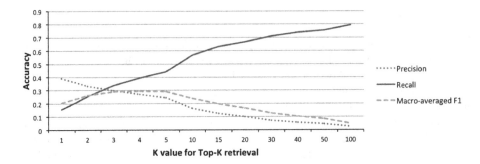

Fig. 5. Recall, precision and macro-averaged F1 evaluated for a different number K of returned scores, on the ITA50 corpus [5].

retrieval over K values, which can be viewed as the probability to find the entire set of right codes within the first K results.

Evaluation on the CMC corpus has been carried out using transfer learning from Wikipedia English (articles title and body) and from the Centers for Medicare and Medicaid Services (abbreviated and full descriptions in dictionary). As for the accuracy of strict TC classifiers, the accuracy of soft classifiers depends on the number of classes involved, as shown in the top-k experiment on the CMC corpus. Considering a SERP of 10 results, the probability of getting all the right codes in the first SERP is quite different in the two datasets: this probability is 97.3 % for the 45 codes of the CMC corpus (Fig. 6) and 56.7 % for the 3,259 codes in *ITA50*.

ICD code retrieval is a soft classifier in which it returns k classes sorted by probability of relevance, therefore no thresholding strategy is defined. Conversely, the CMC challenge systems were hard classifiers, returning a definite set of classes for each sample of the testing set. In order to compare a soft classifier with hard classifiers we defined two elementary thresholding:

– Fixed K: K is fixed to 1, i.e. only the first class is retrieved. Threshold is fixed for all samples of testing set, this can be seen as the worst case scenario.

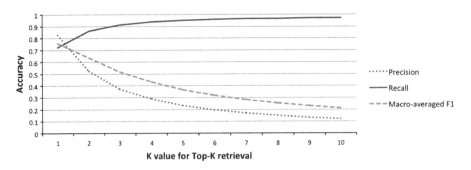

Fig. 6. Recall, precision and macro-averaged F1 evaluated for a different number K of returned scores, on the CMC corpus [17].

– Perfect K_s: for each sample s of the testing set, the top K_s are retrieved, where K_s is the exact number of labels for the sample s. This emulates an ideal thresholding strategy, therefore can be seen as the best case scenario.

Table 2. Final results for top 8 submission of CMC challenge [1], sorted by macro-averaged F1, in comparison with ICD Code Retrieval scores in the two different thresholding settings.

Team/System	Ma-F1	Challenge Rank	Approach
ICD Code Retrieval (Perfect K)	**0.806**		**BM25 + Transfer learning.**
LMCO-IS & S	0.776	5	N/A
Szeged [7]	0.7691	1	Rule based + C4.5 + Maximum entropy classifier
ICD Code Retrieval (Fixed K)	**0.756**		**BM25 + Transfer learning.**
LLX	0.7343	21	N/A
GMJ_JL	0.7334	6	N/A
SULTRG	0.7322	7	N/A
University at Albany [8]	0.7291	2	Rule-based + synonyms from www.icd9data.com
PENN [3]	0.721	4	Rule-based + synonyms from MeSH
University of Turku [20]	0.7034	3	SVM-like (RLS) + concepts from UMLS

Knowing the right number K of codes for each instance in the testing set, we selected the top-K codes from our implementation, thus yelding a macro-averaged F1 of 80.6 %, which is higher than the best scoring rule-based system in the challenge (macro-averaged F1 76.9 % [7]). Even setting a global fixed K to 1, the resulting macro-averaged F1 is 75.6 %, which is slightly lower than the best system, but still higher than any machine-learning approach in literature [19,20]. As shown in Fig. 6, we then evaluated precision, recall and F1 for each globally fixed K between 1 and 10 (Table 2).

6   Conclusion and Future Work

We have presented and evaluated a complete approach for assisting users in diseases coding. Our approach consider two related problems of ICD computer assisted coding systems: the low accuracy in automated TC for large labels space and the lack of balanced, well coded labeled samples.

The low accuracy problem is first established by surveying related works, showing that the accuracy of multi-label TC algorithms is strongly affected by the number of target classes. In order to overcome the difficulty, we have proposed an end-user oriented approach that aims at maximizing the recall of returned results, allowing the user to select the right labels in the smallest possible set of best-scoring matches. In the worst case, when the selected target subset of ICD is bigger than a few hundred codes, navigation through more than one results page could be necessary.

The unavailability of an adequate training set has been tackled through Transfer Learning techniques: the proposed incremental learning strategy allows to bootstrap with an acceptable search engine, which then improves its accuracy through machine learning on users selection feedback. We have shown the substantial benefit of using a combination of multiple sources with respect to a single source (e.g. training labeled samples).

Analysis of unreviewed labeled data coming from italian hospitals has provided a deeper understanding of the real problem hardness, addressing research towards more realistic solutions. Evaluation on the CMC corpus shown evidence of the accuracy of the proposed approach in comparison to the best-scoring systems in literature.

Future work will investigate hierarchical implementations of the proposed soft classifier, in order to leverage the taxonomy of the ICD-9-CM for improved accuracy. A more solid validation must be carried out on a large labeled corpus to show the effectiveness of the proposed approach. A period of expert usage is needed to assess the improvement of the system over time through the learning to rank process.

References

1. Results: Medical nlp challenge, computational medicine center (2007). https://web.archive.org/web/20080111141103/, http://www.computationalmedicine.org/challenge/res.php
2. Chen, H., Dumais, S.: Bringing order to the web: Automatically categorizing search results. In: Proceedings of the SIGCHI Conference on Human Factors in Computing Systems, pp. 145–152. ACM (2000)
3. Crammer, K., Dredze, M., Ganchev, K., Talukdar, P.P., Carroll, S.: Automatic code assignment to medical text. In: Proceedings of the Workshop on BioNLP 2007: Biological, Translational, and Clinical Language Processing, pp. 129–136. Association for Computational Linguistics (2007)
4. Debole, F., Sebastiani, F.: An analysis of the relative hardness of reuters-21578 subsets. J. Am. Soc. Inf. Sci. Technol. 56(6), 584–596 (2005)
5. Fabbri, A., Montesi, D., Rizzo, S.G.: ITA50 corpus of 50 thousands icd-9 labeled medical text (2015). http://smartdata.cs.unibo.it/ITA50/
6. Fan, R.E., Lin, C.J.: A study on threshold selection for multi-labelclassification. Department of Computer Science, National Taiwan University,pp. 1–23 (2007)
7. Farkas, R., Szarvas, G.: Automatic construction of rule-based ICD-9-CM codingsystems. BMC Bioinform. 9(Suppl 3), S10 (2008)
8. Goldstein, I., Arzumtsyan, A., Uzuner, Ö.: Three approaches to automatic assignment of icd-9-cm codes to radiology reports. In: AMIA Annual Symposium Proceedings. vol. 2007, p. 279. American Medical Informatics Association (2007)
9. Jansen, B.J., Spink, A.: How are we searching the world wide web? a comparison of nine search engine transaction logs. Inf. Process. Manag. 42(1), 248–263 (2006)
10. Larkey, L.S., Croft, W.B.: Automatic assignment of icd9 codes to discharge summaries. Technical report (1995)
11. LIU, T.Y., Yang, Y., WAN, H., ZENG, H.J., CHEN, Z., MA, W.Y.: Support vector machines classification with a very large-scale taxonomy. ACM SIGKDD Explor. Newsl. 7(1), 36–43 (2005)
12. Liu, T.Y., Yang, Y., Wan, H., Zhou, Q., Gao, B., Zeng, H.J., Chen, Z., Ma, W.Y.: An experimental study on large-scale web categorization. In: Special Interest Tracks and Posters of the 14th International Conference on World Wide Web, pp. 1106–1107. ACM (2005)

13. Lussier, Y.A., Shagina, L., Friedman, C.: Automating icd-9-cm encoding using medical language processing: A feasibility study. In: Proceedings of the AMIA Symposium, p. 1072. American Medical Informatics Association (2000)
14. Martinez-Alvarez, M., Yahyaei, S., Roelleke, T.: Semi-automatic Document Classification: Exploiting Document Difficulty. In: Baeza-Yates, R., de Vries, A.P., Zaragoza, H., Cambazoglu, B.B., Murdock, V., Lempel, R., Silvestri, F. (eds.) ECIR 2012. LNCS, vol. 7224, pp. 468–471. Springer, Heidelberg (2012)
15. Nigam, K., Lafferty, J., McCallum, A.: Using maximum entropy for text classification. In: IJCAI-99 Workshop on Machine Learning for Information Filtering, vol. 1, pp. 61–67 (1999)
16. Pan, S.J., Yang, Q.: A survey on transfer learning. IEEE Trans. Knowl. Data Eng. **22**(10), 1345–1359 (2010)
17. Pestian, J.P., Brew, C., Matykiewicz, P., Hovermale, D., Johnson, N., Cohen, K.B., Duch, W.: A shared task involving multi-label classification of clinical free text. In: Proceedings of the Workshop on BioNLP 2007: Biological, Translational, and Clinical Language Processing, pp. 97–104. Association for Computational Linguistics (2007)
18. Sandu Popa, I., Zeitouni, K., Gardarin, G., Nakache, D., Métais, E.: Text categorization for multi-label documents and many categories. In: Twentieth IEEE International Symposium on Computer-Based Medical Systems. CBMS 2007, pp. 421–426. IEEE (2007)
19. Sujeevan, A., Youns, B.: Semi-structured document categorization with a semantic kernel. Pattern Recogn. **42**(9), 2067–2076 (2009)
20. Suominen, H., Ginter, F., Pyysalo, S., Airola, A., Pahikkala, T., Salanter, S., Salakoski, T.: Machine learning to automate the assignment of diagnosis codes to free-text radiology reports: a method description. In: Proceedings of the ICML/UAI/COLT Workshop on Machine Learning for Health-Care Applications (2008)
21. Yang, Y., Liu, X.: A re-examination of text categorization methods. In: Proceedings of the 22nd Annual International ACM SIGIR Conference on Research and Development in Information Retrieval, pp. 42–49. ACM (1999)

Medical Research Applications

Integration of Multimodal Neuroimaging and Electroencephalography for the Study of Acute Epileptiform Activity After Traumatic Brain Injury

Andrei Irimia[1], Sheng-Yang M. Goh[1], Paul M. Vespa[2], and John D. Van Horn[1(✉)]

[1] Laboratory of Neuro Imaging, Institute for Neuroimaging and Informatics,
University of Southern California, Los Angeles, CA, USA
{andrei.irimia,matthew.goh,jack.vanhorn}@loni.usc.edu
[2] Brain Injury Research Center and Departments of Neurology and Neurosurgery,
University of California, Los Angeles, CA, USA
pvespa@mednet.ucla.edu

Abstract. The integration of multidimensional, longitudinal data acquired using the combined use of structural neuroimaging [e.g. magnetic resonance imaging (MRI), computed tomography (CT)] and neurophysiological recordings [e.g. electroencephalography (EEG)] poses substantial challenges to neuroinformaticians and to biomedical scientists who interact frequently with such data. In traumatic brain injury (TBI) studies, this challenge is even more severe due to the substantial heterogeneity of TBIs across patients and to the variety of neurophysiological responses to injury. Additionally, the study of acute epileptiform activity prompted by TBI poses logistic, analytic and data integration difficulties. Here we describe our proposed solutions to the integration of structural neuroimaging with neurophysiological recordings to study epileptiform activity after TBI. Based on techniques for TBI-robust segmentation and electrical activity localization, we have developed an approach to the joint analysis of MRI/CT/EEG data to identify the foci of seizure-related activity and to facilitate the study of TBI-related neuropathophysiology.

Keywords: Magnetic resonance imaging · Computed tomography · Electroencephalography · Traumatic brain injury · Big data · Segmentation · Seizure · Neurophysiology

1 Introduction

The advent and proliferation of multimodal neuroimaging approaches for the study of brain structure and function have greatly facilitated both clinical and basic science advances. With such progress, however, has also come the necessity to accommodate, share, process and analyze very large amounts of data. Neuroimaging scans acquired using techniques such as magnetic resonance imaging (MRI) and computed tomography (CT) have the advantage of relatively high spatial resolution, though simultaneously the potential disadvantage of requiring large amounts of data storage and of computationally-intensive algorithms for their analysis. Techniques such as functional MRI (fMRI)

© Springer International Publishing Switzerland 2015
N. Ashish and J.-L. Ambite (Eds.): DILS 2015, LNBI 9162, pp. 165–179, 2015.
DOI: 10.1007/978-3-319-21843-4_13

involve the acquisition of four-dimensional (4D) data (3 spatial dimensions and time), leading to even higher demands from the standpoint of data storage and computation. On the other hand, neurophysiological recordings acquired using methods such as electroencephalography (EEG) benefit from high temporal resolution (on the order of milliseconds), though they suffer from relatively poor spatial resolution compared to MRI. Nevertheless, the use of anatomically-informed inverse localization procedures [1] has greatly widened the horizon of applicability for EEG, though at the expense of compounded, multiplicative increases in data storage allocation and computational time requirements. For these reasons, improved approaches to the problems of storage, management, sharing and analysis of combined MRI/CT/EEG recordings are necessary.

The task of multimodal neuroimaging data integration and joint analysis is particularly challenging in studies of traumatic brain injury (TBI), where the structural profile of the brain can change dramatically over the days and even hours following injury. In TBI patients, large alterations in the biochemical, neurophysiologic and metabolic activity of the brain can occur very rapidly and may require immediate clinical intervention and monitoring. For this reason, neuroimaging the TBI brain to inform clinical decision-making can necessitate frequent acquisition of CT and MRI scans to monitor injury evolution and to formulate appropriate treatments. What is more, TBI is a very heterogeneous condition because the spatiotemporal profiles of brain lesions are extremely difficult to quantify without substantial input from neuroimaging technologies.

Electrophysiological recordings via continuous EEG (cEEG) are used routinely in neurointensive care units to identify changes in the baseline electrical activity of the brain as well as neuropathophysiological manifestations such as epileptiform spiking, seizures, and more serious conditions such *status epilepticus* [2]. Other monitoring techniques which are used routinely in neurointensive care units include magnetic resonance spectroscopy (MRS), blood assays, depth electrode recordings, positron emission tomography (PET), etc. The integration, analysis, and interpretation of data being made available from so many sources can pose substantial challenges not only to clinicians but also to biomedical researchers who aim to integrate, analyze and translate basic findings about TBI into information which has broad bedside relevance and applicability.

In this paper, we aim to describe our proposed solutions to the task of integrating structural neuroimaging with neurophysiological recordings to study epileptiform activity prompted by TBI. Based on techniques which we and our collaborators have pioneered for the purpose of TBI-robust segmentation and electrical activity localization, we have developed a set of approaches for the joint analysis of MRI/CT/EEG data acquired from TBI patients. The integration of these methods across modalities can facilitate the study of TBI-related neuropathophysiology by identifying and analyzing the spatiotemporal properties of seizure-related activity and can contribute to the formulation of TBI patient-tailored interventions and treatments.

2   Methodologies

In what follows, a series of integrated techniques for the acquisition, analysis and interpretation of MRI/CT/EEG data acquired from TBI patients are illustrated.

The approaches described below have resulted from over half a decade of collaborative research between the Laboratory of Neuro Imaging (LONI) and Institute for Neuroimaging and Informatics (INI) at the University of Southern California and the Brain Injury Research Center (BIRC) at the University of California, Los Angeles. In addition to detailed descriptions of the analysis steps involved, we outline some of our numerous challenges and potential solutions for the integration of vastly different neuroimaging modalities in the attempt to combine knowledge of brain structure with information provided by neurophysiology techniques.

2.1 Neuroimaging Data Acquisition

Before studies are conducted, each patient or her/his legally-authorized representative provides informed written consent as required by the Declaration of Helsinki, U.S. 45 CFR 46. Neuroimage volume acquisition is conducted with the approval of the local ethics committees at the research institution where data are acquired. Brain imaging data sets are fully anonymized and stored on the LONI Image Data Archive (IDA), and no linked coding or keys to subject identity are maintained.

One important feature of the approach we use for neuroimaging data integration is that it accommodates multimodally-acquired data. This is very helpful in studies of TBI, where more than one MRI acquisition sequences are often required to identify the nature and extent of pathology. In our own studies, MRI volumes are acquired at 3.0 T using a Trio TIM scanner (Siemens Corp., Erlangen, Germany), although various field strengths, voxel sizes and sequence parameters can be used. The acquisition protocol is designed to optimize the amount of information which can be inferred from multimodal MRI, while minimizing the amount of time which the patient must spend in the scanner. The protocol itself consists of magnetization prepared rapid acquisition gradient echo (MP-RAGE) T_1-weighted imaging, fluid attenuated inversion recovery (FLAIR), turbo spin echo (TSE) T_2-weighted imaging, gradient recalled echo (GRE) T_2-weighted imaging and susceptibility-weighted imaging (SWI; see Fig. 1). For T_1-weighted volumes, typical acquisition parameters include a repetition time (TR) of 1900 ms, an echo time (TE) of 3.52 ms, a flip angle (FA) of 9 degrees, an inversion time (TI) of 900 ms, a voxel size of 1 mm^3, a phase field of view (FOV) of 100 %, a matrix size of $256 \times 256 \times 256$ and 100 % sampling. A detailed list of typical parameters for the other sequence types is provided in [2]. For diffusion tensor imaging (DTI), volumes with up to 68 diffusion gradient directions are typically acquired using a 12-channel coil and a sequence with the following parameters: $TR = 9.4$ s, $TE = 88$ ms, flip angle $= 90°$, voxel size $= 2$ mm^3, acquisition matrix $= 128 \times 128 \times 128$. Two non-diffusion weighted volumes are usually acquired for each patient (B_0 values: 0 s/mm^2 and 1,000 s/mm^2). Conventional computed tomography (CT) scans are also obtained. Continuous electroencephalographic (cEEG) measurements are acquired and monitored continuously at the patient's bedside starting immediately after admission to the neurointensive care unit (NICU).

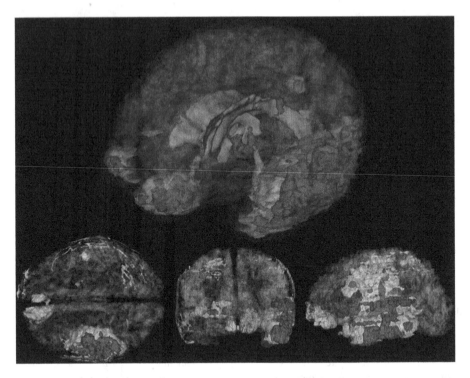

Fig. 1. Visualization of a TBI brain, showing healthy-appearing GM/WM (translucent), the ventricular system (blue), edema (green), and hemorrhage (red) (Color figure onlilne).

2.2 MRI Processing

Prior to any analysis, MRI, CT and DTI volumes are co-registered using a 12-parameter affine registration. Image processing is performed using the LONI Pipeline environment (pipeline.loni.usc.edu), including operations such as bias field correction, skull stripping, and multimodal volume co-registration. Hemorrhagic tissues are segmented from SWI and GRE T_2-weighted volumes, whereas edematous tissues are segmented from TSE T_2-weighted and FLAIR volumes (see Fig. 1). The details of the procedure for pathology identification are detailed elsewhere [4]. FreeSurfer (freesurfer.net) is utilized to segment healthy-appearing white matter (WM), grey matter (GM), and cerebrospinal fluid (CSF) from T_1-weighted volumes, as well as to perform regional parcellation [5, 6]. Briefly, the cortical surface of each patient is reconstructed as a triangular tessellation with an average inter-vertex distance of ~1 mm to produce a high-resolution, smooth representation of the WM/GM interface [7]. At each tessellation vertex, cortical thickness is measured as the distance between the cortical surface and the WM/GM boundary. A total of 74 cortical structures (gyri and sulci) are identified and parceled using a probabilistic atlas [8]. Neuroanatomical labels are assigned to voxels based on probabilistic information estimated from a manually-labeled training set; this method uses the previous probability of a tissue class occurring at a specific atlas location as well as the probability of the local spatial configuration of labels given each tissue class. The technique is comparable in accuracy with manual labeling [9].

TBI-related lesions are segmented from GRE/SWI/FLAIR volumes as outlined elsewhere [10, 11], the scalp is segmented from T_1–weighted MRI, and hard bone is segmented from CT volumes. Eyes, muscle, cartilage, mucus, nerves, teeth, and ventriculostomy shunts are labeled based on T_1/T_2 MRI. 3D models for all tissue type are generated in 3D Slicer (slicer.org), which is also used to generate 3D models and visualizations of TBI-related pathology and of healthy-appearing tissues. Manual correction of segmentation errors is performed by three experienced users with training in neuroanatomy.

2.3 DTI Processing

For DTI, eddy current correction is first applied to each volume, which is subsequently processed using TrackVis (trackvis.org) as well with the Diffusion ToolKit to reconstruct fiber tracts using deterministic tractography. A brain mask is first created using FSL [12] to minimize extra-cerebral noise, and TrackVis is then used to reconstruct and to render fiber tracts, which can subsequently be loaded and viewed in 3D Slicer or using other tractography visualization software. Fiber bundles shorter than 1.5 cm are discarded. Fiber tracts which do not intersect pathology-affected regions can be discarded. To reconstruct tracts of specific interest, seed regions can placed in particular locations (such as the brain stem and the internal capsule in the case of the corticospinal tract, CST), and the WM tracts intersecting these regions can then be isolated (Fig. 2).

2.4 Longitudinal Structural Analysis

Importantly, longitudinal studies can be accommodated in our approach. For example, in a typical study, scanning sessions are held both several days (acute baseline) as well as 6 months (chronic follow-up) after TBI, and the same MRI scanner and acquisition parameters are used in both cases. Lesion volumes are measured in cubic centimeters based on pathology models created in 3D Slicer or ITKSnap (itksnap.org). The percentages of longitudinal volumetric changes in pathology as well as in healthy-appearing WM and GM are calculated as $(v_{i+1} - v_i)/v_i$, where v_i and v_{i+1} are the volumes of the respective structures at times i and $i + 1$, respectively (Fig. 4).

Several ways to analyze longitudinal changes in WM connections are available in our environment. To quantify the manner and extent to which fibers are affected by pathology, the sum over the lengths of fibers intersecting pathology-affected regions can be divided by the sum of the lengths of fibers in the whole brain, thereby yielding the percentage of WM connections in the brain which intersect the primary injury. This is useful because it provides useful information on how broadly DAI may have affected each patient. Alternatively, changes in connectivity strength between different regions can be investigated to determine how severely the wiring of the brain has been affected by TBI. Finally, changes in the ratio of T1 to T2-weighted image intensities can provide a surrogate measure of axonal demyelination [13], which allows us to study long-term effects of brain injuries (Fig. 3).

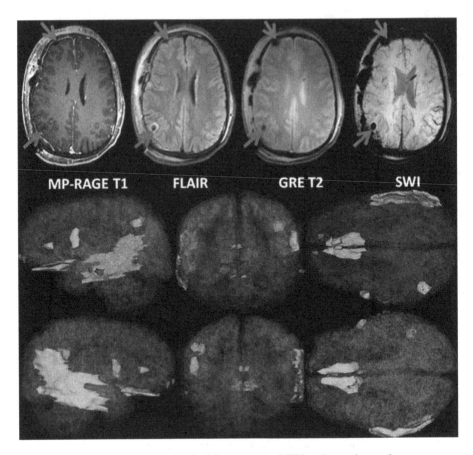

Fig. 2. (A) Sample MRI slices acquired from a typical TBI patient using various sequences. Arrows indicate the locations of primary injuries. (B) Translucent models of the WM and GM (as reconstructed based on the segmentation) with edema (cyan) and hemorrhage (red) shown using opaque 3D models. Note the fronto-temporal spatial distribution of the injuries, typical in TBI (Color figure onlilne).

2.5 EEG Forward Modeling

Integrating structural MRI, CT and DTI data with neurophysiological recordings poses daunting complexities in the context of TBI research. Nevertheless, the advantages of such an integration are manifold because it can allow the high spatial resolution of MRI/ DTI to be combined with the high temporal resolution of EEG and, thereby, to take advantage of all techniques simultaneously (Fig. 5).

The primary sources of EEG potentials are typically currents within the apical dendrites of cortical pyramidal cells [14]; for this reason, EEG generators are assumed to be dipolar currents whose orientations are perpendicular to the cortical surface [15]. In the first step of EEG modeling, finite element method (FEM) models are created by discretizing the head volume of each subject into linear hexahedral isoparametric elements using information provided by the MRI-derived segmentation. A grid-based

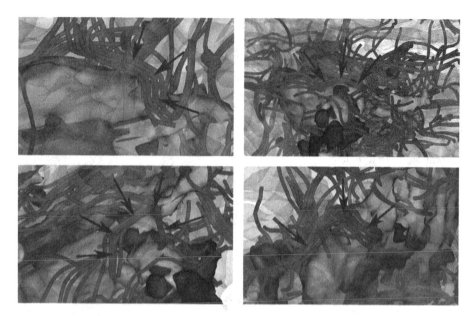

Fig. 3. Detailed views of WM tract deformation (red arrows) due to primary TBI (edema: cyan; hemorrhage: red). Because of the mechanical forces exerted by injuries, WM fibers are subjected to stretching and shearing which lead to diffuse axonal injury (DAI) (Color figure onlilne).

mesh with a mean edge length of ~2 mm, with ~450,000 linear elements and ~400,000 nodes is then generated. After co-registration of the head and sensor locations, the presence of scalp electrodes arranged in the standard 10–10 montage is taken into account and as many as 25 tissue types with distinct conductivity values σ are included.

A TBI-tailored version of the METUFEM software package [16, 17] is used to compute the forward matrix $\mathbf{A}$ of dimensions $m \times n$, where m and n are the number of sensors and sources, respectively. In each volume element within the head, the electric potential Φ is computed using linear interpolation functions [16]. For a given sensor i and cortical source j, the matrix element a_{ij} of $\mathbf{A}$ specifies Φ as recorded by sensor i due to a dipolar source of unit strength which is active at the location of source j. Row $\mathbf{a}_i$ of $\mathbf{A}$ is the so-called 'lead field' (LF) of sensor i, which indicates how each current dipole contributes to the signal recorded by sensor i. Leting J_p denote the primary electric current density of sources in the brain, the solution to the forward problem of electrical source imaging is provided by solving for Φ subject to the boundary conditions

$$\nabla \cdot (\sigma \nabla \Phi) = \nabla \cdot J_p \text{ in } V \tag{1}$$

$$\sigma \partial_n \Phi = 0 \text{ on } S \tag{2}$$

where V and S are the head volume and surface, respectively, $\mathbf{n}$ is the unit normal vector on the surface S, and σ denotes the local tissue conductivity. A point source model [18] is used to assign the desired locations of dipoles within the head. An equivalent discretized model is then constructed for each finite element using Galerkin's weighted

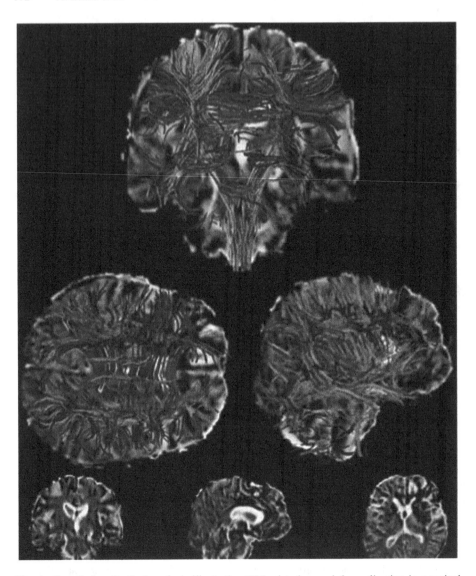

Fig. 4. Sample longitudinal analysis illustrating TBI-related axonal demyelination in a typical patient. Shown are demyelination maps with important WM tracts superimposed. The maps themselves are shown in the bottom row, illustrating substantial demyelination (brighter areas) throughout the brain, especially in peri-ventricular and fronto-temporal areas (Color figure onlilne).

residuals method, and each element contribution is assembled to construct a system of equations whose numerical solution yields the values of Φ [16].

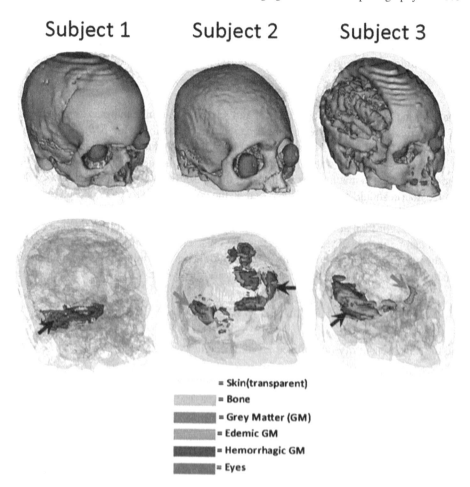

Fig. 5. 3D models of the head for a sample TBI patient. In addition to the full model which includes all tissue types (first row), lesions are shown as well (second row). Hemorrhagic lesions are indicated by blue arrows, while edematous regions are indicated by green arrows. Note the large craniotomy over the right hemisphere of Subject 3, which can be more easily modelled within the FEM formalism as opposed to the boundary element method (BEM) formalism, which requires closed surfaces when approximating the shape of the head (Color figure onlilne).

2.6   EEG Inverse Modeling

The framework for source localization employed here involves a minimum-norm inverse linear operator previously described and widely used [19]. Briefly, one can start from the matrix linear equation

$$\mathbf{x} = \mathbf{As} + \mathbf{n}, \tag{3}$$

where $\mathbf{x}$ is the EEG measurements vector, $\mathbf{A}$ is the EEG forward matrix, $\mathbf{s}$ is a vector containing the direction and orientation of each source, and $\mathbf{n}$ specifies the sensor noise.

To identify **s** from **x** using a linear approach, an inverse operator **W** can be calculated such that the mean difference $\langle ||\mathbf{Wx} - \mathbf{s}||^2 \rangle$ between the estimated and true inverse solutions is minimal. If **n** and **s** are normally distributed with zero mean, **W** is of the form

$$\mathbf{W} = \mathbf{RA}^T \left(\mathbf{ARA}^T + \mathbf{C}\right)^{-1} \tag{4}$$

where **C** and **R** denote the sensor noise and source covariance matrices, respectively [19]. Normally-distributed white noise can often be assumed for both sources and sensors, such that **R** and **C** are within a constant multiplying factor of the identity matrix.

In EEG inverse localization, the primary interest is in identifying cortical activity whose magnitude is much larger than that of the noise. Because of this, each row of the inverse matrix should be normalized based on the noise sensitivity of **W** at each location [19]. This allows activity at locations with relatively low noise sensitivity to be assigned a greater weight than at locations with higher noise sensitivity. Noise sensitivity estimation can be implemented by projecting the noise covariance estimate onto **W**, such that the noise sensitivity-adjusted inverse operator is pre-multiplied by a diagonal noise sensitivity matrix **T** whose matrix elements t_{ii} are specified by

$$t_{ii} = \left[\mathrm{diag}\left(\sqrt{\mathbf{WCW}^T}\right)\right]^{-1} \tag{5}$$

and the noise sensitivity-normalized inverse becomes

$$\tilde{\mathbf{W}} = \mathbf{TW}. \tag{6}$$

Applying the noise-normalized inverse operator to the acquired EEG signals produces a matrix of inversely-localized signals whose rows correspond to cortical locations, whose columns correspond to time points in the EEG recording, and whose units are nAm (electric current dipole strengths). Upon noise normalization, the values of the signals localized on the cortex follow a T distribution with a very large number of degrees of freedom (d. f.) which approaches a normal distribution in the limit d. f. → ∞. For any given cortical location, the value of the t statistic associated with that location indicates the likelihood that the neuronal source positioned there is electrically active. Cortical maps of t statistics are generated using purpose-built software in order to visualize and identify the cortical areas whose activation is most likely to have produced the EEG signals recorded during each epileptiform discharge.

2.7   Epileptiform Signal Analysis

Epileptic seizures are detected by an NICU nurse or by a neurointensivist within the first week post-injury either online, during EEG screening, or via the total power trend seizure detection approach [3]. To identify interictal epileptiform events, cEEG recordings are examined by a neurophysiologist using custom software. For the purpose of most studies, epileptiform discharges are defined as high-frequency (>80 Hz), high-amplitude (>100 mV) bursts or runs of interictal activity which are not consistent with EEG artifacts due to the following causes: (1) electromyographic activity (20–80 Hz), (2) glossokynetic movement, (3) ocular movement, (4) electrocardiographic activity,

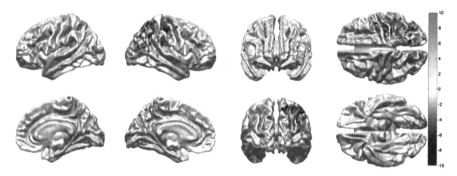

Fig. 6. Example of inversely-localized epileptiform activity in a sample TBI patient. Shown are values of the *t* statistic, as overlayed on the cortical surface. Each *t* statistic indicates the likelihood that the cortex is electrically active at that location. A negative value indicates that the electric current is oriented into the cortex, while a positive value indicates the converse. In this particular case, the presence of a cortical locus of epileptiform electrical activity is found over right parietal cortex.

(5) blood vessel pulsation, (6) respiration, (7) scalp-localized perspiration, (8) electrode disconnection, (9) alternating currents (ACs), and (10) environment-related movement.

Upon identification, all EEG recording segments related to interictal epileptiform events are isolated for subsequent analysis and detrended. Short (~3 s) portions of EEG recordings which either precede or follow each interictal epileptiform event are also saved separately and treated as baseline activity which is used to compute the noise covariance matrix for inverse localization, as described in previous sections. Following the calculation of the noise-normalized inverse operator $\hat{W}$, all EEG-recorded neural activity is localized and the cortical location(s) which are most likely to have generated each epileptiform discharge (i.e. their foci) is/are identified by thresholding the cortical map of *t* statistics which had been generated as previously described.

After identifying epileptiform focus locations, the distance(s) between each of these and the location(s) of primary TBI is/are computed. In the first step, a 3D model of each hemorrhagic or edematous lesion is generated based on the MRI-derived segmentation. In the second step, the shortest Euclidian distance D between each focus and the 3D boundary of each lesion is calculated. In the third step, the location of each epileptiform activity focus is labeled as either intra-, peri- or non-lesional based on the distance between it and the lesion(s) (Fig. 6).

2.8   Accommodation of Semantic Conflicts

Implementation of this project has required substantial accommodation of semantic conflicts between data types to support the process of dynamic reconciliation. To provide interoperability between MRI, CT, DTI and EEG data organization systems, semantic reconciliation was provided by integrating data specifications related to the spatial dimension of the structural data (MRI, CT, DTI) with the temporal dimension provided by the neurophysiological data (EEG). Structural and representational differences were found to occur particularly at the interface between approaches to information organization and mismatched domains. The process of data integration has involved both static schema integration (mapping heterogeneous schemas to a global representation, accounting for context dependencies as precedence relationships during the reconciliation process), as well as dynamic integration (dynamically building appropriate precedence relationships based on already-acquired semantic knowledge).

3   Discussion

From the standpoint of structural neuroimaging data integration, using multimodal data sets which were acquired using different sequences can pose difficulties in several ways. Firstly, due to logistic or technical considerations, imaging volumes cannot always be acquired at the same resolution (i.e. voxel size), which implies that voxel-based multi-modal analysis may require 3D interpolation. Secondly, volumes acquired using different modalities may occasionally cover different—though mostly overlapping—FOVs within the brain. From the standpoint of 3D co-registration, this can pose a challenge because the spatial domains containing data to be registered do not feature an identical extent of head coverage. This problem is often compounded when longitudinal scans of the same patient are acquired, typically because the position of the patient's head within the MRI scanner differs across data acquisition sessions. Thirdly, because the problem of patient motion in the scanner is greater for TBI patients than in most other patient populations, motion-related artifacts can be more difficult to correct and thus highly-robust motion correction algorithms and/or scanning sequences are very useful in TBI neuroimaging. Fourthly, because distinct sequences can feature widely different voxel intensity profiles (e.g. in FLAIR vs. SWI), intensity normalization both across modalities and across time points must be implemented with greater care than in other studies. For example, the presence of lesions can be associated with regions of substantial hyper- or hypo-intensities across imaging modalities, which makes the use of histogram-matching algorithms problematic. In our studies, the challenges described above are typically addressed using sophisticated, TBI-tailored interpolation algorithms available within the LONI Pipeline environment which are described in detail elsewhere [20–22].

Integration of structural MRI data with DTI to study TBI in a longitudinal context is challenging because, in addition to substantial changes in overall shape, the TBI brain can also undergo appreciable deformations throughout the WM. Teasing out such deformations from WM losses can be very difficult because the deformation field which indicates how each point in the brain changes its location cannot always be determined with precision. Ideally, a spatially-resolved deformation field which specifies how each point in the brain has moved from one time point to the next should be available. Nevertheless, because some brain changes are diffeomorphic whereas others are not, the deformation field cannot always be determined with accuracy. Additionally, pathology may appear or disappear between time points, which complicates the task even further. As a result, substantial future efforts are required to formulate TBI-robust registration and segmentation methods.

Though there are numerous advantages to the integration of structural (MRI, CT, DTI) neuroimaging with neurophysiological techniques (EEG in the present case), there are substantial difficulties associated with the fusion of such characteristically different types of data. As in our case, overcoming these barriers can involve the use of sophisticated, anatomically-informed methods for inverse localization of electric potentials. Such methods have been in common use by scientists who investigate the healthy brain, though not as common for the study of acute diseases of the brain, and virtually unheard of—until recently—for the study of TBI. Of crucial importance for the successful integration of EEG with structural neuroimaging is the accuracy of the forward models which are used to calculate the inverse localization operator, primarily because the propagation of electric currents which generate the scalp EEG is highly sensitive upon the electric conductivity profile of the head. Thus, it is important to create realistic geometric models of both healthy-appearing and TBI-affected tissues in order to localize epileptiform activity with spatial accuracy. Currently, no automatic algorithms exist for the segmentation of certain tissue types such as fat, muscle, cartilage, connective tissue, or hard/soft bone, which can make the task of creating accurate EEG forward models both difficult and time-consuming. For this reason, renewed efforts by computer scientists and bioengineers are needed in order to develop new or improved methods for the segmentation of various anatomic structures in addition to those located inside the brain.

4   Conclusion

Although potentially difficult, the integration of structural neuroimaging data with neurophysiologic recordings is very useful for studying a variety of disorders and pathologies, including TBI. The use of multimodal neuroimaging of brain injury is very useful—and indeed, essential—to identify, classify and quantify injury types and to generate realistic models of the TBI head which can be used for EEG modeling and inverse localization. Though epileptiform electrical activity is common in the acute stage of TBI, little research has been devoted to understanding the underlying mechanisms of interictal discharges, which may have an important role in the development of post-traumatic epilepsy. The reason for this lack of information is partly due to the difficulty of integrating EEG recordings with other types of neuroimaging which have comparatively higher spatial resolution, such as MRI, CT, DTI and PET. The techniques we have outlined for such integration have provided the ability to obtain useful insights into TBI-related neuropathophysiology, although substantial additional research is needed to develop automatic methods for TBI segmentation as well as for the automatic classification of tissues which play important roles in the accurate inverse localization of electric potentials.

Acknowledgments.   This work was supported by the National Institutes of Health, grants 2U54EB005149-06 "National Alliance for Medical Image Computing: Traumatic Brain Injury – Driving Biological Project" to J. D. V. H., and R41NS081792-01 "Multimodality Image Based Assessment System for Traumatic Brain Injury", sub-award to J. D. V. H, and by the National Institute of Neurological Disorders and Stroke, grant P01NS058489 to P.M.V. We wish to thank the dedicated staff of the Institute for Neuroimaging and Informatics at the University of Southern California. The authors declare no actual or perceived competing conflict of interest.

References

1. Dale, A.M., Sereno, M.I.: Improved localizadon of cortical activity by combining EEG and MEG with MRI cortical surface reconstruction: a linear approach. J. Cogn. Neurosci. **5**, 162–176 (1993)
2. Brophy, G.M., Bell, R., Claassen, J., Alldredge, B., Bleck, T.P., Glauser, T., Laroche, S.M., Riviello Jr., J.J., Shutter, L., Sperling, M.R., Treiman, D.M., Vespa, P.M.: Neurocritical care society status epilepticus guideline writing, C.: guidelines for the evaluation and management of status epilepticus. Neurocrit. Care **17**, 3–23 (2012)
3. Vespa, P.M., Nuwer, M.R., Nenov, V., Ronne-Engstrom, E., Hovda, D.A., Bergsneider, M., Kelly, D.F., Martin, N.A., Becker, D.P.: Increased incidence and impact of nonconvulsive and convulsive seizures after traumatic brain injury as detected by continuous electroencephalographic monitoring. J. Neurosurg. **91**, 750–760 (1999)
4. Irimia, A., Chambers, M.C., Alger, J.R., Filippou, M., Prastawa, M.W., Wang, B., Hovda, D.A., Gerig, G., Toga, A.W., Kikinis, R., Vespa, P.M., Van Horn, J.D.: Comparison of acute and chronic traumatic brain injury using semi-automatic multimodal segmentation of MR volumes. J. Neurotrauma **28**, 2287–2306 (2011)
5. Dale, A.M., Fischl, B., Sereno, M.I.: Cortical surface-based analysis – I. segmentation and surface reconstruction. NeuroImage **9**, 179–194 (1999)
6. Fischl, B., Sereno, M.I., Dale, A.M.: Cortical surface-based analysis - II: inflation, flattening, and a surface-based coordinate system. Neuroimage **9**, 195–207 (1999)
7. Fischl, B., Salat, D.H., Busa, E., Albert, M., Dieterich, M., Haselgrove, C., van der Kouwe, A., Killiany, R., Kennedy, D., Klaveness, S., Montillo, A., Makris, N., Rosen, B., Dale, A.M.: Whole brain segmentation: automated labeling of neuroanatomical structures in the human brain. Neuron **33**, 341–355 (2002)
8. Destrieux, C., Fischl, B., Dale, A., Halgren, E.: Automatic parcellation of human cortical gyri and sulci using standard anatomical nomenclature. Neuroimage **53**, 1–15 (2010)
9. Fischl, B., Salat, D.H., van der Kouwe, A.J., Makris, N., Segonne, F., Quinn, B.T., Dale, A.M.: Sequence-independent segmentation of magnetic resonance images. NeuroImage **23**(Suppl 1), S69–S84 (2004)
10. Irimia, A., Chambers, M.C., Alger, J.R., Filippou, M., Prastawa, M.W., Wang, B., Hovda, D.A., Gerig, G., Toga, A.W., Kikinis, R., Vespa, P.M., Van Horn, J.D.: Comparison of acute and chronic traumatic brain injury using semi-automatic multimodal segmentation of MR volumes. J. Neurotrauma **28**, 2287–2306 (2011)
11. Irimia, A., Chambers, M.C., Torgerson, C.M., Filippou, M., Hovda, D.A., Alger, J.R., Gerig, G., Toga, A.W., Vespa, P.M., Kikinis, R., Van Horn, J.D.: Patient-tailored connectomics visualization for the assessment of white matter atrophy in traumatic brain injury. Front. Neurol. **3**, 10 (2012)
12. Jenkinson, M., Beckmann, C.F., Behrens, T.E., Woolrich, M.W., Smith, S.M.: Fsl. Neuroimage **62**, 782–790 (2012)
13. Glasser, M.F., Van Essen, D.C.: Mapping human cortical areas in vivo based on myelin content as revealed by T1- and T2-weighted MRI. J. Neurosci. **31**, 11597–11616 (2011)
14. Dale, A., Sereno, M.: Improved localization of cortical activity by combining EEG and MEG with MRI cortical surface reconstruction: a linear approach. J. Cogn. Neurosci. **5**, 162–176 (1993)

15. Irimia, A., Van Horn, J.D., Halgren, E.: Source cancellation profiles of electro encephalography and magnetoencephalography. Neuroimage **59**, 2464–2474 (2012)
16. Acar, Z., Gencer, N.: An advanced BEM implementation for the forward problem of electro-magnetic source Imaging. Phys. Med. Biol. **49**, 5011–5028 (2004)
17. Acar, Z., Makeig, S.: Neuroelectromagnetic forward head modeling toolbox. J. Neurosci. Methods **190**, 258–270 (2010)
18. Yan, Y., Nunez, P.L., Hart, R.T.: Finite-element model of the human head: scalp potentials due to dipole sources. Med. Biol. Eng. Comput. **29**, 475–481 (1991)
19. Liu, A.K., Dale, A.M., Belliveau, J.W.: Monte Carlo simulation studies of EEG and MEG localization accuracy. Hum. Brain Mapp. **16**, 47–62 (2002)
20. Wang, B., Prastawa, M., Irimia, A., Chambers, M.C., Vespa, P.M., Van Horn, J.D., Gerig, G.: A patient-specific segmentation framework for longitudinal MR images of traumatic brain injury. In: Proceedings of Spie 8314 (2012)
21. Wang, B., Prastawa, M., Irimia, A., Chambers, M.C., Sadeghi, N., Vespa, P.M., van Horn, J.D., Gerig, G.: Analyzing imaging biomarkers for traumatic brain injury using 4d modeling of longitudinal MRI. In: I S Biomed Imaging, pp. 1392–1395 (2013)
22. Wang, B., Prastawa, M., Awate, S.P., Irimia, A., Chambers, M.C., Vespa, P.M., van Horn, J.D., Gerig, G.: Segmentation of serial MRI of TBI patients using personalized atlas construction and topological change estimation. In: 2012 9th IEEE International Symposium on Biomedical Imaging (Isbi), pp. 1152–1155 (2012)

SVI: A Simple Single-Nucleotide Human Variant Interpretation Tool for Clinical Use

Paolo Missier[1]([envelope]), Eldarina Wijaya[1], Ryan Kirby[1], and Michael Keogh[2]

[1] School of Computing Science, Newcastle University, Newcastle upon Tyne, UK
{paolo.missier,eldarina.wijaya,ryan.kirby}@ncl.ac.uk
[2] Institute of Genetic Medicine, Newcastle University, Newcastle upon Tyne, UK
michael.keogh@newcastle.ac.uk

Abstract. The rapid evolution of Next Generation Sequencing technology will soon make it possible to test patients for genetic disorders at population scale. However, clinical interpretation of human variants extracted from raw NGS data in the clinical setting is likely to become a bottleneck, as long as it requires expert human judgement. While several attempts are under way to try and automate the diagnostic process, most still assume a specialist's understanding of the variants' significance. In this paper we present our early experiments with a simple process and prototype clinical tool for single-nucleotide variant filtering, called SVI, which automates much of the interpretation process by integrating disease-gene and disease-variant mapping resources. As the content and quality of these resources improve over time, it is important to identify past patients' cases which may benefit from re-analysis. By persistently recording the entire diagnostic process, SVI can selectively trigger case re-analysis on the basis of updates in the external knowledge sources.

1 Introduction

1.1 Background and Motivation

Whole-exome and whole-genome sequencing (WES, WGS) are increasingly utilised in clinical diagnostics. As the cost of sequencing a human genome continues to decrease [1], and with the number of DNA base pairs sequenced per $ unit reportedly doubling every five months [2], WGS-based genetic testing is poised to become a routine diagnostic technique that can be deployed on a large scale [3]. At the same time, allocating the computation resources needed to process the data is also becoming increasingly affordable. Large initiatives like the 100,000 Genome Project in the UK[1], with specific focus on cancer and rare diseases, promise to deliver genetic testing at population scale within the next few years. As genetic diseases affect about 8 % of the UK population (5 million people), the potential societal benefits in this country alone are substantial.

---

[1] http://www.genomicsengland.co.uk/.

© Springer International Publishing Switzerland 2015
N. Ashish and J.-L. Ambite (Eds.): DILS 2015, LNBI 9162, pp. 180–194, 2015.
DOI: 10.1007/978-3-319-21843-4_14

The diagnosis of genetic disorders based on WGS data consists of two main stages: variant calling and variant interpretation. Variant calling includes processing the patients genome, or the exome [4,5], using a well-established sequence of computational steps, arranged into a pipeline. This results in a large set of variants, or single-nucleotide mutations and indels. The pipeline incorporates bioinformatics tools chosen from a growing pool of publicly available distributions [6]. The second stage involves analysing the variants based on a clinical hypothesis established from the patients phenotype, with the goal to identify variants that support the hypothesis.

The increasing volume of genomes to be processed, along with the widespread adoption of genetic testing in the clinic, call for scalable solutions for both phases. The *Cloud-e-Genome* project, a collaboration between the Institute of Genetic Medicine and the School of Computing Science at Newcastle University, was funded in 2013[2] to investigate such solutions.

In this paper we focus specifically on the variant interpretation phase, while a separate strand of work is concerned with the exploitation of cloud infrastructure to address scalability of the NGS data processing pipeline [7]. A first scalability issue concerning interpretation is that, although the gap between research and clinical exploitation of genetic diagnostic tools is narrowing, variant interpretation remains a knowledge-intensive decision process, especially for the diagnosis of rare disorders [8]. Diagnosis often requires the expertise of a geneticist, a scarce and expensive resource, for all but the most common cases. This makes the process difficult to scale, as larger number of patients are enrolled for testing.

A second scalability issue is more subtle. Diagnosis relies upon a combination of knowledge, i.e. variant-disease associations, and bioinformatics tools, which compose the exome/genome processing pipeline. Incomplete knowledge and limitations in the tools still result in both false positives and false negatives, or in inconclusive diagnosis, with success rate reported as low as 25 % [9]. As both these elements evolve over time, however, there is an expectation that accuracy will improve, suggesting that it may beneficial to periodically revisit certain old cases that may have not been fully solved at the time they were first addressed. The choice of which cases to revisit depends on the combination of knowledge sources and tool selection used to process the original data, and the type of updates that become available, i.e., either in a variant database or in the pipeline. As these cases add to the volume, it is important to ensure that they are chosen accurately.

1.2   Goals

With these premises, in this project we explore two hypotheses. Firstly, that it is possible to automate much of the diagnostic process, by capturing its most common elements into a simple-to-use tool which integrates with a number of external knowledge sources. And secondly, that by recording all details of each

---

[2] Funding for Cloud-e-Genome comes from the NIHR (National Institute for Health and Research) and Biomedical Research Centre in the UK.

patient investigation, from variants to diagnosis, it becomes possible to selectively identify old cases that might benefit from re-analysis, in light of knowledge and/or technology advances.

1.3 Contributions

As our first contribution we have studied a cohort of five patients, seen by the Institute of Genetic Medicine (IGM) in Newcastle since 2012, to determine how the temporal evolution of variant-disease associations in the ClinVar[3] variation database affected the ability to diagnose their phenotypes (Sect. 2). This small study supports our hypothesis that complete traceability and reproducibility of the diagnostics process is an important requirement, as it enables past patient cases to be selectively revisited based on their original outcome and following updates in the knowledge base.

Our second contribution is the design of a process for single-nucleotide variant interpretation, which reflects emerging practice in the research lab while aiming to bridge the knowledge gap between genetic research and clinical diagnosis. The process is described in Sect. 3.

Thirdly, based on such process we have been implementing a variant interpretation user tool that simplifies the decision process by integrating multiple external knowledge sources to assist in the diagnosis. The tool, code-named SVI and still currently under development, is described in Sect. 4. SVI currently integrates OMIM[4] and ClinVar as its main external knowledge sources. However, the architecture is designed to accept additional sources of disease-variant associations as those may become available.

The SVI tool is still under active development, in collaboration with researchers at the IGM.

1.4 Related Work

To the best our knowledge, most of the tools available for variant interpretation cater more to geneticist researchers than to clinicians. One example is the Exomiser [10,11], which computes variant prioritisation according to a number of user-defined criteria, which partially overlap with those used in SVI. Pathogenicity prediction comes from the dbNSFP database [12]. Although the online tool offers a simple input interface, its output would be difficult for non-specialist clinicians to interpret.

Qiagen's Ingeniuty Variant Analysis is a mature tool that benefits from the HGMD variant-disease association knowledge base[5]. While it purportedly does target variant interpretation in the clinic, it is a commercial product that plays a role in the genetic diagnostics market.

---

[3] http://www.ncbi.nlm.nih.gov/clinvar/.

[4] http://www.ncbi.nlm.nih.gov/omim.

[5] http://www.hgmd.cf.ac.uk/.

In contrast, Extasy [13] is a research product, derived from the Annotate-it tool [14], which relies on a combination of multiple predictions from different sources. We see this tool as a possible additional source of predictive knowledge of pathogenicity, which we may try to integrate into SVI in the future. Once again, however, its output is designed to be consumed by specialists.

1.5   Recording the Diagnostic Process

One novel feature of SVI is the tracking of the entire diagnostic process, for each patient case, including human decisions as well as the dependencies amongst the data consumed and produced at each step, from user input to diagnosis (which may be inconclusive). This form of systematic provenance tracking aims to bring a number of additional benefits to users. Firstly, provenance tracking provides a way to fulfill one of our main goals, namely to determine which past cases should be revisited, in view of updates to any of the knowledge bases involved in the process (or when a new one is added).

Secondly, it provides both accountability and the ability to explain the decision process in detail. This is important not only because of the sensitivity of the process domain (clinical diagnostics), but also because of the sensitivity of the process itself. These include, amongst others, the version of external data sources, as well as the parameters used for variant filtering, as briefly described in Sect. 4.

Finally, as the collection of provenance traces grows and it is stored persistently, SVI provides support for a variety of analytical functions that cut across patient cases, different clinicians, and also range over time. For example, one common use case for this capability is to establish associations amongst independent cases, based on commonalities amongst the data involved in each of their processes. In turn, this has the potential to make investigators more efficient by allowing them to selectively share their cases with other group members.

1.6   Choosing a Primary Variant Database

It is broadly accepted within the genetic research community that no single variant database is sufficient to cover a broad range of pathologies. We have chosen to use ClinVar, NCBI's human genomic variations database, as our primary source for integration into SVI, on account of its fast growth and good overall coverage, as well as based on availability considerations. While several other variant repositories are available, not all of them are freely accessible (e.g. HGMD, mentioned earlier, which requires a license), and those that are tend to focus on specific phenotypes, or sub-specialties of clinical practice, or are exposed to false negatives due to incompleteness. Two prominent examples are the family of Locus Specific Mutation Databases (LSDB)[6], hosted on the LOVD (Leiden Open Variation Database) platform[7], and the Decipher project [15].

---

[6] http://grenada.lumc.nl/LSDB_list/lsdbs.
[7] http://www.lovd.nl/.

LSDB. As each LSDB is locus-specific, investigations that focus on specific phenotypes require that the appropriate databases be selected within the family. Although their common LOVD interface facilitates integration through programmatic access, their coverage is unpredictable and on a number of cases they have proven unreliably incomplete for the purpose of clinical diagnosis. Consider for instance the NM_020745.3 single nucleotide variant on Gene AARS2 (c.1774C>T). This variant has been described as being highly likely to be pathogenic, as described in the next section. ClinVar records the variant as *Likely Pathogenic* with a known associated condition, which was last evaluated in Aug. 2014, and cites the relevant support literature [16]. Searching for AARS2 variants across the LOVD network returns hits in three additional databases: the LOVD shared installation (LUMC - NL), LOVD at University of Melbourne, and the Mitochondrial Disease MSeqDR-LSDB (Massachusetts). However, of these only MSeqDR-LSDB reports the variant, and it actually cites ClinVar as the source. Other pathogenic variants on AARS2, listed on ClinVar, are missing from the entire network at the time of writing.

Decipher is a recent project aimed at sharing knowledge of genotype-phenotype associations, following the rationale that "accurate diagnosis of human genetic disorders in a clinical setting requires the identification of other patients that share the same/similar genomic variants and comparison of their phenotypes" [15]. The are two main reasons why Decipher is not a suitable choice for our investigations. Firstly, it is once again focused on specific phenotypes, namely developmental delay disorders in children. Such phenotypes are not common in the clinical setting from which our test cases were obtained, which specialises on rare mitochondrial diseases and degenerative disorders. Secondly, it relies on submission of anonymised patient data. In contrast, privacy and patient consent must be considered before uploading large scale individual genetic data in the clinical or research setting. Decipher remains, however, one of the best examples of international collaborative phenotype-genotype consortia. In the future we may be able to engage with similar initiatives in the area of adult rare disease, such as GEM.app[8].

2   A Small-Scale Time-Travel Experiment

We now present a study on 5 WES patient cases, all of them with the same phenotype (*multiple mitochondrial respiratory complex deficiency*), which were solved by our geneticist researchers in October 2012. The aim of this study is manifold. We want to determine whether or not a diagnosis can be reached using a limited number of external knowledge sources, such as OMIM and Clinvar. We are also interested in tracking, albeit at an anedoctal level, how the diagnostic power of those sources changes over time, and how it compares with a diagnostic process based solely on published literature research. Finally, we have used the study experience to help design the process that forms the basis for our tool.

---

[8] https://genomics.med.miami.edu/.

Table 1. Variants identified in Clinvar based on records in November 2014.

Patient	Gene name	Variant	Clinvar 2014	Date submitted
1	C12orf65	Hom c.210delA:p.P70fs	Pathogenic	22-Nov-13
2	RMND1	Hom. c.1349G>C:p.*450Serext*32	Pathogenic	04-Aug-14
3	AARS2	Het c.1774C>T:p.Arg592Trp	Pathogenic	04-Aug-14
4	MTO1	Hom. c.1232C>T:p.Thr411Ile	Not found	
5	VARS2	Het c.1045G>A:p.Ala349Thr	Not found	

The study involved "going back in time", in this case to 2012, to see whether the knowledge that was available then was sufficient to produce a diagnosis, either by an expert, who would be using direct research from phenotypic or investigational search terms relevant for each case within literature search databases such as PubMed, or by an automated process using ClinVar. Our findings are summarised in Table 1, while the charts in Fig. 1 give a sense of progress in ClinVar content over time, by reporting on the number of variants of interest available in 2012 and in 2014.

As the cases were indeed solved with a positive diagnosis, we benefit from the ground truth consisting of the actual variants found by the researchers. Our first finding is that none of these variants were recorded in the 2012 version of ClinVar, while only three out of five appear in the 2014 version. When they do appear, their clinical significance is reported as Pathogenic/Likely pathogenic, confirming the early researchers' diagnosis. This seems to support, at least anecdotally, the hypothesis that the relevance of a variant databases like ClinVar does increase over time, complementing and possibly eventually replacing experts' knowledge.

Next, we focused on articles that could have been used at different points in time as reference to solve the cases. We recorded the number of papers available at the time of diagnosis, which are related to the patient phenotype, as well as the number papers published before the date of diagnosis. Our findings, reported in Table 2, indicate that of the five cases, only two could have been solved using literature support. One additional case (patient 5) was solved using direct researchers' knowledge of association between the VARS2 gene and the multiple mitochondrial complex deficiency phenotype.

Despite these successes, it is often the case that genetic diagnosis cannot be reached. To illustrate, we have analysed a further patient, which to date is still an unsolved case. Researchers manually identified eight candidate variants for this patient in 2012, however none of those appeared in ClinVar at the time, or could otherwise be confirmed as pathogenic. Using the 2014 version of ClinVar, only one of the variants (c.242G>A:p.Arg81Gln on gene TYMP) was found to be benign, while the others remain unknown. No additional literature has so far emerged (to the best of our knowledge) to support the diagnosis.

3   Variant Interpretation for Genetic Diagnosis

We now describe the process of single-nucleotide variant interpretation that underpins our clinical tool, SVI. In a clinical setting, the interpretation process

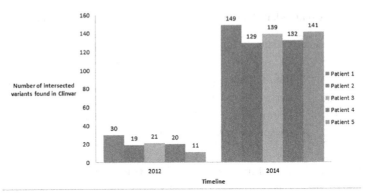

(a) Variants on patients' genes filtered for their relevant phenotype

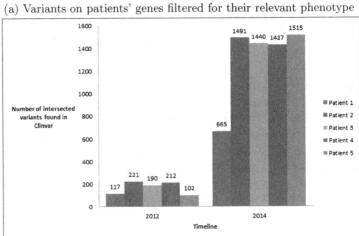

(b) Variants on patients' genes, no phenotype filtering

Fig. 1. ClinVar evolution relative to the variants of interest for sample patients

Table 2. Number of publications in Pubmed concerning the gene of interest for a specific variant, prior to date of diagnosis in 2012 and in 2014.

Patient	Gene name	Variant	Pubmed publications (2014)	Year reference paper published	Pubmed publications (before 2012)	Solvable before 2012?
1	C12orf65	Hom c.210delA:p.P70fs	9	2010	2	Yes
2	RMND1	Hom. c.1349G>C:p.*450Serext*32	6	2012	3	No
3	AARS2	Het c.1774C>T:p.Arg592Trp	4	2011	1	Yes
4	MTO1	Hom. c.1232C>T:p.Thr411Ile	48	2012	29	No
5	VARS2	Het c.1045G>A:p.Ala349Thr	14	NA	11	No

is normally driven by a *disease hypothesis*, specified by the clinician on the basis of factual observations. The goal of the process is to find variants in the patient's exome, amongst those called by the upstream pipeline, which have either previously been reported to be associated conclusively with similar phenotypes, or conform to the appropriate inheritance pattern, and disease population frequency and occur in genes either known to cause a similar phenotype, or affect similar biological functions. In addition, in silico software tools provide a mechanism of inferring the biological effect of the mutation. The diagnosis is considered inconclusive (on the basis of the variants alone) if no such variants can be found.

Genome variant interpretation has been described as a "needle in the bunch on needles" problem [17], as the target variants are a tiny proportion, typically no more than ten, of the more than 20,000 variants that are detected by a typical pipeline. The vast majority of variants are benign, such as common polymorphisms, which do not affect a patients health. Ideally, the variants of interest lie at the intersection between two subsets of the overall patient's variants, namely (i) deleterious variants, i.e., protein altering and splice site altering mutations, and (ii) variants that are known from the literature to play a role in the target phenotype. As we will see, however, it is not always possible to identify variants that lie precisely in this intersection. Our selection process therefore aims at segregating variants into classes, depending on the amount of available evidence to support the hypothesis that they are indeed the basis for a disease diagnosis. The process consists of three phases, which we describe next: (i) restricting the investigation to a specific set of genes (phenotype and variant scoping), (ii) variant filtering aimed at identifying deleterious variants, and (iii) variant classification. The overall process is depicted in Fig. 2.

3.1   Phenotype and Variant Scoping

In this phase, user input terms are mapped to genes. Users may specify the disease hypothesis at varying levels of precision, ranging from free text keywords, to terms from the OMIM vocabulary[9] or from the Human Phenotype Ontology [18] (HPO[10]). The latter provides a more precise characterisation of the phenotype (so called *deep phenotyping* [19,20]). OMIM and HPO both provide standard reference taxonomies of phenotype terms. In addition, we normalise all input formats to OMIM, which also offers phenotype-to-gene mapping. HPO provides a direct mapping to OMIM, and free text keywords are simply mapped to OMIM terms through string matching. The resulting OMIM terms are then mapped to a set of genes, which define the initial scope of the investigation, in the next phase.

As genetic testing in clinics tends to specialise on specific disorder areas, the scope can be further restricted to a set of genes that are known to be implicated in phenotypes in that area. Thus, when using the tool the clinician may also optionally provide a more precise characterisation of the scope of the investigation, by directly specifying a list of target genes of interest. This process,

---

[9] http://www.omim.org/.
[10] http://www.human-phenotype-ontology.org/.

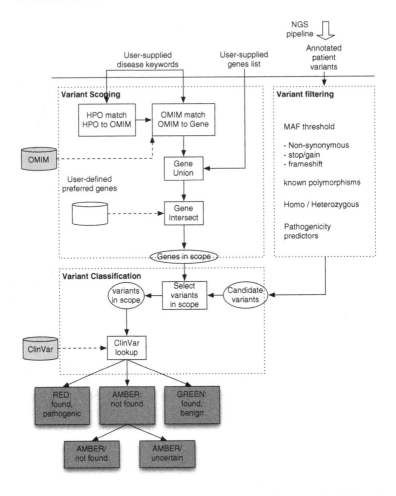

Fig. 2. Variant interpretation process as implemented in SVI.

depicted on the top left in Fig. 2, produces a final set of *genes in scope*. Only the subset of candidate variants found in phase II (variant filtering), which lie on the scope genes, will be considered for classification.

3.2   Variant Filtering for Identification of Deleterious Variants

This phase relies on variant annotations, provided by the well-known Annovar annotation service [21]. SVI implements an extensible set of filters, reflecting emerging pratice in the lab. Currently, variants are filtered according to the following conditions.

- Identification of polymorphisms. Variants that are recorded as polymorphisms in the dbSNP database are excluded, as these are common mutations which occur at higher frequencies than the disease phenotype in the population, and are known to be non-deleterious.

- Coverage test. We check that variants are called at 30x fold or more, as this is a de facto standard for confidence in a read. Also, we check the exome coverage percentage (i.e. what fraction of the exome is covered to 30 fold), and distribution of % coverage across the exome, if this information is available.
- *Synonymous* variants are removed, as those are non-protein altering or splice site altering. Only non-synonymous, stop/gain, frameshift mutations are retained.
- Variants with MAFs (Minor Allele Frequency) greater than 0.01 are also discarded. Ideally, MAF should be checked separately against international controls as well as local control patients. For instance, harmless mutations that are rare within the general population (low MAF) may be incorrectly included, although a localised patients control database would reveal a higher frequency in the patients area of origin. No such localised databases are currently available to us, however.
- When performing trio genetic testing (typically involving parents and affected child), remove all variants which do not conform to pedigree, i.e., remove potentially pathogenic heterozygous variants due to their observation in an unaffected parent, and the detection of de novo variants. Also, determine whether the presence of the same variants is consistent with Mendelian inheritance, as indicated for instance in [22].
- User-defined thresholds on a variety of individual or aggregate pathogenicity predictors [23], including PolyPhen[11] and others that are available through Annovar annotations.

The outcome of this phase is denoted as *candidate variants* in Fig. 2.

3.3 Variant Classification

At this stage we have isolated variants with the following properties: (i) they are likely to be deleterious, and (ii) they lie in genes that are broadly related to the target phenotype, via OMIM mapping. The uncertainty associated with the filtering process, combined with the broad nature of OMIM disease-gene mapping, suggest that these conditions are still too weak to provide conclusive evidence in support of the hypothesis. Indeed, at this stage hundreds of variants are still under consideration, mostly false positives.

Definite evidence can only be provided by research on specific disease-variant associations. As mentioned, we have chosen ClinVar as our initial reference source, with the intention to extend the knowledge base to other sources in the future. To each known single nucleotide variant, ClinVar associates a clinical significance that is simple to interpret (Likely benign/Likely pathogenic/Uncertain) along with the condition associated with a pathogenic significance (using OMIM terms). Importantly for us, in view of the tracking capabilities of our tool, ClinVar also provides metadata about the review status of the entry, with timestamps of the latest update. As shown in the bottom part of Fig. 3, we exploit the ClinVar output to create a simple separation of the candidate variants, into three

---

[11] http://genetics.bwh.harvard.edu/pph2/.

classes: Red, Amber, and Green, using a "traffic light" metaphor that clinicians
are likely to find simple and useful.

Red variants are those that are recorded as pathogenic in ClinVar. Considering the prior filtering and scoping, these provide conclusive evidence for a
positive diagnosis.

Amber variants are those that are in scope but either not known to Clin-
Var, denoted Amber/unknown, or recorded in ClinVar with Uncertain significance (Amber/uncertain). Variants `c.4132A>G:p.Ser1378Gly` on gene LRP-
PRC and `c.842G>A:p.Gly281Asp`on PARK2 are examples of Amber/unknown
and Amber/Uncertain variants, respectively. These variants provide weaker evidence than the Red ones, yet they cannot be dismissed, as absence from ClinVar
may simply mean that research is still be ongoing or that curation efforts have
not yet brought recently published research into database.

Finally, **Green** variants are those that are found in ClinVar, reported as
likely benign.

This simple user output is designed to reduce the clinician's decision process,
by separating the "easy" cases which reveal Red variants, from all others.
Cases where Amber but no Red variants are found can be referred to specialist
researchers for further investigation.

In SVI, these are the prime candidates for re-analysis when updates to Clin-
Var become available, or when new variant databases are integrated.

4   A Provenance-Aware Diagnostic Tool

We have implemented the process into SVI, a Web-based user tool designed to
be used by clinicians. Evaluation of the tool is still ongoing, both in terms of
effectiveness of the variant filtering, and in terms of usability. We define effectiveness as the ability to reproduce benchmark diagnostics decisions obtained
by experts. While our results are still preliminary, as an example we report the
effect of filtering on the five test patients used in the study described in Sect. 2.
In all cases, from generic user input expressing the patients' common phenotype
(*multiple mitochondrial respiratory complex deficiency*) SVI identified between
7 and 11 Red variants, as indicated in Fig. 3 and in Table 3. In all cases, the Red
variants include those listed in Table 1 on page 6.[12]

In addition to supporting the filtering process, SVI provides complete tracing
of the process itself. The underlying data model (implemented using the Mon-
goDB DBMS) is centred around the main concept of an *Investigation* (Fig. 4).
An investigation is part of a case about a patient. A case is owned by an investigator (the clinician/user), and it may consists of multiple investigations, each
containing full details of one individual search. These details include a reference
to the patient, user input (keywords, HPO, OMIM terms) along with their mapping to genes, the variants selected at each stage in the process, and the "traffic
light" classification of each variant. Annotations made by the user in support

---

[12] Experts were not available to confirm whether any of the other Red variants had
also been detected.

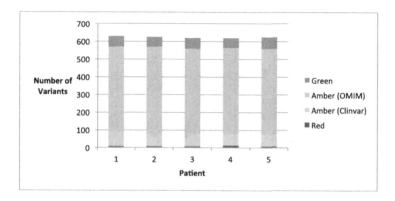

Fig. 3. Distribution of variants amongst the Red/Amber/Green classes for out patients sample (Color figure online)

Table 3. Effect of variant filtering in SVI for a specific phenotype

Patient	Candidate variants	Present in ClinVar	Red	Amber (uncertain)	Amber (unknown)	Green
1	631	149	10	77	482	62
2	625	129	7	65	496	57
3	622	139	7	69	483	63
4	618	132	11	67	486	54
5	627	141	8	65	486	68

of a decision, at the level of individual variants, are also captured. Finally, an investigation records the versions of all external data sources used for filtering.

An investigation provides a persistent provenance trace of each user execution. We are currently in the process of implementing a number of added value features on top of this provenance database. These include:

- The ability to selectively trigger new analysis of old cases, when changes occur anywhere in the knowledge sources (or indeed in the pipeline upstream). Specifically, when an Amber variant in an investigation appears or changes status in ClinVar, it moves from the Amber class to either the Green or the Red class, possibly resulting in the case being revisited by the clinician. This process can be automated through a simple *diff* process whenever a new version of ClinVar becomes available.
- Analyse historical investigations to determine possible implicit associations between independent cases. For instance, cases that exhibit a substantial overlap in the gene scope or the variant scope may be linked, so that whenever a problem/solution is found in one, the other can be flagged up for further consideration.
- Query the investigation database across multiple dimensions (patients, phenotype, investigator, time). Examples of queries include: "find all patients

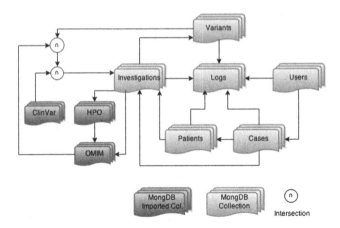

Fig. 4. Data model centred on investigations, designed for provenance support. The arrows indicate one-to-many or many-to-many relationships

annotated with shared HPO terms, who also share variants or have variants on the same genes", and "determine how many patients with the same variant have the same HPO matching terms".

Most importantly, the provenance database provides accountability over the entire decision process. This is important not only for audit purposes, but also to allow third party clinicians, who have not been involved in the case, to fully understand how the investigator reached important decisions, which potentially affects a patient's quality of life.

5   Conclusions and Current Work

NGS-based genetic diagnosis is rapidly coming of age. As NGS technology matures, the new bottleneck is likely to be the clinical interpretation of the lists of human variants extracted from the raw WGS data, which remains a knowledge-intensive activity requiring expert human judgement. Making sure that the diagnostic process scales with the increasing volume of patient cases requires automation of this activity. In this paper we have presented an initial attempt at addressing this issue. We have been experimenting with a simple variant filtering process and tool, code-named SVI, which automates most of the process by relying on integration of variant databases. In this initial effort, we have chosen ClinVar as the exemplar variant database, as its content and curation appear to progress rapidly, increasing the chances to identify relevant pathogenic variants. The tool includes full traceability of the diagnostic process.

Our work is progressing in several directions. Firstly, we are now evaluating the effectiveness of SVI in terms of false positives/negatives relative to the expert judgment on a testbed of real patient cases. Secondly, we are working to integrate additional sources of variant-disease associations, such as those on the LOVD platform. Finally, as the number of investigations increases, we expect to be able to perform interesting analysis on the provenance database.

References

1. Wetterstrand, K.: DNA sequencing costs: data from the NHGRI Genome Sequencing Program (GSP) (2015)
2. Stein, L.D.: The case for cloud computing in genome informatics. Genome Biol. **11**, 207 (2010)
3. Xuan, J., Yu, Y., Qing, T., Guo, L., Shi, L.: Next-generation sequencing in the clinic: promises and challenges. Cancer Lett. **340**, 284–295 (2013)
4. Worthey, E.A., Mayer, A.N., Syverson, G.D., Helbling, D., Bonacci, B.B., Decker, B., Serpe, J.M., Dasu, T., Tschannen, M.R., Veith, R.L., Basehore, M.J., Broeckel, U., Tomita-Mitchell, A., Arca, M.J., Casper, J.T., Margolis, D.A., Bick, D.P., Hessner, M.J., Routes, J.M., Verbsky, J.W., Jacob, H.J., Dimmock, D.P.: Making a definitive diagnosis: successful clinical application of whole exome sequencing in a child with intractable inflammatory bowel disease. Genet. Med. Official J. Am. Coll. Med. Genet. **13**, 255–262 (2011)
5. Yang, Y., Muzny, D.M., Reid, J.G., Bainbridge, M.N., Willis, A., Ward, P.A., Braxton, A., Beuten, J., Xia, F., Niu, Z., Hardison, M., Person, R., Bekheirnia, M.R., Leduc, M.S., Kirby, A., Pham, P., Scull, J., Wang, M., Ding, Y., Plon, S.E., Lupski, J.R., Beaudet, A.L., Gibbs, R.A., Eng, C.M.: Clinical whole-exome sequencing for the diagnosis of mendelian disorders. N. Engl. J. Med. **369**, 1502–1511 (2013)
6. Pabinger, S., Dander, A., Fischer, M., Snajder, R., Sperk, M., Efremova, M., Krabichler, B., Speicher, M.R., Zschocke, J., Trajanoski, Z.: A survey of tools for variant analysis of next-generation genome sequencing data. Briefings in bioinformatics (2013). doi:10.1093/bib/bbs086
7. Cala, J., Xu, Y.X., Wijaya, E.A., Missier, P.: From scripted HPC-based NGS pipelines to workflows on the cloud. In: Proceedings of C4Bio Workshop, Co-located with the 2014 CCGrid Conference. IEEE, Chicago (2013)
8. Shashi, V., McConkie-Rosell, A., Rosell, B., Schoch, K., Vellore, K., McDonald, M., Jiang, Y.H., Xie, P., Need, A., Goldstein, D.B., Goldstein, D.G.: The utility of the traditional medical genetics diagnostic evaluation in the context of next-generation sequencing for undiagnosed genetic disorders. Genet. Med. Official J. Am. Coll. Med. Genet. **16**, 176–182 (2014)
9. Atwal, P.S., Brennan, M.L., Cox, R., Niaki, M., Platt, J., Homeyer, M., Kwan, A., Parkin, S., Schelley, S., Slattery, L., Wilnai, Y., Bernstein, J.A., Enns, G.M., Hudgins, L.: Clinical whole-exome sequencing: are we there yet? Genet. Med. Official J. Am. Coll. Med. Genet. **16**, 717–719 (2014)
10. Zemojtel, T., Kohler, S., Mackenroth, L., Jager, M., Hecht, J., Krawitz, P., Graul-Neumann, L., Doelken, S., Ehmke, N., Spielmann, M., Oien, N.C., Schweiger, M.R., Kruger, U., Frommer, G., Fischer, B., Kornak, U., Flottmann, R., Ardeshirdavani, A., Moreau, Y., Lewis, S.E., Haendel, M., Smedley, D., Horn, D., Mundlos, S., Robinson, P.N.: Effective diagnosis of genetic disease by computational phenotype analysis of the disease-associated genome. Sci. Transl. Med. **6**, 252ra123 (2014)
11. Robinson, P.N., Köhler, S., Oellrich, A., Wang, K., Mungall, C.J., Lewis, S.E., Washington, N., Bauer, S., Seelow, D., Krawitz, P., Gilissen, C., Haendel, M., Smedley, D.: Improved exome prioritization of disease genes through cross-species phenotype comparison. Genome Res. **24**, 340–348 (2014)
12. Liu, X., Jian, X., Boerwinkle, E.: dbNSFP: a lightweight database of human non-synonymous SNPs and their functional predictions. Hum. Mutat. **32**, 894–899 (2011)

13. Sifrim, A., Popovic, D., Tranchevent, L.C., Ardeshirdavani, A., Sakai, R., Konings, P., Vermeesch, J.R., Aerts, J., De Moor, B., Moreau, Y.: eXtasy: variant prioritization by genomic data fusion. Nat. Meth. **10**, 1083–1084 (2013)
14. Sifrim, A., Van Houdt, J.K., Tranchevent, L.C., Nowakowska, B., Sakai, R., Pavlopoulos, G.A., Devriendt, K., Vermeesch, J.R., Moreau, Y., Aerts, J.: Annotate-it: a Swiss-knife approach to annotation, analysis and interpretation of single nucleotide variation in human disease. Genome Med. **4**, 73 (2012)
15. Swaminathan, G.J., Bragin, E., Chatzimichali, E.A., Corpas, M., Bevan, A.P., Wright, C.F., Carter, N.P., Hurles, M.E., Firth, H.V.: DECIPHER: web-based, community resource for clinical interpretation of rare variants in developmental disorders. Hum. Mol. Genet. **21**, R37–44 (2012)
16. Götz, A., Tyynismaa, H., Euro, L., Ellonen, P., Hyötyläinen, T., Ojala, T., Hämäläinen, R.H., Tommiska, J., Raivio, T., Oresic, M., Karikoski, R., Tammela, O., Simola, K.O.J., Paetau, A., Tyni, T., Suomalainen, A.: Exome sequencing identifies mitochondrial alanyl-tRNA synthetase mutations in infantile mitochondrial cardiomyopathy. Am. J. Hum. Genet. **88**, 635–642 (2011)
17. Cooper, G.M., Shendure, J.: Needles in stacks of needles: finding disease-causal variants in a wealth of genomic data. Nat. Rev. Genet. **12**, 628–640 (2011)
18. Robinson, P.N., Mundlos, S.: The human phenotype ontology. Clin. Genet. **77**, 525–534 (2010)
19. Hennekam, R.C.M., Biesecker, L.G.: Next-generation sequencing demands next-generation phenotyping. Hum. Mutat. **33**, 884–886 (2012)
20. Köhler, S., Doelken, S.C., Mungall, C.J., Bauer, S., Firth, H.V., Bailleul-Forestier, I., Black, G.C.M., Brown, D.L., Brudno, M., Campbell, J., FitzPatrick, D.R., Eppig, J.T., Jackson, A.P., Freson, K., Girdea, M., Helbig, I., Hurst, J.A., Jähn, J., Jackson, L.G., Kelly, A.M., Ledbetter, D.H., Mansour, S., Martin, C.L., Moss, C., Mumford, A., Ouwehand, W.H., Park, S.M., Riggs, E.R., Scott, R.H., Sisodiya, S., Van Vooren, S., Wapner, R.J., Wilkie, A.O.M., Wright, C.F., Vulto-van, S.A.T., de Leeuw, N., de Vries, B.B.A., Washingthon, N.L., Smith, C.L., Westerfield, M., Schofield, P., Ruef, B.J., Gkoutos, G.V., Haendel, M., Smedley, D., Lewis, S.E., Robinson, P.N.: The Human Phenotype Ontology project: linking molecular biology and disease through phenotype data. Nucleic Acids Res. **42**, D966–D974 (2014)
21. Wang, K., Li, M., Hakonarson, H.: ANNOVAR: functional annotation of genetic variants from high-throughput sequencing data. Nucleic Acids Res. **38**, e164–e164 (2010)
22. Keogh, M.J., Daud, D., Chinnery, P.F.: Exome sequencing: how to understand it. Pract. Neurol. 1–9 (2013)
23. Thusberg, J., Olatubosun, A., Vihinen, M.: Performance of mutation pathogenicity prediction methods on missense variants. Hum. Mutat. **32**, 358–368 (2011)

Quality Control Considerations for the Effective Integration of Neuroimaging Data

Sumiko Abe, Andrei Irimia, and John Darrell Van Horn[(✉)]

Laboratory of Neuro Imaging, Institute for Neuroimaging and Informatics, University of Southern California, Los Angeles, CA, USA
{sabe,andrei.irimia,jack.vanhorn}@loni.usc.edu

Abstract. Ensuring image quality control (QC) for data acquired in a multi-modality context offers substantial advantages for both multi-level and multi-point analysis. Although a variety of neuroimage analysis algorithms exist, the tasks of multimodal neuroimaging data QC and integration remain challenging because image quality can be affected by numerous factors. Here, we discuss the challenges of the QC and integration of neuroimaging data and provide two examples of often-neglected and potentially under-appreciated problems related to the QC of diffusion tensor imaging (DTI) data and to their integration with other modalities. Specifically, we illustrate the challenges of (1) DTI/MRI co-registration and (2) scanner vibration artifacts, both being representative examples of difficulties involving both data QC and its integration. Additionally, we highlight the need for automatic methods which can address neuroimaging data QC which allows for its successful integration.

Keywords: Neuroimaging · Data quality control · Data integration · Diffusion tensor imaging · 3D visualization

1 Introduction

The heterogeneity of neuroimaging data can render their integration challenging, particularly in the case of diffusion tensor imaging (DTI), where sophisticated post-acquisition processing can be required for such data to become amenable to integration with other imaging data types, such as T_1-weighted magnetic resonance imaging (MRI), functional MRI (fMRI) and positron emission tomography (PET). Figure 1 illustrates several common neuroimaging artifacts affecting study quality which (a) indicate that data would be a challenge to integrate, and (b) likely imply the necessity of discarding experimental subjects so affected from further analyses. What is more, during the image acquisition process, under-appreciated and occasionally-neglected issues may arise. During DTI scans, artifacts due to scanner vibration may occur and these can translate into undesired tractography results, with certain types of MRI scanners being more prone to vibration artifacts than others. The purpose of this paper is to discuss the potential challenges of multimodal neuroimaging data integration and quality control (QC).

© Springer International Publishing Switzerland 2015
N. Ashish and J.-L. Ambite (Eds.): DILS 2015, LNBI 9162, pp. 195–201, 2015.
DOI: 10.1007/978-3-319-21843-4_15

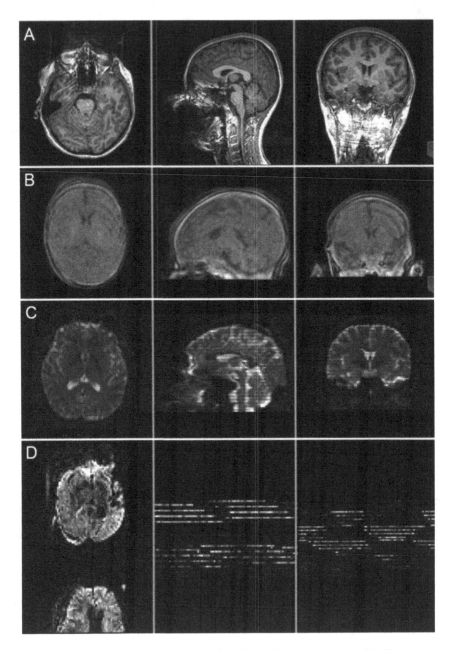

Fig. 1. Commonly encountered examples of artifacts affecting image quality (in transverse, saggital, and coronal planes): (A) a dental appliance resulting in T1 image distortion, (B) ghosting artifact, (C) echo-planar susceptibility artifacts, and (D) T_2-weighted image volume slice misalignment.

2   QC as a Requirement for Multimodal Integration

Beyond the obvious QC issues shown in Fig. 1, two representative examples of often unappreciated challenges are provided for illustration purposes. The first is the scenario where volumes acquired using distinct modalities have different spatial resolutions, which suggests the need for implementing three-dimensional (3D) interpolation during co-registration prior to data integration and analysis. The application of such operations is often accompanied by numerical errors which can affect the quality of DTI tractography, and the detailed effects of co-registration/interpolation methods should be quantified carefully during QC and data integration. Secondly, we illustrate the under-appreciated problem related to QC and to data integration, which involves the occasional presence of systematic vibration artifacts in DTI. Specifically, because large gradient lobes are employed during data acquisition, the accompanying vibrations of the patient table can lead to substantial disruption of diffusion measures, particularly in occipital areas. QC metrics which can identify and quantify such effects automatically would be very useful, as would their resolution using image processing methods which can be applied prior to integrating DTI data with other neuroimaging modalities.

2.1   Accounting for Differences in Spatial Resolution

Neuroimaging data can be acquired using a variety of different modalities which often have distinct spatial resolutions. For example, T_1-weighted MRI volumes are often acquired at relatively high spatial resolution because they are used to quantify structural properties of the brain, whereas DTI and PET volumes may have lower resolutions than structural MRI due to the various challenges of acquiring high-resolution volumes using these modalities for water diffusion and metabolic measurements, respectively. For multimodal neuroimaging data integration, however, it is often necessary to scale data to the same resolution because many analysis are performed at the voxel level.

Various methods for the co-registration of DTI volumes to MRI volumes exist. In a very common approach, the DTI B_0 volume is registered and interpolated to the resolution of the T_1-weighted volume, whereafter each DTI gradient volume is registered and interpolated to the already-interpolated B_0 volume. Though common in practice, this method requires two registration and interpolation steps and appreciable differences in the end result can exist depending on which interpolation and registration algorithms are used, possibly resulting in propagated errors.

An alternative approach involves reconstructing the diffusion tensors in the native space of the DTI volume. Specifically, FA volume and eigenvectors are calculated first and the FA volume is then registered to the T_1-weighted volume. The same transformation matrix can then be applied to the other volumes, and this approach requires only one registration operation. Additionally, the operation of eigenvector normalization can avoid the cancellation of fiber directions information which may result from eigenvector interpolation.

Figure 2 illustrates DTI tractography differences which are due to the use of various interpolation methods. As the figure suggests, different interpolation methods can yield vastly different tractography results. Given these substantial differences, it results that reducing the number of times that interpolation is implemented is desirable because it reduces the amount of propagated interpolation error.

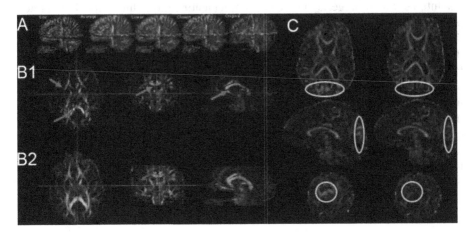

Fig. 2. (A) Effects of applying several DTI data interpolation techniques, namely sinc, average, linear and closest neighbor can lead to substantial differences in tractography results. (B) Eigenvector normalization (B2) is found to improve data quality over the scenario where this operation is not performed (B1). (C) Correction of an artifact due to scanner table vibration. The first row illustrates the artifact, and the second row shows corrected images.

This example illustrates the fact that the use of alternative methods for co-registering and then integrating neuroimaging data may inadvertently result in substantially different results, which can also pose problems from the standpoint of QC. When the alternative approach for data integration is applied as described in the previous paragraph, the implementation of eigenvector normalization is found to result in improved quality of the interpolation due to the fact that this operation is only applied once (Fig. 2).

2.2 Accounting for Scanner Vibration Artifacts

Frequently, scanner vibration artifacts in DTI data are insufficiently appreciated. Although such artifacts have been identified in data acquired from many sites, it is not clear how widespread this problem is and whether all MRI scanners are affected. Such artifacts are due to the vibration of the patient table during gradient data acquisition and can affect DTI recordings, particularly in occipital brain white matter regions. These artifacts can disrupt DTI image quality and can be controlled via a linear correction method, which has been found to be effective (Fig. 2). This figure illustrates that, after using the linear method for the reduction of artifacts due to scanner motion, the effect of the latter is greatly reduced, confirming the improvement in image quality and suggesting that the effects of this artifact can be addressed satisfactorily. For QC purposes, it would be useful to develop methods which identify this type of artifact and which can then signal the researcher that an appropriate correction should be implemented during the process of pre-processing DTI volumes.

Figure 3 illustrates a suggested data integration workflow for MRI/DTI/PET co-registration and analysis, which can be implemented after accounting for problems such as differences in image resolutions and scanner vibration artifacts. Figure 4 shows the results of multimodal integration of MRI/DTI/PET data, as visualized simultaneously.

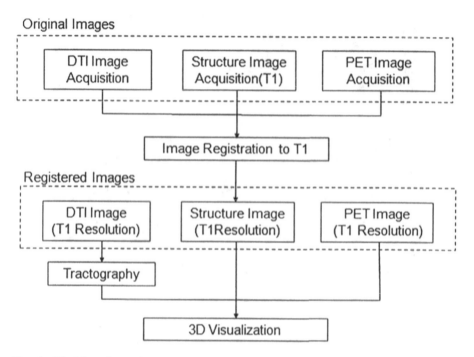

Fig. 3. Workflow for multiple modality image registration. Each of the steps involved in multimodal registration can present challenges due to the presence of artifacts, resulting in the need for image QC.

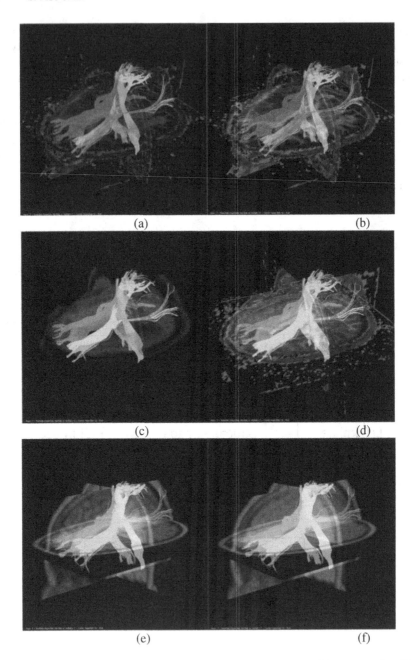

Fig. 4. DTI/PET/T1-weighted MRI data integration. (A) RGB map with tractography; (B) FA map with tractography; (C) PET image with tractography; (D): PET, FA map with tractography; (E) T1 image with tractography; (F) T1, PET image with tractography.

3   Conclusions

In this paper, we discussed several basic challenges of multimodal image QC and integration of neuroimaging data. We provide two examples of often-neglected and potentially under-appreciated problems related to the QC of diffusion tensor imaging (DTI)
data and to their integration with other modalities. The usefulness of minimizing the
number of interpolations when registering DTI data to structural MRI was illustrated,
in addition to the need to account for scanner vibration artifacts prior to htfidelity data
integration. Additionally, we discussed several challenges of multimodal image QC and
of neuroimaging data integration. For vibration artifacts, MRI scanners may occasionally induce vibration artifacts during DTI scans due to the nature of pulse sequence
designs for this modality.

In conclusion, we provided examples of often-neglected and potentially under-
appreciated problems related to the QC of diffusion tensor imaging (DTI) data and to
their integration with other modalities. The usefulness of minimizing the number of
interpolations when registering DTI data to structural MRI was illustrated, in addition
to the need to account for scanner vibration artifacts prior to DTI tractography and
analysis. Image QC is a necessary step in advance of high-fidelity data integration.

References

1. Poline, J.B., Breeze, J.L., Ghosh, S., Gorgolewski, K., Halchenko, Y.O., Hanke, M.,
   Haselgrove, C., Helmer, K.G., Keator, D.B., Marcus, D.S., Poldrack, R.A., Schwartz, Y.,
   Ashburner, J., Kennedy, D.N.: Data sharing in neuroimaging research. Front. Neuroinformatics
   6, 9 (2012)
2. Abe, S., Preda, A., Turner, J., Keator, D., Potkin, S.: FBIRN. DTI Co-registration method
   comparison based on DTI tractography analysis in the human brain. In: Annual Meeting of the
   Organization for Human Brain Mapping (2009)
3. Gallichan, D., Scholz, J., Bartsch, A., Behrens, T.E., Robson, M.D., Miller, K.L.: Addressing
   a systematic vibration artifact in diffusion-weighted MRI. Hum. Brain Mapp. **31**, 193–202
   (2010)

Integration of Behavioral, Structural, Functional, and Genetic Data for the Study of Autism Spectrum Disorders

Carinna M. Torgerson, Andrei Irimia, S.-Y. Matthew Goh, and John D. Van Horn[✉]

Laboratory of Neuro Imaging, Keck School of Medicine, USC Mark and Mary Stevens Neuroimaging and Informatics Institute, University of Southern California, Los Angeles, USA
{ctorgers,jack.vanhorn,andrei.irimia,
matthew.goh}@loni.usc.edu

Abstract. Pursuant to its commitment to cultivating a greater understanding of mental illness, the National Institutes of Health (NIH) have created the National Database for Clinical Trials, where data from a wide variety of NIH-funded studies are deposited in the hope that as many qualified researchers as possible can examine these data. As the designated Data Coordinating Center in the Autism Center of Excellence (ACE) network, the Laboratory of Neuro Imaging (LONI) is faced with the task of efficiently organizing data from behavioral assessments, magnetic resonance imaging (MRI), functional MRI (fMRI), diffusion tensor imaging (DTI), electroencephalography (EEG), and whole-genome analysis. To encourage fusion of data across modalities, we have integrated a direct National Database for Autism Research (NDAR) data sharing capability into the LONI Pipeline processing environment, which allows users to create workflows by mixing and matching analytic tools from a library of common neuroimaging, genetics, and statistical software packages.

Keywords: Diffusion tensor imaging · Functional magnetic resonance imaging · Genetics · Autism spectrum disorder · Pipeline processing

1 Introduction

Autism spectrum disorders (ASDs) seem to result from a multitude of contributing factors – from genes to neurotransmitters to structural abnormalities to altered connectivity (Atkinson and Braddick 2011, McPartland et al. 2011). It is this heterogeneity which has made understanding this assortment of linked disorders particularly challenging, and which makes it ripe for multi-modal examination. Existing research has led to a variety of proposed treatments, with inconsistent results across different types of autism cases. The National Autism Center (NAC; www.nationalautismcenter.org) reports that a myriad of biomedical and neuropsychological data are needed to adequately assess an individual's disease severity before an effective treatment plan can be formulated (National Autism Center 2011). Such necessary information may come from evaluating genomics data, biographical information, co-morbid conditions,

© Springer International Publishing Switzerland 2015
N. Ashish and J.-L. Ambite (Eds.): DILS 2015, LNBI 9162, pp. 202–207, 2015.
DOI: 10.1007/978-3-319-21843-4_16

neuroimages, the onset and latency of the disorder, the type of treatment, and many other factors.

As the National Institutes of Health (NIH) increase their efforts to make the data produced by its funding freely available, its data repositories have come to hold more and more types of data. Meanwhile, the Autism Centers of Excellence (ACE) network grants awarded by the NIH seek to facilitate a broader understanding of a very nuanced spectrum of disorders, and thereby to encourage the acquisition, integration and analysis of heterogeneous data. Our laboratory functions as the Data Coordinating Center (DCC) for one such ACE network, i.e. the Multimodal Developmental Neurogenetics of Females with ASD Collection. (https://ndar.nih.gov/edit_collection.html?id=2021). As of January 2015, our site alone had collected behavioral, structural, functional, and genetic information from 135 children. Analysis of such a wide array of data would be severely limited if it were then only analyzed uni-modally.

One substantial advantage of multi-modal neuroimaging data is their ability to facilitate the creation of more insightful pictures of the brain (Van Horn and Ball, 2008, Van Horn, Dobson, et al. 2006, Van Horn and Gazzaniga, 2002, Van Horn and Gazzaniga, 2012, Van Horn and Ishai, 2007). Unfortunately, most neuroimaging and genetics techniques have only become widely available within the last couple of decades. At the current rate of scientific progress, it may soon become nearly impossible for anyone to become an expert in each of the collection and analysis methods which are considered vital for understanding mental illness. In our role as the DCC, we sought to overcome this barrier partly by using the LONI Pipeline processing environment, where researchers can create simple data analysis workflows by utilizing some of the most common analytic tools available today, and then sharing these workflows with others. A workflow can easily be customized by the expert analyst, or can simply be re-executed by someone who wants to incorporate an neuroimaging modality into their analysis without having to learn the details of the analysis technique itself, e.g. in the case of an EEG researcher who wishes to measure individual brain activation differences as measured using fMRI. By combining a massive multi-modal database and a processing environment which can handle a wide variety of data types, our project has aimed to make data integration the least difficult component of multi-modal studies.

2   Accessing the NDAR Database

Neuroimaging data stored in the National Database for Clinical Trials is subdivided into smaller databases according to research type. The National Database for Autism Research (NDAR) repository allows researchers from qualified institutions to download data from the numerous ACE and ACE network grants. The first step toward gaining such access is to acquire a username and password by completing the NDAR access application. Investigators must be registered with the eRA Commons (https://commons.era.nih.gov) and must secure local institutional approval (see http://ndar.nih.gov/ndarpublicweb/access.html for details on the access request process). Upon approval by NIH officials (http://ndar.nih.gov/policies_data_access_committee.html), researchers can search NDAR contents, create data packages of useful de-identified data sets, and download them for further examination. One can even search for pertinent details from the experimental protocol of the study or studies in which certain data were collected, such as pertaining to artifact detection algorithms or data inclusion criteria.

Once approved, one can use the available 'Query' tool in order to filter data by type, age, gender, number of subjects, etc. A 'Download Data' button leads to a new webpage which allows the user to select the types of data they wish to download for their cohort of interest. Then, these results can be bundled using a 'Create Package' functionality. Once the user requests this, the system asks her/him to name the package. The NDAR system generates a numerical package ID as well, which can be used to reference the package in other locations, such as the LONI Pipeline interface.

The NDAR Download Manager is a program which facilitates the download of collections to researchers' local storage, thereby enabling them to have data delivered locally. Conversely, users may prefer not to download data at all, but instead to reference these NDAR package IDs directly within data processing workflow tools located on remote computing systems, clusters, or 'in the cloud' using NDAR's 'Mini-NDAR' or 'miNDAR' capabilities (http://ndar.nih.gov/cloud_get_started.html).

Integrating data collected by someone else can be complex. Some information may be difficult to communicate within a file. NDAR also utilizes the link-out capability within PubMed and is now issuing Digital Object Identifiers (DOIs) for shared studies, so that a simple search can direct researchers to the actual data used in their references. This feature has vast potential for comparative and replication studies, as well as for following up on particular directions for future research, as suggested by the authors of past studies. In this way, NDAR interactivity with the LONI Pipeline can help to formulate hypotheses and to fill knowledge gaps in our understanding of ASD. Conversely, within the NDAR website, one can search for data based on the laboratory with which a study is associated, or be directed to all publications associated with a specific cohort. In this way, autism researchers can investigate how certain data were used in the past, which can help them to formulate or modify scientific hypotheses for future studies and analyses conducted using the LONI Pipeline.

3 LONI Pipeline Processing Environment

Scientific workflow methodologies can enable the creation of heterogeneous processing chains which can be executed on parallel computing systems. Various workflow systems exist and have been used successfully in neuroimaging (Stef-Praun et al. 2007, Gorgolewski, Burns et al. 2011). The LONI Pipeline workflow environment is a graphical framework for constructing workflows and for implementing high-throughput analysis (Dinov et al. 2009, Dinov et al. 2010). This program, now in version 6.0 (as of March 2015), is freely available (http://pipeline.loni.usc.edu) and provides processing modules from well-known neuroimaging software programs, as well as end-to-end protocols for performing image-processing tasks. Employing the LONI Pipeline can help standardize processing methodologies within or between research groups, and such exact replication of methods can improve the accuracy of reported data processing provenance (MacKenzie-Graham et al. 2008, Mackenzie-Graham et al. 2008). Additionally, it can prevent researchers from implementing the same data analysis twice, or from executing a set of analysis steps in an improper order, a safety feature which has been notoriously lacking in the neuroimaging community (Kennedy 2012). The LONI Pipeline is also available through the Neuroimaging Tools and Resource Clearinghouse (NITRC; http://www.nitrc.org) (Luo et al. 2009), which enables researchers to locate, install, and compare resources for functional and structural neuroimaging analyses, as well as to collect and point to standardized information about tools for performing such analyses. Users can interact with the LONI Pipeline client within the Windows, Mac, or Linux operating systems to design and execute workflows which are physically executed on a Pipeline-enabled computer cluster through the use of a remote connection. LONI itself maintains a large-scale cluster with over 3,500 compute nodes dedicated to supporting thousands of simultaneous Pipeline workflow submissions. The Pipeline is also available as an Amazon-EC2 service (http://pipeline.loni.usc.edu/products-services/pipeline-server-on-ec2/) and via the NITRC Compute Environment (NITRC-CE) (http://www.nitrc.org/projects/nitrc_es).

4   NDAR Access Through LONI Pipeline

Within the Pipeline program there exists the means for directly logging into the NDAR cloud storage and accessing previously defined data package IDs (see 'Accessing the NDAR Database' above). Once an NDAR data package is specified on the NDAR login screen, a three-component set of modules is automatically generated. These modules download the compressed data packages, unzip their contents, and convert them to any one of three commonly utilized neuroimaging file formats: Analyze, MINC, or the modules' default file type, i.e. the NIfTI (.nii) file format (http://nifti.nimh.nih.gov/). Additional modules are available in the Pipeline Server Library, and can be easily added to the NDAR download modules. Alternatively, the library also offers fully-developed workflows for an array of common processing tasks including FSL, FreeSurfer, Brain-Suite, and Diffusion Toolkit. Lastly, modules defined for user-built executables can also be inserted to generate unique workflows.

5   Role of the DCC

The DCC has two primary goals. Firstly, the site is expected to screen incoming data from each collection site to ensure that all data are readable, formatted correctly, labeled properly, and organized together with all other data for each subject. Contributors to the NDAR database are recommended not to convert their imaging data in any way, but to send the original DICOM output files from their MRI scanner. This rule was implemented to prevent the loss of metadata, which is often stripped away during conversion to more compact formats. Having all data in the same format is critical for streamlining the process of downloading large cohorts of data directly to a processing environment. Another critical piece of our role is ensuring that datasets do not lack any of the pieces of necessary information for data analysis. For example, an fMRI data file is useless without information provided in another file to indicate the time points where stimuli were presented, and DTI data require matrices specifying magnetic field gradients in each direction of data acquisition.

6   Conclusion

With a library of most commonly-used analytic tools for each modality, the LONI Pipeline allows researchers to branch out into the analysis of data types which they may not have investigated before. Providing members of our collaborative network with the ability to perform analyses which follow identical steps across sites—especially when experience in a particular acquisition modality is lacking at a particular site—will hopefully allow researchers to acquire deeper insights into the many facets of ASD. Whereas almost any study could benefit from the inclusion of additional data types, the investigation of mental illnesses – which are famously complex and heterogeneous – could greatly benefit from a higher preponderance of both multi-modal studies as well as integrated analyses using these modalities. In the *status quo*, integrated analyses are typically possible only for the most experienced researchers with expertise across data types, or for collaborations involving researchers with different areas of expertise who join efforts. Our hope, however, is that these efforts to integrate neuroimaging and genetics data from the NDAR database with leading scientific workflow technology will greatly expand the breadth of researchers able to perform rigorous, comprehensive, and insightful analyses on patients diagnosed with ASD.

References

Atkinson, J., Braddick, O.: From genes to brain development to phenotypic behavior: 'dorsal-stream vulnerability' in relation to spatial cognition, attention, and planning of actions in Williams syndrome (WS) and other developmental disorders. Prog. Brain Res. **189**, 261–283 (2011)

Dinov, I., Lozev, K., Petrosyan, P., Liu, Z., Eggert, P., Pierce, J., Zamanyan, A., Chakrapani, S., Van Horn, J., Parker, D.S., Magsipoc, R., Leung, K., Gutman, B., Woods, R., Toga, A.: Neuroimaging study designs, computational analyses and data provenance using the LONI pipeline. PLoS ONE **5**(9), e13070 (2010)

Dinov, I.D., Van Horn, J.D., Lozev, K.M., Magsipoc, R., Petrosyan, P., Liu, Z., MacKenzie-Graham, A., Eggert, P., Parker, D.S., Toga, A.W.: Efficient, distributed and interactive neuroimaging data analysis using the LONI pipeline. Front. Neuroinform. **3**, 1–10 (2009)

Gorgolewski, K., Burns, C.D., Madison, C., Clark, D., Halchenko, Y.O., Waskom, M.L., Ghosh, S.S.: Nipype: a flexible, lightweight and extensible neuroimaging data processing framework in python. Front Neuroinform **5**(3) (2011)

Kennedy, D.N.: The benefits of preparing data for sharing even when you don't. Neuroinformatics **10**(3), 223–224 (2012)

Luo, X.-Z.J., Kennedy, D.N., Cohen, Z.: Neuroimaging informatics tools and resources clearinghouse (NITRC) resource announcement. Neuroinformatics **7**(1), 55–56 (2009)

McPartland, J.C., Coffman, M., Pelphrey, K.A.: Recent advances in understanding the neural bases of autism spectrum disorder. Curr. Opin. Pediatr. **23**(6), 628–632 (2011)

MacKenzie-Graham, A.J., Payan, A., Dinov, I.D., Van Horn, J.D., Toga, A.W.: Neuroimaging data provenance using the LONI pipeline workflow environment. In: Freire, J., Koop, D., Moreau, L. (eds.) IPAW 2008. LNCS, vol. 5272, pp. 208–220. Springer, Heidelberg (2008a)

Mackenzie-Graham, A.J., Van Horn, J.D., Woods, R.P., Crawford, K.L., Toga, A.W.: Provenance in neuroimaging. Neuroimage 42(1), 178–195 (2008b)

National Autism Center: Evidence-based Practice and Autism in the Schools. Randolph, Massachusetts (2011)

Stef-Praun, T., Clifford, B., Foster, I., Hasson, U., Hategan, M., Small, S.L., Wilde, M., Zhao, Y.: Accelerating Medical Research using the Swift Workflow System. Stud. Health Technol. Inform. 126, 207–216 (2007)

Van Horn, J.D., Ball, C.A.: Domain-specific data sharing in neuroscience: what do we have to learn from each other? Neuroinformatics 6(2), 117–121 (2008)

Van Horn, J.D., Dobson, J., Woodward, J., Wilde, M., Zhao, Y., Voeckler, J., Foster, I.: Grid-based computing and the future of neuroscience computation. In: Senior, C., Russell, T., Gazzaniga, M.S. (eds.) Methods in Mind, pp. 141–170. MIT Press, Cambridge (2006)

Van Horn, J.D., Gazzaniga, M.S.: Databasing fMRI studies - toward a 'discovery science' of brain function. Nat. Rev. Neurosci. 3(4), 314–318 (2002)

Van Horn, J.D., Gazzaniga, M.S.: Why share data? Lessons learned from the fMRIDC. Neuroimage 63, 1353–1363 (2012)

Van Horn, J.D., Ishai, A.: Mapping the human brain: new insights from FMRI data sharing. Neuroinformatics 5(3), 146–153 (2007)

Reverse Engineering Measures of Clinical Care Quality: Sequential Pattern Mining

Hsuan Chiu[1(✉)] and Daniella Meeker[2]

[1] Department of Computer Science, University of California, Los Angeles, USA
cherylautumn@cs.ucla.edu
[2] Department of Preventive Medicine, University of Southern California,
Los Angeles, USA
dmeeker@usc.edu

Abstract. Pattern mining has been applied to classification problems. However, detection and analysis of frequently occurring patterns in clinical data is less studied. Instead, data-driven measures of the quality of clinical care are based on abstractions from clinical guidelines, and often are not validated on the basis of outcomes. We hypothesize that by using outcomes as a training signal, we can discover patterns of treatment that lead to better or worse than expected outcomes. Because clinical data is often censored, traditional classification algorithms are inappropriate. In addition, it is difficult to infer the latent meanings of patterns in clinical data if frequency is the only explanation. In this paper, we present a framework for discovering critical patterns in censored data. We evaluate this framework by comparing the patterns we detect with guidelines. Our framework can improve the accuracy in survival analysis and facilitate discovery of patterns of care that improve outcomes.

Keywords: Sequential pattern mining · Survival analysis

1 Introduction

The increased adoption of electronic health records (EHRs) creates new opportunities for both medical discovery and measurement of the quality of care. These activities have largely been conducted in parallel with little dialogue between researchers. The intent of this work is to describe a framework for discovering patterns of care that lead to better or worse than expected outcomes.

1.1 Electronic Clinical Quality Measures

The widespread adoption of electronic health records has led to a corresponding interest in using information capture in these applications to measure the quality of patient care. The Federal Meaningful Use program is an incentive program to healthcare providers and hospitals to encourage adoption of EHRs. They have released over 100 such measures that have been developed by expert consensus. These measures operationalize clinical guidelines into metrics that are based on transactional data

© Springer International Publishing Switzerland 2015
N. Ashish and J.-L. Ambite (Eds.): DILS 2015, LNBI 9162, pp. 208–222, 2015.
DOI: 10.1007/978-3-319-21843-4_17

elements in structured fields in the EHRs. These electronic clinical quality measures (eCQMs) are generally reported as the ratio of patients that have received high quality of care to those that have not given that a guideline applies. If a guideline is applicable to a particular patient he is in the "denominator" of the ratio- the inclusion and exclusion criteria for measure denominators are defined on the basis of EHR documentation. The measure numerator is usually either a clinical outcome (e.g. lab test results indicate good control of diabetes) or a clinical process (treatment with beta blockers). Like most metrics from transactional databases, the data elements in a quality measure come in the form of time-stamped events – most commonly the time stamp is a data entry event, but potentially also a reported time of an event, as in the history of a heart attack.

While some eCQMs are based on very complicated patterns that define a sequence of inclusion and exclusion criteria intended to increase the specificity of the applicable populations, some guidelines that have been operationalized into electronic quality measures are more straightforward. Furthermore, many quality measures that are abstracted from clinical guidelines have not been shown to have predictive validity on the basis of certain outcomes [1]. These characteristics make many eCQMs poor candidates for evaluating our framework, but also demonstrate the need for a framework that links process of care to outcomes. Some of the simplest eCQMs are represented by known Drug-Drug-Interactions (DDIs) – patients concurrently exposed to two drugs known to interact are likely to have worse outcomes than similar patients that were not exposed to both drugs. The knowledgebase of DDI is standardized and well-developed, with the denominator population easily defined on the basis of exposure to one of two drugs known to interact. For these reasons, we can assess the face validity of our results on the basis of our ability to detect DDIs.

1.2   Methods for Mining Clinical Data

Large observational datasets provide a valuable compliment to the gold standard of randomized clinical trials. It has often been pointed out that clinical trials have a careful selection of uncomplicated subjects that may not reflect real-world exposures [2, 3]. A less frequently acknowledged value conferred by observational analyses is a richer complexity of treatment histories and combinations of exposures to multiple therapies. Therefore, some data mining approaches like text mining [4], temporal pattern mining [5, 6] or sequential pattern mining (SPM) [7, 8] have been applied to medical data with the expectation of accelerating novel knowledge discovery. However, some new issues are raised after these general data mining techniques are directly applied to medical data.

Data mining in medicine is differentiated from other fields insofar as the notion of "comprehensibility" plays an important role [9], and hypothesis-generating studies such as these must also have external validity and comport with clinical models. Because observational studies cannot control for selection bias, they must be conducted and interpreted carefully for purposes of causal inference [10]. Therefore, one big issue raised from data mining results, such as sequential pattern mining, is the interpretation difficulty because results are mined according to frequency, which not only generates too many similar patterns but also hard to explain these patterns' latent meaning.

Outside of biomedical literature, sequential pattern mining has been more broadly adopted to solve classification problems. For example, Cheng et al. [11, 12] applied the discriminative pattern mining on software failure detection and trajectories on road network classification. While classifiers, such as logistic regression or SVM [13] are commonly used tools in biomedical literature and data mining, important methods in a clinical data analyst's arsenal are survival analyses.

Survival analysis accounts for censoring – the lack of complete follow up on outcomes used to train classification algorithms. Most clinical data where outcomes can only be observed after extended time has elapsed have this limitation. Censoring means the precise survival time cannot be fully captured by the observational data. For example, suppose two patients who entered our dataset at age 90, one of which was observed for 8 years before he died and the other was observed for 6 months before becoming lost to follow up. At the end of the study, we do not know the actual survival time of the patient followed up to 6 months because his outcome, death, is not observed. In terms of modeling censored data, survival analysis is better than classification because survival analysis accounts not only for the likelihood of outcomes and exposure of interest, but also for the likelihood that each subject could have been observed given the observation length. Using binary classification to model censored data has several drawbacks. First, we cannot simply classify patients as "alive" or "dead" because some actual outcomes may not be observed. Second, the number of observed events is typically significantly undersized in the population, leading to a skewed dataset.

So far, discovering critical patterns in censored data is less studied. Mining critical patterns help researchers identify which patterns play key roles in the survival probability. For purposes of causal inference, it is also important to interpret the latent meanings of patterns, such as their relative influence upon the survival probability.

Considering the problems mentioned above, we will solve two problems in this paper. First, we discover a set of critical sequential patterns, which have stronger relationships with the survival outcome after an incident diagnosis from the censored data. For example, if we incorporate these patterns as covariates into survival analysis, such as *Cox proportional hazard regression model* [14], these patterns should perform as reliable predictors. Secondly, we expect the latent meanings of these critical patterns to be interpretable, such as to what extent these critical patterns influence the survival outcome. To the best of our knowledge, mining the critical sequential patterns in the censoring data for survival analysis is are yet to be studied.

The rest of the paper is structured as follows: In Sect. 2, we discuss related work about data mining in health data. Our framework about how to discover reliable frequent patterns as covariates is introduced in Sect. 3. In Sect. 4, we present the experimental evaluations. Lastly, we conclude the paper with study limitation and future work in Sect. 5.

2   Related Work

2.1   Care Pathways, Treatment Patterns, and Outcomes in Healthcare Databases

Treatment guidelines and care pathways are currently developed primarily by deliberative expert consensus to promote the practice of "evidence based medicine". The evidence under consideration is typically in the form of a systematic review of the literature, with higher 'evidence value' being placed on randomized clinical trials that may or may not have ecological validity. These care pathways are often operationalized into quality indicators and performance metrics as process measures that inform policy and, in turn, practice. Despite this careful attention to evidence in the literature, and acknowledgement of the importance of predictive validity by organizations such as the National Quality Forum, there have been few studies investigating whether pathways and patterns in quality indicators are indeed associated with better outcomes in the real world after adjusting for underlying risk factors. We argue that there is not only a need to bolster the evidence that "evidence-based medicine" is effective, but also that there may be undiscovered patterns and pathways that lead to *better than expected* outcomes that exploratory analysis might surface as candidates for quality indicators.

By contrast, there has been extensive attention to *worse than expected* outcomes for drug treatments in the field of pharmacovigilance [15]. These studies, while originally focused on adverse event reporting databases, soon extended to include analysis of the same data sources that are being used to compute performance metrics – administrative claims and electronic medical records. These studies have fallen into two categories – (1) post-market surveillance in the form of risk-adjusted hypothesis testing (with a focus on specific drugs and outcomes) and (2) exploratory data mining to potentially identify new patterns. While the first category of work has generated substantial innovations in risk-adjustment methods that are relevant to addressing selection bias [16] (a primary limitation of observational data analysis), we are more interested in the second category for the purposes of this work. In addition to conventional association mining between a single drug and a single outcome in the form of disproportionality analysis, there have been studies that have explored combinations and sequences to generate new hypotheses about combinations of drugs [17] and methods for detecting interesting temporal patterns [18]. Similar to genome-wide association studies, this type of exploratory analysis requires insuring against spurious correlations and multiple comparisons [9, 19].

2.2   Pattern Mining in Medical Domain

Currently, applying data mining to medical data is a growing trend and most data mining applications in medical fields are directly using the state of art approaches like classical classifier, clustering or association rules to derive results [20]. However, directly applying these generalized methods to health data still cannot achieve satisfied expectations. In health studies, survival analysis is one of the most important statistical approaches. Since the health data is often censored due to the termination of a study or the failure to follow-up observation subject, usually the outcome of interest in survival analysis is the time-to-event data. Thus far, there are only a few works studied in the relationship between frequent sequential treatment patterns and survival time. Silva et al. [8] studied how to evaluate the relationship between survival time with sequential treatment patterns. They used Kaplan Meier [21] to estimate the median survival time among a set of patients who have the same treatment patterns and further pruned out patterns with shorter median survival time. In our work, we further examine how each sequential treatment pattern will influence the survival probability. Malhotra et al. [7] also used a sequential pattern mining technique to retrieve frequent sequential treatment patterns for Glioblastoma Multiforme (GBM). They formulate their problem as a classification problem, and use these sequential treatment patterns as additional features to predict whether a patient can survive longer than the median survival period or not. In our work, we consider using Cox proportional hazard regression instead of classification to model the survival problem since most health data contains censored issues.

3   Framework

3.1   Data Description

Source of Data. The primary source of data for this study was administrative claims submitted to insurance companies by healthcare providers to receive reimbursement for services. Administrative claims lack the clinical detail that might be present in electronic health records, but have the benefit of capturing care and outcomes across all of the healthcare providers from whom a patient has received care. These administrative data sets were aggregated and cleaned by the Innovation in Medical Evidence Development and Surveillances (IMEDS) lab [22] hosted by Reagan-Udall Foundation for the FDA. This clinical data is translated into standardized vocabularies containing all of the medical code sets, terminologies, vocabularies and ontologies taxonomies. Drugs are also coded with RxNorm, which is a drug reference terminology maintained by the National Library of Medicine (NLM), and conforms to the Observational Medical Outcomes Partnership (OMOP) Common Data Model originally developed by the Foundation for the National Institutes of Health (http://omop.fnih.org).

Clinical Population. We randomly sampled 42,365 patients from a total of 1,027,339 patients diagnosed with Congestive Heart Failure (CHF) between January 1, 2003 and March 31, 2003. Among these 42,365 patients, 1,599 death events were observed. We used gender, Deyo's Charlson Comorbidity Index Variables, [23] and the age at CHF index diagnosis date as a part of patient features. Summary statistics are listed in Table 1. We used random samples of 42,365 patients to run the experiments due to computational constraints. This approach is valid for the following reasons: (1) We wished to verify whether frequent patterns can perform as reliable predictors in censored data, and (2) We want to ascertain whether the latent meaning of frequent patterns can be discovered through our method. Our experiments show that our framework has potential for achieving these goals.

Table 1. Population description.

Covariate	Proportion (%)
Male	54.04
Myocardial Infarction	8.90
Peripheral Vascular Disease	3.05
Cerebrovascular Disease	12.27
Dementia	0.28
Chronic Pulmonary Disease	27.53
Rheumatologic Disease	4.24
Peptic Ulcer Disease	2.11
Mild Liver Disease	1.75
Diabetes	33.42
Diabetes with Chronic Complications	9.10
Hemiplegia or Paraplegia	1.07
Renal Disease	10.08
Moderate or Severe Liver Disease	5.86
AIDS	0.43

Covariate	Min	Max	Mean	Std
Age on Index Date (years)	0	89	53	11.5

3.2   Framework Overview

We briefly introduce our framework and then illustrate details in each section. Initially, we set a censored date and randomly sample a set of patients with demographic, disease and drug information. Then, we construct two types of features for each patient. The first are baseline characteristics composed of demographic and health status at index diagnosis, and another is the treatment feature type derived from sequential pattern mining. Because the quantity of treatment features may grow to more than 5,000, when we relax the support threshold, we screen out those inactive features before we incorporate them into Cox regression model. Thus, we take two screening strategies to do the ranking. We select only top-K treatments after controlling for baseline health status and age in the Cox model. We hypothesize that the screening strategy can reliably bring predictive patterns into the model.

3.3   Feature Generation

In our study, we generate two types of feature for patients. The first are baseline characteristics that cannot be changed during the course of medical care, such as age at index diagnosis, sex and comorbidity diseases listed in Table 1. For each patient, the first date that s/he was diagnosed with CHF is referred to as index date. The comorbid disease features are based on Charlson Comorbidity Index Indicators [23] – 13 diseases coded by ICD9 (International Classification of Diseases and Related Health Problem, v9) such as renal disease, liver disease and HIV. For example, if a CHF patient also has liver disease and heart disease before the index date, we will assign a binary value 1 in these two features. By controlling for these covariates we will detect patterns that arise independent of health status.

The covariates of interest in this work (treatment covariates) are the treatment sequence after the index date. We build treatment covariates by using sequential pattern mining to extract patterns from patients' drug history after the index date. We view patients' drug history as a transaction database D which contains a set of tuples (pid, tid, Itemset), where pid is a patient id, tid is a transaction id based on the prescription time, and Itemset is a set of drugs prescribed on the same day. All these tuples with the same pid can be regarded as a sequence of itemsets ordered by increasing tid. Thus, we can leverage the state-of-the-art sequential pattern mining algorithm to generate a set of frequent sequential patterns as treatment patterns.

In this work, we leverage SPADE [24] and VMSP [25] as our sequential pattern mining approach. The difference between SPADE and VMSP is that the former generates a complete set of frequent patterns while the latter generates maximum length frequent patterns. Treatment covariates are denoted as binary value. If a frequent pattern occurs in a patient's sequence, we assign it as true; otherwise we label it as false.

3.4   Feature Screening

So far, we generate a feature set including patients' demographic information, given health conditions and a set of frequent sequential treatment patterns. When the number of patterns is massive, only critical patterns are necessary for building a regression model. Most regression models leverage feature selection strategy by adding a specific penalty function into the regression model. When the quantity of covariates and the sample size are large, high computational cost makes this method inefficient. In this work, we are focusing on how to effectively select critical patterns before we use them to train a regression model. We also do not want to limit the feature selection strategy for a certain type regression model. Here we provide two approaches to achieve pruning.

Model-free Screening. To estimate the discriminative power of a feature, we leverage the novel feature screening method proposed by Zhu et al. [26]. The most distinguishable point of their method, Model-free screening (MFS), is that the ranking procedure widely covers many parametric and semi-parametric models, such as linear regression, logistic regression and Cox proportional hazard regression. When the number of covariates is huge and the information about the underlying model is limited, MFS provides a great flexibility to rank these features.

In MFS, covariates $\mathbb{Z} = (Z_1, Z_2, \ldots, Z_p)^T$ are classified into two sets, active predictors with non-zero coefficient, $\mathbb{Z}_A$, and inactive predictors with zero coefficients $\mathbb{Z}_I$. Their method claims that $\mathbb{Z}_A$ can be consistently ranked before $\mathbb{Z}_I$.

Given a sample with size n, they use $\widehat{w_k}$ as a natural estimator for measuring the marginal utility of the k'th element in $\mathbb{Z}$, where

$$\widehat{w_k} = \frac{1}{n}\sum\nolimits_{j=1}^{n}\{\frac{1}{n}\sum\nolimits_{i=1}^{n}\mathbb{Z}_{ik}I(Y_i < Y_j)\}^2$$

with assumptions $\frac{1}{n}\sum_{i=1}^{n}\mathbb{Z}_{ik} = 0$ and $\frac{1}{n}\sum_{i=1}^{n}\mathbb{Z}_{ik}^2 = 1$. By ranking $\widehat{w_k}$ in descending order, their approach is claimed to consistently screen out inactive predictors. To implement their ranking method, the first step is to rank tuples in the sample set according to the outcome variable Y in ascending order. Next, calculating $\widehat{w_k}$ for each covariate is through scanning $\mathbb{Z}_k$ value in n tuples. Lastly, order the p covariates by $\widehat{w_k}$ in descending sequence. The complexity requires $O(n\log n + np + p\log p)$.

Maximized Coverage Screening. We can observe that when the sample size n goes large, the complexity of MFS will be dominated by $O(np)$. In this work, we provide another heuristic strategy to rank these features in a more efficient way.

Our basic idea is to choose the feature with maximized coverage of data points in each round. At the first step, we rank sequential patterns by supports in descending order. Then, we pick the one with the widest coverage rate, which means the largest number of individuals who own this feature. If more than one feature contain the same highest coverage rate, we choose the feature with the highest support. After we select a feature, all individuals having this feature will be eliminated. In the next iteration, the identical choosing strategy is applied, but to a smaller set of individuals. When all individuals are eliminated, we recover all individuals back and we continue the selection procedure until all features are ranked.

In order to efficiently select the feature with the highest coverage rate, we use the bitmap representation to denote how a sequential pattern distributes among individuals in the sample dataset. Initially, we have an empty bitmap, BM_{all}, with length $|BM_{all}| = n$ and all bits in the BM_{all} are set to zero. For each sequential pattern i, a bitmap BM_i is created and the index of each bit in a bitmap represents each individual in the dataset. If a sequential pattern i occurs in individual j's sequence, the j'th bit will be set to one in i's bitmap, $BM_i(j) = 1$; otherwise, $BM_i(j) = 0$. We apply BM_i ANDNOT BM_{all}, and then counting the cardinality of BM_i, meaning the number of new individuals are covered by the feature i in current iteration. After the highest coverage sequential pattern h derived in current iteration, we simply use BM_h OR BM_{all} to represent how many individuals are already covered so far. Then in the next round, we use the updated BM_{all} to discover the next candidate among the rest sequential patterns. Once all bits in BM_{all} are set to one, we reset the BM_{all}. The ranking process is continued until all sequential patterns are ranked. Since computing the coverage rate can be regarded as constant time by implementing in bitmap, the total cost is bounded by $O(p^2)$.

Algorithm. Maximize Coverage Screening

```
Input: Frequent sequential_pattern_set F
Output: An ordered selected pattern set Fₛ
Sort patterns in F according to support in descending order.
currentCoverage←0
maxCoverage←0
BMₐₗₗ ←clear each bits
BMₘₐₓ ←clear each bits
While F is not null
   For each pattern p in F, do
      BMₚ.ANDNOT(BMₐₗₗ)
        currentCoverage← |BMₚ|
        if currentCoverage > maxCoverage
         maxCoverage=currentCoverage;
          BMₘₐₓ = BMₚ
    if BMₘₐₓ is not null
      BMₐₗₗ.OR(BMₘₐₓ)
      F.remove(pattern max)
      Fₛ.add(pattern max)
    else BMₐₗₗ ←clear each bits
 end
 return Fₛ
```

3.5   Feature Construction

In our study, we leverage both immutable covariates and treatment covariates as features in the Cox model. After we rank treatment covariates either by MFS or by Maximized Coverage, only top-K patterns will be incorporated into the regression model. The reason that we need to include immutable covariates is we do not want to incorrectly assume people are dying because of the drug rather than the illness. We set a censored date as the termination of the observation, and we set the event as death. Finally, we leverage immutable covariates, treatment covariates and outcomes to train the Cox model.

4 Experimental Evaluation

In this section, we evaluate the performance of the Cox model incorporated with frequent patterns. All experiments are conducted on 8 EC2 Compute Units (4 virtual cores with 2 EC2 Compute Units each) with 15 GB of main memory, running on Linux 64-bit platform.

Our goal in this study is to select critical sequential patterns as covariates in the Cox regression adjusted for underlying risk. We expect that the selected sequential patterns can be sufficient enough to perform as reliable predictors in the Cox regression. In our evaluation, as the response variable of Cox regression contains both binary and continuous variable which associate with time, we chose to use RisksetAUC [27] as our main measurement.

4.1 Approaches for Comparison

We compare three different ranking mechanisms to order sequential patterns and we apply the greedy forward selection to iteratively pick top-K sequential patterns as Cox regression covariates. For each Cox regression, we measure the RisksetAUC value as the performance. The benchmark ranking method is to order sequential patterns by the support value from high to low. The other two ranking methods are MFS and Maximized coverage.

The experiment data is extracted randomly from IMEDS with medical records ranging from January 1, 2003 to March 31, 2013 among 1,027,339 CHF patients. Initially we set censored date on October 10, 2014 and we randomly selected 42,365 patients. Next, we apply both SPADE and VMSP in package spmf [28], with setting minimum support threshold 0.1, 0.05 and 0.025. Table 2 shows the number of sequential patterns generated in dataset DS2014.

Table 2. The number of features generated.

Method	SPADE			VMSP		
Threshold	0.1	0.05	0.025	0.1	0.05	0.025
Number of Patterns	85	643	5162	59	373	2,750

4.2 Results

Accuracy of Survival Analysis Controlling for Charlson Index Indicators in Absence of Treatment Covariates. Table 3 shows coefficients of Cox model trained with patients' immutable features in dataset DS2014. Positive coefficient represents a patient that has that feature, and his hazard ratio is expected to increase. We can see that most coefficients are positive and this result is reasonable since comorbid diseases denoted in Charlson index indeed have the potential to increase the risk among each other.

Table 3. Coefficients and accuracy of immutable features.

	Coef	p-value
Gender	0.002	0.278
Myocardial Infarction	0.205	0.013
Peripheral Vascular Disease	0.050	0.699
Cerebrovascular Disease	−0.004	0.958
Dementia	−0.231	0.609
Chronic Pulmonary Disease	0.369	0
Rheumatologic Disease	0.313	0.002
Peptic Ulcer Disease	0.308	0.019
Mild Liver Disease	1.070	0
Diabetes	0.058	0.323
Diabetes with Chronic Complications	0.217	0.008
Hemiplegia or Paraplegia	0.926	0
Renal Disease	0.884	0
Moderate or Severe Liver Disease	0.619	0
AIDS	0.949	0
Age on Index Date	0.035	0
AUC	0.648	

Accuracy Results. Since the feature set of the Cox model can be formed by three ranking mechanisms, (support, MFS and Maximized coverage), we compare how these ranking methods affect the Cox model accuracy when we incorporate top-K features into the model. In each figure, we list the total number of patterns generated by the pattern mining algorithm associated with a threshold. For example, the main title, SPADE_0.1, in Fig. 1a means we apply SPADE with threshold 0.1 to generate frequent patterns and we obtain total 85 patterns in this case. The accuracy depicted in all figures starts from the base AUC, 0.648.

In some cases, including all patterns into the model is allowable, such as Fig. 1a and d. However, in some other cases, not all patterns are suitable to be fully incorporated due to the large number of patterns, such as Fig. 1c and f. Thus, the feature screen strategy is important in the latter scenarios. For example, in Fig. 1c, if we select only 10 % of features into the Cox model and attain higher than 85 % accuracy, this implies that these features are sufficient to play as reliable predictors for the dataset.

From Fig. 1 we can observe that the base accuracy is enhanced significantly when we bring these patterns into the model initially, and then the accuracy grows stable until all features are included. Compare to MFS and Maximized coverage, we also observe that the support ranking strategy does not effectively choose reliable predictors into top-K feature set in most cases because the RisksetAUC of support does not show competitive accuracy until we include all features into the Cox model, such as Fig. 1a and d. This implies that patterns chosen by support may not be sufficient enough to explain the outcome unless we apply all patterns to describe it. Next, we can view that features filtered by MFS provide highest accuracy when we include only a few of them into the model. When we incorporate more covariates, Maximized coverage is able to support equal or higher discriminative ability. This observation delivers flexibility of choosing the ranking strategy from MFS or Maximized coverage. For example, if we want to preserve just a few features, such as the number is less than 100, MFS will be a good option for feature screening. However, if we want to keep more features at the beginning because the size of frequent pattern is large (such as more than 5000), Maximized Coverage serves as a better choice. The reason is that Maximized Coverage not only saves more computation time, especially when the number of features and the number of tuples are massive, but also attains equal or higher accuracy than MFS.

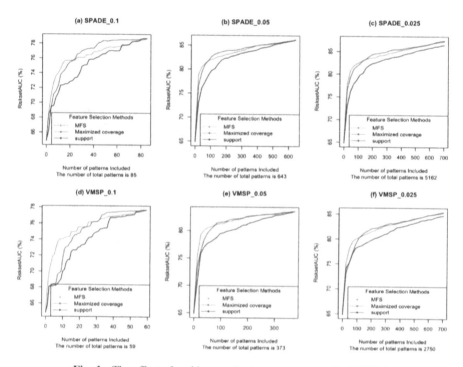

Fig. 1. The effect of ranking mechanism on accuracy for DS2014.

Empirical Validation. In this section, we want to ascertain the validity of our selected critical patterns, and we use drug-drug interaction (DDI) as our sanity check. We run a simple validation as following. For each Cox model, we apply Benjamin Hochberg method to adjust each feature's p-value for reducing false discovery rate, and then we select positive coefficient feature with adjusted p-value less than 0.05. The latent meaning of the selected feature is: (1) this feature is significantly related to the outcome, and (2) if a patient has this feature, his hazard ratio is expected to increase. Next, we use external knowledgebase [29] to see whether this selected pattern contains known DDI. The external knowledgebase classifies DDI into two levels, moderate and severe. If the selected pattern contains DDI, we list it in the results.

We use Cox models trained from DS2014 to run the DDI validation. Frequent patterns are generated by VMSP with threshold 0.05, and patterns are ordered by support, MFS and Maximized Coverage, respectively. Due to space constraints, we only list distinct patterns detected with DDI in Table 4. For example, in Table 4, when the Cox model incorporating top 120 patterns, ranked by MFS, as covariates, the pattern {Acetaminophen → Warfarin} is significant and this pattern with positive coefficient is also verified as having severe DDI. We observe that our proposed framework has potential to select truly critical patterns and some of their latent meanings can be verified. For the other significant patterns, they might be candidates in new medical knowledge discovery after further investigation with medical domain experts.

Table 4. Verified DDI patterns mined by VMSP

	PtnN	DDI	Coef	adjP	Drug sequence
Support	48	Moderate	0.353	0.001	Furosemide → Albuterol
	84	Moderate	0.450	0.000	salmeterol fluticasone
	132	Moderate	0.343	0.049	Azithromycin → Prednisone
	228	Severe	0.350	0.044	Acetaminophen → Warfarin
	348	Moderate	0.408	0.041	Lisinopril → Furosemide
MFS	120	Severe	0.349	0.001	Acetaminophen → Warfarin
	132	Severe	0.324	0.018	Furosemide → Warfarin
	288	Moderate	0.384	0.040	Albuterol → Prednisone
	300	Severe	0.384	0.045	Azithromycin → Levofloxacin
	312	Moderate	0.520	0.000	salmeterol fluticasone
	336	Moderate	0.396	0.047	Lisinopril → Furosemide
Maximized coverage	60	Moderate	0.216	0.039	salmeterol fluticasone
	72	Moderate	0.303	0.008	Lisinopril → Furosemide
	96	Moderate	0.228	0.049	Furosemide → Albuterol
	132	Moderate	0.351	0.023	Albuterol → Prednisone

5 Conclusion

In this paper, we proposed a framework to efficiently discover critical sequential patterns as reliable predictors in censored data. We used Cox regression to model the censored data in order to avoid the skewed data problem in classification. We applied SPM to generate frequent patterns and we provide two feature-ranking methods, MFS and Maximized coverage, to select important patterns. Our main contribution is to accurately screen out those insignificant but frequent sequential patterns. In experiments, we demonstrated that the discovered sequential patterns are able to improve the prediction accuracy, and we also showed that the Cox regression model provides a better way to explain the latent meaning of sequential patterns.

The framework we adopted has some limitations that might be addressed in future work. By adopting an epidemiological framework that holds fixed the disease state at the index date of CHF diagnosis, we are not addressing the dynamic nature of disease evolution and the challenges associated multi-morbid patients and complex interactions between disease, side-effects, and treatments. In future work, we might consider Bayesian networks to help disentangle some of these confounding effects and incorporate knowledge that has been generated in hypothesis-driven research. This approach would help resolve confounding concerns between drugs used to treat conditions that evolve after the index date and indications that may be side-effects.

References

1. Mant, J.: Process versus outcome indicators in the assessment of quality of health care. Int. J. Qual. Heal. Care **13**, 475–480 (2001)
2. Delen, D., Walker, G., Kadam, A.: Predicting breast cancer survivability: A comparison of three data mining methods. Artif. Intell. Med. **34**(2), 113–127 (2005)
3. D'Agostinio, R.S., D'Agostinio, R.J.: Estimating treatment effects using observational data. J. Am. Med. Assoc. **297**(3), 314–316 (2007)
4. Shetty, K.D., Dalal, S.R.: Using information mining of the medical literature to improve drug safety. J. Am. Med. Inform. Assoc. **18**(5), 668–674 (2011)
5. Nor, G.N., Bate, A., Hopstadius, J., Star, K., Edwards, I.R.: Temporal Pattern Discovery for Trends and Transient Effects: Its Application to Patient Records, pp. 963–971. ACM, New York (2008)
6. Norén, G.N., Hopstadius, J., Bate, A., Star, K., Edwards, I.R.: Temporal pattern discovery in longitudinal electronic patient records. Data Min. Knowl. Disc. **20**, 361–387 (2010)
7. Malhotra, K., Chau, D.H., Sun, J., Hadjipanayis, C., Navathe, S.B.: Temporal event sequence mining for glioblastoma survival prediction. In: KDD 2014 Workshop on Health Informatics (HI-KDD 2014) (2014)
8. Silva, A., Meira Jr., W., Queiroz, O., Cherchiglia, M.: Sequential medical treatment mining for survival analysis. In: SBBD 2009, pp. 166–180 (2009)
9. Bellazzi, R., Zupan, B.: Predictive data mining in clinical medicine: Current issues and guidelines. Int. J. Med. Inform. **77**(2), 81–97 (2008)
10. Fisher, E.S., Wennberg, D.E., Alter, D.A., Vermeulen, M.J.: Analysis of observational studies in the presences of treatment selection bias: Effects of invasive cardiac management on AMI survival using propensity score and instrumental variable methods. J. Am. Med. Assoc. **297**(3), 278–285 (2007)
11. Lee, J.G., Han, J., Li, X., Cheng, H.: Mining discriminative patterns for classifying trajectories on road networks. IEEE Trans. Knowl. Data Eng. **23**(5), 712–726 (2011)
12. Lo, D., Cheng, H., Han, J., Khoo, S.C., Sun, C.: Classification of software behaviors for failure detection: A discriminative pattern mining approach. In: Proceedings of the 15th ACM SIGKDD International Conference on Knowledge Discovery and Data Mining, vol. 73, no. 2, pp. 557–565 (2009)
13. Cortes, C., Vapnik, V.: Support-vector networks. Mach. Learn. **20**, 273–297 (1995)
14. Cox, D.R.: Regression models and life tables. J. R. Stat. Soc. Ser. B **34**(2), 187–220 (1972)
15. Liu, M., Matheny, M.E., Hu, Y., Xu, H.: Data mining methodologies for pharmacovigilance. SIGKDD Explor. Newsl. **14**, 35–42 (2012)

16. Schneeweiss, S., Rassen, J.A., Glynn, R.J., Avorn, J., Mogun, H., Brookhart, M.A.: High-dimensional propensity score adjustment in studies of treatment effects using health care claims data. Epidemiology **20**(4), 512–522 (2009)

17. Tatonetti, N.P., Denny, J.C., Murphy, S.N., Fernald, G.H., Krishnan, G., Castro, V., Yue, P., Tsau, P.S., Kohane, I., Roden, D.M., Altman, R.B.: Detecting drug interactions from adverse-event reports: interaction between paroxetine and pravastatin increases blood glucose levels. Clin. Pharmacol. Ther. **90**(1), 133–142 (2011)

18. Jin, H., Chen, J., He, H., Williams, G.J., Kelman, C., O'Keefe, C.M.: Mining unexpected temporal associations: Applications in detecting adverse drug reactions. IEEE Trans. Inf Technol. Biomed. **12**(4), 488–500 (2008)

19. Mazlack, L.J.: Using association rules without understanding their underlying causality reduces their decision value, pp. 312–319 (2004)

20. Esfandiari, N., Babavalian, M.R., Moghadam, A.-M.E., Tabar, V.K.: Knowledge discovery in medicine: Current issue and future trend. Expert Syst. Appl. **41**(9), 4434–4463 (2014)

21. Kleinbaum, G.D., Klein, M.: Survival Analysis: A Self-Learning Text. Statistics for Biology and Health, 3rd edn. Springer, New York (2011)

22. IMED. http://imeds.reaganudall.org/

23. Deyo, R.A., Cherkin, D.C., Ciol, M.A.: Adapting a clinical comorbidity index for use with ICD-9-CM administrative databases. J. Clin. Epidemiol. **45**(6), 613–619 (1992)

24. Zaki, M.: SPADE: An efficient algorithm for mining frequent sequences. Mach. Learn. **42**(1), 31–60 (2001)

25. Fournier-Viger, P., Wu, C.-W., Gomariz, A., Tseng, V.S.: VMSP: Efficient vertical mining of maximal sequential patterns. In: Sokolova, M., van Beek, P. (eds.) Canadian AI. LNCS, vol. 8436, pp. 83–94. Springer, Heidelberg (2014)

26. Zhu, L.-P., Li, L., Li, R., Zhu, L.-X.: Model-free feature screening for ultrahigh-dimensional data. J. Am. Stat. Assoc. **106**(496), 1464–1475 (2011)

27. Heagerty, P.J., Zheng, Y.: Survival model predictive accuracy and ROC curves 1. Biometrics **61**(March), 92–105 (2005)

28. spmf. An Open-Source Data Mining Library. http://www.philippe-fournier-viger.com/spmf

29. Healthline. http://www.healthline.com/druginteractions

Inference and Verification of Probabilistic Graphical Models from High-Dimensional Data

Yinjiao Ma[1], Kevin Damazyn[2], Jakob Klinger[2], and Haijun Gong[2]($\boxtimes$)

[1] Department of Biostatistics, Saint Louis University, St. Louis, MO, USA
[2] Department of Mathematics and Comptuer Science, Saint Louis University,
220 N Grand Blvd, St. Louis, MO, USA
hgong2@slu.edu

Abstract. Probabilistic graphical modelling technique has been widely used to infer the causal relations in the network from high-dimensional data. One of the most challenging biological questions is the inference and verification of biological network, for example, gene regulatory network and signaling pathway, from high-dimensional omics data. Conditionally dependent genes and undirected network can be inferred from the independently and identically distributed static data, while the time series data can help reconstruct a directed network which is more important to our understanding of the complex biological system. Due to the curse of dimensionality and network sparsity, statistical inference algorithm alone is not efficient and realistic to infer and verify large networks. In this work, we propose a novel technique, which applies the dimensionality reduction, network inference and formal verification methods together to reconstruct some regulatory networks from the static and time-series microarray data. A graphical lasso algorithm is first applied to learn the structure of Gaussian graphical models from static data and infer some conditionally dependent genes. Then, an extended dynamic Bayesian network method is applied to reconstruct some weighted and directed networks from the time series data of selected genes, and also generate symbolic model verification code for model checking. Finally, we apply this technique to reconstruct and verify some regulatory networks in yeast and prostate cancer in response to stress and irradiation respectively for illustration.

Keywords: Dimensionality reduction · Gaussian graphical model · Graphical lasso · Dynamic Bayesian network · Model checking · Microarray · Prostate cancer

1 Introduction

High-dimensional data, including the static and time-series types, provide abundant and important information to help us understand the dynamic and temporal properties in the complex system. One of the most challenging biological questions is the inference and verification of complex biological network, for example,

© Springer International Publishing Switzerland 2015
N. Ashish and J.-L. Ambite (Eds.): DILS 2015, LNBI 9162, pp. 223–239, 2015.
DOI: 10.1007/978-3-319-21843-4_18

gene regulatory network and signaling pathway, from high-dimensional omics data. Correctly deciphering the gene regulatory networks can elucidate some fundamental biological processes in the cell and pathogenesis of some diseases. A number of machine learning and statistical inference algorithms [18,26,28], including the graphical model methods [5,6,16], have been proposed to study the gene regulatory networks (GRN) from microarray data, where, each node represents a variable, and the edge connecting two nodes indicates a possible causal relationship.

Since the chemical reactions in the regulatory network are stochastic processes, probabilistic graphical model methods have been widely used to describe the conditional dependence between two random variables in the network. Two nodes in the graph are connected if and only if they are conditionally dependent given the other variables. Gaussian graphical model (GGM) has attracted a lot of attention from computational biologists to learn network structures from static microarray data. In the Gaussian graphical models, the random variable vector X follows a multivariate Gaussian distribution with mean-vector μ and covariance matrix Σ. In the undirected graph, a missing edge implies a conditional independence between two random variables given the rest. So, the problem of inferring a GGM is equivalent to estimating an inverse covariance matrix Σ^{-1}, where the non-zero off-diagnol element indicates the existence of an edge between two nodes. Due to a large number of covariates p (e.g., genes) and insufficient observations ($n << p$), different optimization techniques [2,20], e.g., graphical lasso regularization algorithm [4], have been proposed to estimate the inverse covariance matrix and increase its sparsity through maximizing the L1-penalized log-lihelihood function. However, these techniques could only infer an undirected network, while other important information, such as the positions of genes in the pathway, upstream or downstream, activation or inhibition relationship can not be inferred.

Dynamic Bayesian network (DBN) [6,16,17,22] is a promising learning technique that can reconstruct a directed gene regulatory network with feedback loops from time-series data. Expectation-maximisation algorithm [24] can estimate the parameters in the model. DBN method is based on the first-order Markov chain, and different DBN-based softwares have been developed to increase inference accuracy and reduce computational time. However, most of these softwares can not either infer the "activation" or "inhibition" relationship between different genes in the directed network, or estimate the interaction strength. Moreover, the inferred networks are sensitive to the data discretization policies. Bayesian network inference with Java objects, called Banjo [28] which is based on DBN, can infer an optimal directed and weighted network through calculating an signed (activation or inhibition) influence score for each edge.

Another important aspect in the gene regulatory network learning is the model validation. Previous studies focus on the development of novel inference algorithms to learn a statistically optimal network, and the inferred networks are manually compared with existing database or known models, which is not realistic in the large network verification. Our work has proposed and applied a formal verification technique, called model checking, alone to study some given signaling pathways [10,11,13,14,19] in the cancer cells. Model checking [3] can automatically and exhaustively search the state space to determine whether or not a given system satisfies some desired temporal logic formula. Recently, we proposed a novel procedure [9] to apply the dynamic Bayesian network algorithm with model checking technique to infer and verify a subnetwork from time series data of yeast. In that work, we have to manually select a subset of genes to reconstruct a subnetwork, and also manually prepare the formal verification code to do model checking for each network, which is not realistic for the verification of multiple large networks.

The goal of this work is to integrate the dimensionality reduction, network inference and model checking methods to reconstruct and verify gene regulatory network from high-dimensional static and time-series microarray data. A graphical lasso algorithm is first applied to learn an undirected Gaussian graphical model and identify some conditionally dependent variables from static data. Then, a dynamic Bayesian network inference method (modified Banjo) is applied to reconstruct some directed and weighted regulatory network candidates, and also automatically generate formal verification code for each model. Finally, model checker is applied to automatically verify the inferred networks. We illustrate this technique to reconstruct and verify gene regulatory networks from the microarray data of yeast and prostate cancer.

2   Statistical Learning and Verification Methods

2.1   Dimensionality Reduction with Graphical Lasso

In this section, we assume the observations measuring the expression levels of genes in the static microarray data are independent and follow the Gaussian distribution, that is, the random vectors $\mathbf{X_1}, \ldots, \mathbf{X_n} \sim N(\mu, \Sigma_p)$, where $\mu \in R^p$ is a mean vector (p denotes the number of features or genes) and Σ_p is $p \times p$ covariance matrix. In this work, without loss of generality, we assume $\mu = 0$. The precision matrix $\Theta = \Sigma_p^{-1}$ has been used to represent the conditional independence and dependence relationship among the variables [4] in the Gaussian graphical models (GGM). A non-zero off-diagonal element ($\theta_{ij} \neq 0$) in the precision matrix indicates a dependence between two covariates, while, $\theta_{ij} = 0$ implies a conditional independence between two variables given the rest.

Inference of the GGM is equivalent to estimating the elements in an unknown precision matrix Θ, which are taken as random variables instead of fixed parameters. Then, the problem is to optimize the log-likelihood function, that is, the log of a joint probability density function which is expressed as

$$l(\mathbf{X_1}, \ldots, \mathbf{X_n}, \Theta) = log P(\mathbf{X_1}, \ldots, \mathbf{X_n}|\Theta) + log P(\Theta)$$

$$\propto \frac{n}{2} \log \det \Theta - \frac{n}{2} \text{tr}(\Theta \mathbf{S}) + log P(\Theta), \qquad (1)$$

where $\mathbf{S}$ is an observed or empirical covariance matrix of the data, and it is written as

$$\mathbf{S} = \frac{1}{n} \sum_{i=1}^{n} (\mathbf{X_i} - \bar{X})(\mathbf{X_i} - \bar{X})^T.$$

If we assume the random variables Θ follow Laplacian distribution, that is, the prior

$$\theta_{ij} \sim \frac{\lambda}{2} exp(-\lambda|\theta_{ij}|),$$

then, the likelihood function in Eq. 1 can be written as

$$l(\mathbf{X_1}, \ldots, \mathbf{X_n}, \Theta) \propto \frac{n}{2} \log \det \Theta - \frac{n}{2} \text{tr}(\Theta \mathbf{S}) - \frac{n}{2}\lambda||\Theta||_1, \tag{2}$$

Equation 2 is equivalent to the graphical lasso method which builds undirected graphs by panalizing the off-diagonal elements of Θ with an $L1$ norm proposed by Friedman et al. [4]. The optimization problem is expressed as

$$\underset{\Theta}{\text{maximize}}\ l(\Theta) = \underset{\Theta}{\text{maximize}}\{\log \det \Theta - \text{tr}(\mathbf{S}\Theta) - \lambda||\Theta||_1\}, \tag{3}$$

where λ is a nonnegative tuning parameter controling the sparsity of the matrix, and $||\Theta||_1 = \sum_{ij} |\theta_{ij}|$. That is, we need solve the following equation

$$\frac{\partial}{\partial \Theta}l(\Theta) = \Theta^{-1} - \mathbf{S} - \lambda \cdot sign(\Theta) = 0. \tag{4}$$

Algorithm 1 describes the graphical lasso based on the block-coordinate descent method which can estimate the sparse precision matrix Θ. We will briefly discuss the procedure to solve Eq. 4 proposed in [4]. Each matrix, including $\mathbf{W} = \Theta^{-1}$, Θ, and $\mathbf{S}$, will be partitioned as following:

$$\begin{pmatrix} \mathbf{W_{11}} & \mathbf{w_{12}} \\ \mathbf{w_{12}^T} & w_{22} \end{pmatrix}, \begin{pmatrix} \Theta_{11} & \theta_{12} \\ \theta_{12}^T & \theta_{22} \end{pmatrix}, \begin{pmatrix} \mathbf{S_{11}} & \mathbf{s_{12}} \\ \mathbf{s_{12}^T} & s_{22} \end{pmatrix},$$

where the sizes of $(\mathbf{W_{11}}, \Theta_{11}, \mathbf{S_{11}})$ and $(\mathbf{w_{12}}, \theta_{12}$ and $\mathbf{s_{12}})$ are $(p-1) \times (p-1)$, $(p-1) \times 1$ respectively, w_{22}, θ_{22} and s_{22} are scalars.

Algorithm 1. Graphical lasso based on a block-coordinate descent method

---

Input: Omics Data, $\mathbf{S}, \lambda$
Output: Θ, conditionally dependent variables
Initialization: $\mathbf{W} = \Theta^{-1} = \mathbf{S} + \lambda\mathbf{I}$
while $\mathbf{W}$ *is not converged* **do**
    | Partition of matrix $\mathbf{W}$ into blocks
    | Apply block-coordinate descent approach to solve L1 lasso penalized problem.
    | Update $\mathbf{w_{12}}$
end
Calculate $\theta_{22} = 1/(w_{22} - \mathbf{w_{12}^T}\mathbf{W_{11}^{-1}}\mathbf{w_{12}})$;
Calculate $\theta_{12} = -\theta_{22}\mathbf{W_{11}^{-1}}\mathbf{w_{12}}$.
return Θ;
output conditionally dependent variables.

Then, the elements in the precision matrix Θ can be expressed as $\theta_{12} = -\theta_{22}\mathbf{W}_{11}^{-1}\mathbf{w}_{12}$, and $\theta_{22} = 1/(w_{22} - \mathbf{w}_{12}^T\mathbf{W}_{11}^{-1}\mathbf{w}_{12})$, where $\mathbf{w}_{12} = -\mathbf{W}_{11}\theta_{12}/\theta_{22}$. Graphical lasso method (implemented by the R package GLASSOPATH) applies $L1$ lasso algorithm based on a block-coordinate descent method to estimate the sparse precision matrix.

We can apply the graphical lasso algorithm to infer a sparse undirected probabilistic graphical model which is composed of conditionally-dependent genes. However, biologists are more interested in the directed regulatory network which contains not only the conditional dependence information, but also the activation or inhibition relationship between two genes. Next we will introduce an extended dynamic Bayesian network inference algorithm which can reconstruct directed regulatory networks from the time series data and automatically generate formal verification code for model checking.

2.2   Directed Network Inference

In the time series microarray data, the expression levels of p genes at n different time points can be described by the random vectors $\mathbf{X}_1, \ldots, \mathbf{X}_n$, where $\mathbf{X}_i = (X_{i1}, \ldots, X_{ip})^T$ is defined as the p random variables (e.g., genes) measured at time i, and x_{ij} represents an observation value (expression level) of the random variable X_{ij}. Dynamic Bayesian network (DBN) [6,16,22] has been used to reconstruct a directed network, where each edge can be either activation or inhibition relationship between two nodes. This method is based on the first-order Markov chain assumption that, each random variable at time i is dependent on its parents at time $i - 1$ only. Therefore, a directed network can be graphically represented by a joint distribution of n random vectors over time [16], which is expressed as $P(\mathbf{X}_1, \mathbf{X}_2, \ldots, \mathbf{X}_n) = P(\mathbf{X}_1)P(\mathbf{X}_2|\mathbf{X}_1) \times \ldots \times P(\mathbf{X}_n|\mathbf{X}_{n-1})$, and $P(\mathbf{X}_i|\mathbf{X}_{i-1}) = P(X_{i1}|Par(X_{i1})) \times \ldots \times P(X_{ip}|Par(X_{ip}))$, where $Par(X_{ij})$ represents the gene j's parents at time $i - 1$ [9,16].

In this work, we use the $n \times p$ matrix $\mathbf{X}$ to represent the time-series microarray data which consists of p genes measured at n different time points, and also it is discrete. The goodness of a network is evaluated by the likelihood-equivalence Bayesian Dirichlet (BDe) scoring function proposed in Heckerman et al's work and used by many researchers in the network inference studies [9,15,16,22]. This work will apply the Bayesian network inference with Java objects [28], which is a network learning software, to calculate BDe scores. The idea is to maximize the posterior probability distribution of the network G conditional on the microarray data $\mathbf{X}$, which is written as

$$P(G|\mathbf{X}) \propto P(G, \mathbf{X}) = \int P(G, \mathbf{X}, \Theta)d\Theta = P(G) \int P(\mathbf{X}|G, \Theta)P(\Theta|G)d\Theta,$$

where, $P(G)$ is the prior of the network G, which can be chosen in different ways, for example, Friedman chose $P(G)$ based on the minimal description length (MDL) encoding of G. The BDe score function is based on the following assumptions [15]:

1. The data $\mathbf{X}$ is a multinomial sample dependent on the parameters Θ, that is, $\mathbf{X}|\Theta \sim Multinomial(\Theta)$;
2. The parameters in Θ are globally and locally independent;
3. Given a network G, the parameters in Θ follows Dirichlet distribution with a hyperparameter vector α, that is, $\Theta|G \sim Dirichlet(\alpha)$. The Dirichlet function has been given in [15, 16].
4. Two directed acyclic networks G_1, G_2 are equivalent if they encode the same joint probability distribution;
5. If the network G_1 is equivalent to G_2, the distribution function of Θ will be same in both networks.

The BDe scores for all possible networks will be calculated by the Bayesian network inference with Java objects [28], then, a greedy searching or simulated annealing algorithm proposed by Heckerman will be used to find optimal networks. Learning the activation and inhibition relationship between two genes will help us comprehensively understand the mechanism underlying the gene regulatory network. The influence score proposed in Yu et al.'s work [28] can be used to identify the activation and inhibition relationship and interaction strength. A positive influence score indicates an activation event, while a negative value corresponds to an inhibition event between two nodes. If the influence score is close to 0, the sign can not be identified based on the current time series data. The Bayesian network inference with Java objects [28] used a voting system and the value of a cumulative distribution function to estimate the influence score

$$G_{ijk}(t) = \sum_{l=0}^{k} \omega_{ijl}(t) = \sum_{l=0}^{k} P(X_{ti} = 1|Par(X_{ti}) = j). \tag{5}$$

$G_{ijk}(t)$ describes the probability that, at time t, gene X_{ti} takes a (discrete) value less than or equal to k given its parent gene takes a value of j, where, $\omega_{ijk}(t)$ is the probability that gene X_{ti} takes a value of k given its parent gene $Par(X_{ti})$ takes a value of j. The interested reader could refer to [28] for details. Algorithm 2 shows the procedure of dynamic Bayesian network inference based on BDe metrics and influence score estimation. We modified the Banjo code to search and output top n high-scoring directed networks with influence scores, and automatically generate the weighted SMV formal verification code for each network to do model checking.

Model verification is another aspect to studying the gene regulatory network due to the complexity of biological system. How to verify or falsify the network candidates inferred by the DBN? Recently, we proposed a weighted symbolic model verification (SMV) technique [9] to formally verify the networks. However, in that work [9], the regulatory subnetworks are inferred from a given subset of genes, and they are manually encoded into SMV program for model checking, which is not realistic and efficient to encode multiple large networks.

Besides the dimensionality reduction method is first used to select the conditionally dependent genes intead of manually selecting a subset of genes, another novelty in this work is that, the extended dynamic Bayesian network inference

---

Algorithm 2. Directed graph inference based on dynamic Bayesian network method

---

Input : Conditionally-dependent variables selected by Algorithm 1;
Time series data **X**
Output: Directed networks of top n BDe scores;
Symbolic model verification (SMV) code for each network.

Data Discretization;
for *each network G* **do**
    Evaluate the goodness of a network ;
        Data $\mathbf{X}|\Theta \sim Multinomial(\Theta)$;
        $\Theta|G \sim Dirichlet(\alpha)$;
        Calculate BDe score based on $P(G|\mathbf{X})$;
    Network searching;
        Network sorting based on BDe scores;
        Greedy search or simulated annealing algorithm;
    Estimate influence score;
        for *each edge $(X_i, Par(X_i))$* **do**
            Compute $\omega_{ijk}(t) = P(X_{ti} = k|Par(X_{ti}) = j)$;
            Estimate $G_{ijk}(t) = \sum_{l=0}^{k} \omega_{ijl}(t)$;
            Identify the sign and magnitude of interaction using a vote
        end
    Output top n networks;
    Generate weighted SMV code for each model.
end

---

with Java object method can automatically encode all the inferred network candidates into weighted SMV program for model checking. Next, we will introduce the weighted symbolic model checking technique used for network verification which has been discussed in our recent work [9].

2.3 Network Verification

An inferred network might be trustable only if it is consistent with the existing experiment or knowledge. Previous studies manually compared the inferred network with existing database or known models. Our recent studies [9,14] have demonstrated the power of formal verification technique in the biological studies. Model checking [3] is a powerful and automatic formal verification method, it can check whether or not a given model M satisfies a desired temporal logic formula ψ, denoted by $M \models \psi$. Different model checkers have been developed and successfully applied to verify the hardware and software systems in the past thirty years.

We have discussed the model checking technique in our recent work [9,14], for completeness, we will review some fundamental concepts and algorithms in this work. In formal verification studies, a model is described as a Kripke structure [3,12] $M = (S, s_0, R, L)$ with the initial state $s_0 \in S$, states transition relation R, and a labeling function L. SMV [21] is one of the most popular symbolic model checking tools that are encoded by ordered binary decision diagram

(OBDD) [1]. During model checking process, SMV model checker will automatically and exhaustively search the state transition system M to verify some desired property ψ which is expressed as a computation tree logic (CTL) formula. CTL formula is composed of Boolean logic connectives, temporal operators describing some property on a path and path quantifiers describing the branching structure in the computation tree. Table 1 lists these operators and the corresponding meanings. For example, $\mathbf{AG}(\mathbf{AF})\phi$ means ϕ is globally (finally) true on all paths; $\mathbf{EG}(\mathbf{EF})\phi$ means ϕ will be true always (in the future) on some path. In this work, most CTL formulas are constructed using these 6 operators: $\mathbf{AX}, \mathbf{EX}, \mathbf{AG}, \mathbf{EG}, \mathbf{AF}, \mathbf{EF}$. The interested readers could refer to [3] for more interesting operators. In the CTL syntax, the state formula and path formula are represented by ψ and ϕ respectively, and an infinite sequence of states or a path is denoted by π. The interested readers could refer to [3] for the syntax and semantics of CTL logic, and CTL formulas. After verification, the SMV model checker will output either "True" if the property is satisfied, or "False" with a counter example.

Table 1. Boolean logic connective, temporal operator and path quantifier in CTL formula.

Operators	!	|	&	$\rightarrow$	X	F	G	U	A	E
Meaning	not	or	and	implies	neXt	Future	Globally	Until	All paths	There Exists some path

Algorithm 3 (Part I) presents the weighted symbolic model checking pseudocode of SMV program that can be automatically genetated by the Algorithm 2 for each network, which is an extension of the unweighted model checking method. Similar to the unweighted model checking code, the program should start with "MODULE MAIN", and all the variables are defined and initialized by "VAR" and "init" respectively under the keyword "ASSIGN". The difference is, the state transition update for each variable is not only dependent on its parents' states, but also the *integral* influence score (only integers or Boolean values are allowed in the symbolic model checking), which is calculated by Algorithm 2. SMV model checker will automatically verify all the CTL formulas (encoded by the keyword "SPEC") to find the best models (which could be more than one candidates) satisfying all or most of the properties proposed or desired by the investigators. Part II shows the SMV algorithm based on OBDD data structure [1]. A Boolean function is applied to describe the transition relation between states implicitly. Detailed symbolic model checking algorithm and weighted SMV code have been discussed in [3,9,21].

3   Applications

In this section, we will apply the proposed integrative methods in the Algorithms 1–3 to analyze the static and time series microarray data of yeast and prostate cancer. The graphical lasso method is first applied for dimensionality reduction,

---

Algorithm 3. Weighted symbolic model checking pseudocode and SMV algorithm

---

Part I: Weighted symbolic model checking pseudocode

Input 1   : Inferred regulatory networks M by Algorithm 2;
                Temporal logic formula ψ
Output 1: True or False

for *each network* **do**
>   Variable declaration by "VAR";
>   Variable initialization by "init";
>   State update with the weighted transfer functions by "next";
>   CTL formula specification by "SPEC";
> $M \models \psi$: output True or False.
end

Part II: SMV Algorithm [3]

Input 2: A model M; desired CTL formulas f, g
Check: Take a CTL formula as its argument
Return: OBDD for the set of states that satisfy a given temporal logic formula.
Output 2: A set of states of M, which satisfy the formula.

- – if f is an atomic proposition v_i: return **Check**$(f) = v_i$;
- – if $\neg f$: return **Check**$(\neg f) = \neg$**Check**(f);
- – if $f \vee g$: return **Check**$(f) \vee$ **Check**(g);
- – if **EX**f: return **Check**(**EX**(**Check**(f)));
- – if **E**$[f$**U**$g]$: return **Check**(**EU**(**Check**(f), **Check**(g)));
- – if **EG**f: return **Check**(**EG**(**Check**(f))).

---

infer an undirected Gaussian graph model from the static data, and identify a subset of genes that are conditionally dependent. Then the dynamic Bayesian network inference method is applied to reconstruct some directed networks from the time series data of conditionally dependent genes, which will be verified by the symbolic model checking technique. The graphical lasso, modified Banjo code, and weighted SMV code developed for this work are available at http://cs.slu.edu/~gong/Research/DILS.zip.

3.1   Yeast Data Analysis

The static microarray data (Accession No: GSE19213) of the yeast studies the transcription factor Yap1 which mediates an adaptive response to oxidative stress (e.g., H_2O_2 or thiol-reactive chemicals) by regulating some protective genes [23]. For illustration, only the top around 5000 differently expressed genes (between treatment and control group) in the wild-type strain treated with H_2O_2 will be used in our studies. For simplicity, the expression levels among different probes that map to the same gene were averaged to a single value in our data analysis.

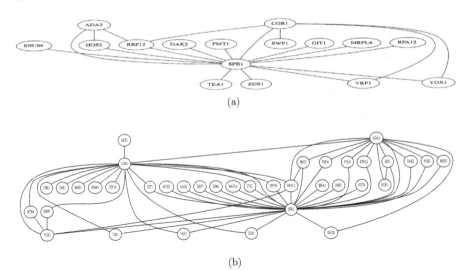

Fig. 1. Conditionally dependent genes and undirected Gaussian graph models inferred from static microarray data of yeast with different values of λ: (a) λ = 0.41, (b) λ = 0.30.

Graphical lasso method is applied with different λ values in order to infer the precision matrices ranging from a dense matrix to a sparse one, it is known that a large λ value will result in a sparse matrix. Figure 1 shows two figures with λ = 0.41 (16 genes) and λ = 0.30 (37 genes) for demonstration. More figures with a wide range of λ value are given in the online supplementary files. It is apparent that Fig. 1(a) is a subnetwork of Fig. 1(b), SPB1 and CGR1 are highly connected genes, which are also called hub genes. Goel et al's work [8] has confirmed the hub protein SPB1's important role in rRNA processing and ribosome biogenesis.

Then, the modified dynamic Bayesian network inference with Java Object is applied to reconstruct directed regulatory networks of high-BDe scores from time series microarray data and automatically output the encoded symbolic model

Table 2. Proposed CTL formulas for the network verification of yeast

	CTL formula
Property 1	A(CGR1 = 1 → AX(RRP12 = 1))
Property 2	EG(TEA1 = 1 → EF(SNU66 ≤ 0))
Property 3	AG(RRP12 = 1 → AF(SNU66 = −1))
Property 4	AG(CGR1 = 1 → AF(MRPL4 < 0 & HOS2 < 0 & VRP1 = 1))
Property 5	EG((SWF1 = 1 | FMT1= 1 → EF(RPA12 = 0 & GIT1 ≥ 0)))
Property 6	AG((SNU66 = 1 → AF(TEA1 = 1)) &(TEA1 = 1 → AF(SNU66 ≤ 0)))

verification (SMV) program for all the network candidates. The time series data (Access No: GSE62120) measure the expression levels of yeast in response to the oxidative stress (H_2O_2) with 11 time points. Only the conditionally dependent genes identified by the graphical lasso in Fig. 1 will be used for the directed network reconstruction. Since the Banjo performs well with a small number of genes, in this work, we select 16 genes for network construction. The goal is to find a network that might regulate the oxidative stress in the yeast.

Figure 2 demonstrates some directed and weighted regulatory network candidates (of top two BDe scores) based on the genes selected in the GGM with $\lambda = 0.41$ and two different discretization policies q2 (a–b) and i2 (c–d). The solid lines with arrows represent an activation event, while the circle-head arrows represent inhibition processes. The integers on the directed edges represent the

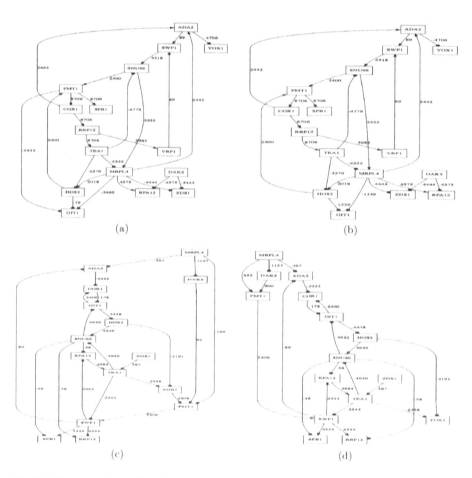

(a)　　　　　　(b)

(c)　　　　　　(d)

Fig. 2. Top two directed and weighted gene regulatory network candidates of yeast based on q2 (a–b) and i2 (c–d) discretization policies with $\lambda = 0.41$. Solid lines with arrows represent an activation event, circle-head arrows represent inhibition processes. The values on the directed edges represent the influence scores.

modified influence scores or weights, which will be used for the weighted symbolic model checking. All these network candidates take the MRPL4 gene as a hub, which plays an important role in the protein synthesis within the mitochondrion.

Figures 1 and 2 demonstrate that, given different values of λ, graphical lasso and dynamic Bayesian network inference methods could generate many statistically optimal undirected and directed network candidates. Compared with our previous work, the novelty of this method is that, the extended dynamic Bayesian network inference method, a modified Banjo, could automatically generate SMV verification code for each network candidate which will be used for model checking. Then, next step, we apply SMV model checker to verify or falsify these inferred networks through checking some putative properties that we defined in the Table 2.

Table 2 summarizes some putative CTL formulas that we assume the inferred networks should satisfy. Each gene or variable can take three possible values: $-1, 0, 1$, which denote inhibited, normal and activated, and the initial state is set to be either 0 or -1. Property 1 indicates that RRP12 might be a downstream gene of CGR1, that is, CGR1's activation will immediately activate RRP12 in the neXt step. Property 2 means, there exist a path on which TEA1's activation will finally inhibit SNU66's expression, while Property 3 means, for all paths, it is globally true that RRP12's activation will finally inhibit SNU66's activity. Property 4 and 5 are similar to property 3 and 2 respectively. Property 5 describes a negative feedback loop between SNU66 and TEA1.

Next, symbolic model checker will automatically verify or falsify all the 4 inferred networks shown in Fig. 2, and output either "True" or "False" if some property is satisfied or not respectively. Table 3 summarizes the verification results of these putative properties in 4 different models. Our methods do not intend to infer and verify only one statistically optimal network (as other researchers' work), however, the model checker will search and find one or a pool of "best-fit" networks from a number of inferred network candidates which satisfies all or most of desired temporal logic properties. Moreover, new evidence or future studies can continue to refine the "optimal" network pool with more properties. In our examples, the inferred networks in Fig. 2 (a–b), which satisfy 4 putative properties, might be better than those in Fig. 2 (c–d). But more temporal properties from the wet lab experiments will be needed to identify a really best-fit network candidate.

Table 3. Network verification results of yeast

	Property 1	Property 2	Property 3	Property 4	Property 5	Property 6
Model a	True	True	True	False	False	True
Model b	True	True	True	False	False	True
Model c	True	True	False	False	False	True
Model d	True	True	False	False	False	True

3.2   Prostate Cancer Data Analysis

The static microarray data of prostate cancer [25] contains 639 tumor samples, including 270 African-American and 369 European American patients, where 517 genes linked with prostate cancer were measured by 1,507 probes (Gene Expression Omnibus accession number GSE41969). The expression levels among different probes that map to the same gene were averaged to a single value for the data analysis. The time series data (GSE770) studied the androgen-independent LNCaP C4-2 human prostate adenocarcinoma cells following irradiation, the RNA was extracted from cells at 1, 2, 4, 6, 8, 12, 16, 20 and 24 h after irradiation, and the untreated control sample was labeled 0. Our goal is to find some networks that might be associated with the prostate cancer in response to irradiation.

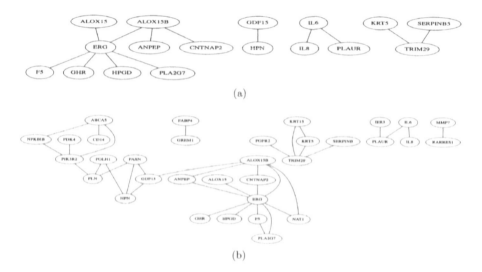

(a)

(b)

Fig. 3. Conditionally dependent genes and undirected Gaussian graph models inferred from static microarray data of prostate cancer with different values of λ: (a) $\lambda = 0.39$, (b) $\lambda = 0.32$.

Similar to the yeast data analysis, we first select some conditionally dependent genes and infer undirected Gaussian graphical models given different values of λ which are shown in the Fig. 3 ((a) $\lambda = 0.39$, (b) $\lambda = 0.32$). The highly connected genes, including ERG, ALOX15B, TRIM29 have been found to be deregulated in the prostate cancer [7]. ERG activation, one of the most common oncogenic alterations, is present in 50–70% of prostate tumors; especially, TRIM29 can negatively regulates p53 via inhibition of Tip60 [27], and it is over-expressed in lung, bladder, pancreatic and endometrial cancers, but opposite in prostate cancer.

Figure 4 shows four optimal directed and weighted network candidates of androgen-independent prostate cancer in response to irradiation based on the

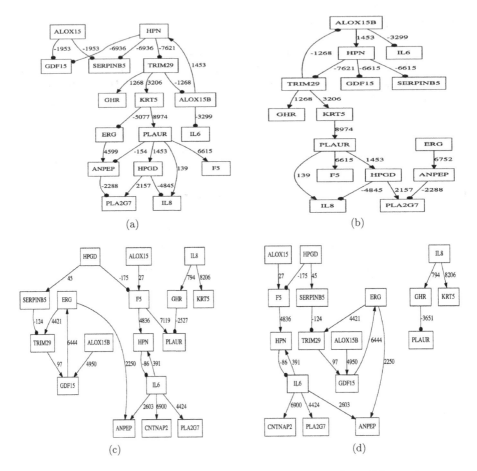

Fig. 4. Top two directed and weighted gene regulatory network candidates of prostate cancer based on $q2$ (a–b) and $i2$ (c–d) discretization policies with $\lambda = 0.39$.

conditionally dependent genes selected by GGM with $\lambda = 0.39$ and two different discretization policies $q2$ (a–b) and $i2$ (c–d) using the modified Banjo software. Besides the verification of desired properties, the model checker could also predict some properties that the future experiments can test. We proposed two predictions which describe two possible feedback loops related to the highly connected gene TRIM29. Prediction 1 incorporates two inhibition events, while Prediction 2 is composed of activation events only. The difference of these two predictions could be observed easily from the Fig. 4, which is a small network, but difficult in the large model. However, the model checker could easily and automatically find this difference in different models through checking the following two properties using the generated SMV formal verification code:

Prediction 1: AG((HPN1 $= 1 \rightarrow$ AF(TRIM29 ≤ 0)) & (TRIM29 $\leq 0 \rightarrow$ AF(ALOX15B ≥ 0)) & (ALOX15B $\geq 0 \rightarrow$ AF(HPN ≥ 0))).

Prediction 2: A((ERG = 1 → AF(TRIM29 = 1)) & (TRIM29 = 1 → AF(GDF15 = 1)) & (GDF15 = 1 → AF(ERG = 1))).

Figure 4(a–b) satisfy both predictions, but Fig. 4(c–d) only satisfy the Prediction 2. The future experiments could help validate these predictions, and help refine the inferred models of prostate cancer cells after irradiation.

4 Conclusions

Correct learning and efficient verification of complex biological networks from high dimensional data is a challenging job in systems biology. In this work, we proposed an integrative technique, which incorporates the graphical lasso, dynamic Bayesian network inference algorithm and weighted symbolic model checker, to analyze both static and time series microarray data of yeast and prostate cancer in response to oxidative stress and irradiation respectively. The graphical lasso first identified some conditionally dependent genes and inferred undirected networks from static microarray data that are associated with the oxidative stress or irradiation; then, DBN is applied to reconstruct the directed and weighted networks from time series data using different data discretization policies and automatically generate formal verification code for model checking. Compared with other researchers' work which learns only one statistically optimal network, this proposed method can both infer and verify several optimal networks that satisfy some desired temporal properties. This method is universal and applicable to any type of static and time series data, which can help us investigate the biological networks implicated in the pathogenesis of some diseases.

Our studies found the Bayesian network inference with Java objects [28] method is very sensitive to the data discretization policies, and it could learn and generate reasonably-connected networks only if the number of genes are not very large. However the gene regulatory network is large in fact and the model checking technique is powerful in the verification of large networks. Our future work will develop new learning algorithms which can handle the inference of large number of variables and take advantage of the verification power in model checking. Moreover, we will develop a GUI version to make the network learning and verification easy and convenient.

5 Contribution

HG proposed the project, YM wrote the glasso code and analyzed the microarray data, KD and JK modified the Banjo code to infer directed network and automatically generate verification code.

Acknowledgment. This work was partially supported by HG's new faculty start-up grant and President Research Fund award (230152) from the Saint Louis University.

References

1. Bryant, R.: Graph-based algorithms for boolean function manipulation. IEEE Trans. Comput. **35**(8), 677–691 (1986)
2. Celik, S., Logsdon, B., Lee, S.: Efficient dimensionality reduction for high-dimensional network estimation. JMLR **32** (2014)
3. Clarke, E.M., Grumberg, O., Peled, D.A.: Model Checking. MIT Press, Cambridge (1999)
4. Friedman, J., Hastie, T., Tibshirani, R.: Sparse inverse covariance estimation with the graphical lasso. Biostatistics **9**(3), 432–441 (2008)
5. Friedman, N., Linial, M., Nachman, I., Pe'er, D.: Using BN to analyze expression data. J. Comp. Biol. **7**, 601–620 (2000)
6. Friedman, N., Murphy, K., Russell, S.: Learning the structure of dynamic probabilistic networks. In: Proceedings of the 14th Conference on the Uncertainty in Artificial Intelligence (1998)
7. Furusato, B., Tan, S., et al.: ERG oncoprotein expression in prostate cancer: clonal progression of ERG-positive tumor cells and potential for ERG-based stratification. Prostate Cancer Prostatic Dis. **13**, 228–237 (2010)
8. Goel, A., Wilkins, M.R.: Dynamic hubs show competitive and static hubs non-competitive regulation of their interaction partners. PLoS One **7**(10), e48209 (2012)
9. Gong, H., Klinger, J., Damazyn, K., Li, X., Huang, S.: A novel procedure for statistical inference and verification of gene regulatory subnetwork. BMC Bioinformatics **16**(Suppl 7), S7 (2015)
10. Gong, H., Zuliani, P., Komuravelli, A., Faeder, J.R., Clarke, E.M.: Computational modeling and verification of signaling pathways in cancer. In: Horimoto, K., Nakatsui, M., Popov, N. (eds.) ANB 2010. LNCS, vol. 6479, pp. 117–135. Springer, Heidelberg (2012)
11. Gong, H., Zuliani, P., Komuravelli, A., Faeder, J.R., Clarke, E.M.: Analysis and verification of the HMGB1 signaling pathway. BMC Bioinformatics **11**(Supp 7), S10 (2010)
12. Gong, H.: Analysis of intercellular signal transduction in the tumor microenvironment. BMC Syst. Biol. **7**, S5 (2013)
13. Gong, H., Feng, L.: Computational analysis of the roles of ER-Golgi network in the cell cycle. BMC Syst. Biol. **8**, S4 (2014)
14. Gong, H., Feng, L.: Probabilistic verification of ER stress-induced signaling pathways. In: Proceedings of IEEE International Conference on Bioinformatics and Biomedicine (2014)
15. Heckerman, D., Geiger, D., Chickering, D.: Learning bayesian networks: the combination of knowledge and statistical data. Mach. Learn. **20**(3), 197–243 (1995)
16. Kim, S., Imoto, S., Miyano, S.: Inferring gene networks from time series microarray data using dynamic Bayesian networks. Briefings Bioinf. **4**, 228–235 (2003)
17. Kim, S., Imoto, S., Miyano, S.: Dynamic Bayesian network and nonparametric regression for nonlinear modeling of gene networks from time series gene expression data. BioSystems **75**, 57–65 (2004)
18. Liang, X., Xia, Z., Zhang, L., Wu, F.: Inference of gene regulatory subnetworks from time course gene expression data. BMC Bioinformatics **13**, S3 (2012)
19. Ma, Y., Feng, L., Guo, Y., Gong, H.: Statistical analysis and probabilistic verification of stress-induced signaling pathways. Int. J. Data Min. Bioinf. (2015)
20. Mazumder, R., Hastie, T.: The graphical lasso: new isights and alternatives. Electron. J. Stat. **6**, 2125 (2012)

21. McMillan, K.L.: Ph.D thesis: Symbolic model checking - an approach to the state explosion problem. Carnegie Mellon University (1992)
22. Ong, I., Glasner, J., Page, D.: Modelling regulatoruypathways in E. coli from time series expression profiles. Bioinformatics **18**, S241–S248 (2002)
23. Ouyang, X., Tran, Q., Goodwin, S., Wible, R., Sutter, C., Sutter, T.: Yap1 activation by H2o2 or thiol-reactive chemicals elicits distinct adaptive gene responses. Free Radic. Biol. Med. **50**, 1–13 (2011)
24. Perrin, B., Ralaivola, L., Mazurie, A., et al.: Gene networks inference using dynamic bayesian networks. Bioinformatics **74**, i138–i148 (2003)
25. Powell, I., Dyson, G., et al.: Genes associated with prostate cancer are differentially expressed in African American and European American men. Cancer Epidemiol. Biomark. Prev. **22**, 891–897 (2013)
26. Rob Smith, R., Ventura, D., Prince, J.: Controlling for confounding variables in MS-omics protocol: why modularity matters. Brief Bioinform. **15**(5), 768–770 (2014)
27. Shoa, T., Tsukiyama, T., et al.: Trim29 negatively regulates p53 via inhibition of Tip60. Mol. Cell Res. **1813**, 1245–1253 (2011)
28. Yu, J., Smith, V., Wang, P., Hartemink, A., Jarvis, E.: Advances to bayesian network inference for generating causal networks from observational biological data. Bioinformatics **20**, 3594–3603 (2004)

SPIRIT-ML: A Machine Learning Platform for Deriving Knowledge from Biomedical Datasets

Srisairam Achuthan$^{(\boxtimes)}$, Mike Chang, and Ajay Shah

Division of Research Informatics and Systems, Department of Information Sciences,
City of Hope National Medical Center, Duarte, CA 91010, USA
sachuthan@coh.org

Abstract. SPIRIT-ML (Software Platform for Integrated Research Information and Transformation - Machine Learning) is a synergistic and flexible machine learning component of integrated research informatics platform, SPIRIT, being developed at City of Hope. SPIRIT-ML is being developed to analyze varied data analysis problems in biomedical and clinical datasets to further translational research. An interactive interface, broad spectrum of data driven learning models, multiple cross-validation techniques, visualization methods and reporting metrics constitute the platform.

Keywords: Machine learning · Translational research · Platform

1 Introduction

Machine learning algorithms have been applied to solve research problems encountered routinely in various biological and clinical settings. They have been applied to identify patient cohorts based on electronic medical record (EMR) data, identify malignant tumors based on image data, and for adverse drug surveillance based on publicly available databases, to name a few [2].

A biomedical dataset containing collection of patterns can be grouped into clusters based on similarity. For example, a cohort of cancer patients can be stratified into distinct clusters based on their demographic, biological and clinical characteristics. In solving a classification problem, we are interested in predicting the outcome (class label) of the dataset by building a model based on a training dataset. Similarly, malignant and benign tumors can be classified based on tumor characteristics from breast cancer patients [3,4]. Bayesian networks can help discover the dependent and independent variables [5] in high throughput molecular dataset consisting of genes and proteins identified in gene regulatory pathways.

Significant effort is spent when various machine learning methods are applied to biomedical and clinical problems using independent one-off deployment of computational pipeline. To address this problem we extended SPIRIT platform to include an interactive interface for applying a comprehensive set of

© Springer International Publishing Switzerland 2015
N. Ashish and J.-L. Ambite (Eds.): DILS 2015, LNBI 9162, pp. 240–250, 2015.
DOI: 10.1007/978-3-319-21843-4_19

machine learning methods. SPIRIT-ML allows normalization and binning of the input data, applies uniform data validation methods and creates reports that allow users to compare results across all the methods. SPIRIT-ML is specifically designed for extracting knowledge from biomedical datasets. SPIRIT-ML comes with a standard set of machine learning algorithms. Additional algorithms can be incorporated efficiently into SPIRIT-ML.

2   Methods

Increasingly, a large number of cloud based machine learning platforms are available for large scale data analysis and predictive analytics. These include, AWS Machine Learning platform [16], H2O [17], Apache Mahout [18] etc. WEKA [19] is an open source application that integrates several machine learning algorithms for data mining tasks. WEKA has been integrated with KNIME data pipelining tool to create data analysis pipeline. Our approach is similar, but singularly focused on biomedical data.

We utilize a commercial data pipelining and scientific informatics platform (Biovia's Pipeline Pilot, [21]) to integrate several machine learning algorithms from R, MATLAB, Huggin etc. One of the advantages of SPIRIT-ML is its ability to utilize a rich source of components in Pipeline Pilot. For example, Pipeline Pilot has an extensive collection of cheminformatics components. These components enable molecular similarity analysis, prediction of toxicology profiles of molecules and molecular database searching. Combing the machine learning algorithms with these cheminformatics algorithms can provide a powerful molecular classification application. Similarly, Pipeline Pilot provides access to a wide variety of computational protocols in bioinformatics. For example, Fig. 1 is a Pipeline Pilot protocol that is available to stratify Acute Lymphoblastic Leukemia (ALL) patients based on gene expression data [1]. Starting from the gene expression data from 32 ALL patients, using pairwise differential expression component along with intensity variation component one can extract the genes that meet the selection criteria. A PCA analysis of the corresponding microarrays is able to identify two clusters of patients as seen in Fig. 2. Pipeline Pilot protocols like this when integrated with machine learning algorithms in SPIRIT-ML increases its utility.

Pipeline Pilot can also be utilized to create machine learning applications for image analysis as well as text analysis. Image segmentation, morphology, transformations, image filtering and enhancement are some of areas within image analysis with multiple Pipeline Pilot protocols potentially available to SPIRIT-ML. For example, Per Object Thresholding component within image segmentation finds a different threshold for each biological cell in an array and successfully segments all arrays. Text analysis orientated Pipeline Pilot protocols can help crawl web pages, can create ontology files from different source formats, perform local searches (by indexing Pubmed for example) etc.

The entire SPIRIT-ML platform is built on top of Pipeline Pilot, a data pipeline software that provides a web interface for accepting user specified

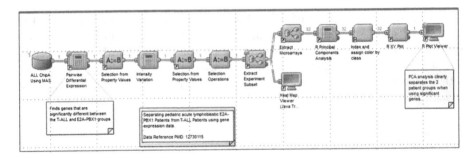

Fig. 1. A Pipeline Pilot protocol based on gene expression data to separate pediatric acute lymphoblastic E2A-PBX1 patients from T-ALL patients

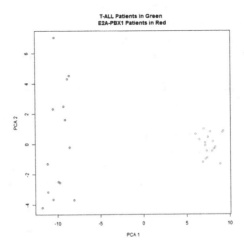

Fig. 2. A PCA of the gene expression data shows two clusters (T-ALL patients in green and E2A-PBX1 patients in red) (Color figure online)

options as well as displaying all the results obtained. Pipeline Pilot uses a data pipeling approach to handle and analyze research data. It uses a data flow framework to describe the processing of data. Algorithms written in R and MATLAB as well as external APIs provided by other scientific software applications like Hugin [20] can be integrated within the Pipeline Pilot environment. Using individual components, the entire data pre-processing, data analysis, visualization and web reporting is handled conveniently within Pipeline Pilot.

Figure 3 presents SPIRIT-ML approach to analyzing biomedical data sets. The data is grouped together as a matrix with columns containing features or attributes and rows containing observations or instances. The raw data is transformed via built-in options such as normalization and binning. Data attributes that are continuous are selected for normalization. Normalization scales the instances of each selected attribute to lie within unit range. The attributes that need to be binned can then be selected with user specified number of bins.

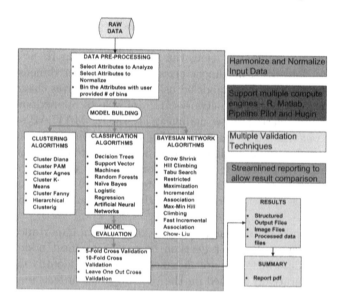

Fig. 3. SPIRIT-ML: The machine learning component of Software Platform for Integrated Research Information and Transformation. The texts in red color were implemented by using the R clustering algorithms implement in Pipeline Pilot version 9.1. The texts in green color were implemented by using different libraries in R. The texts in blue color were implanted using MATLAB (Color figure online).

SPIRIT-ML is a comprehensive framework for clustering, classifying, and deciphering relationships among covariates. It provides three types of data driven learning methods: unsupervised learning algorithms (i.e. clustering), supervised learning algorithms and Bayesian network models.

Clustering methods in SPIRIT-ML includes both hierarchical as well as non-hierarchical algorithms [6]. Agnes algorithm, an agglomerative hierarchical method, and DIANA algorithm, a divisive hierarchical method, are two hierarchical R clustering algorithms included as part of SPIRIT-ML. Non-hierarchical algorithms that are part of the clustering module of SPIRIT-ML include K-means [7], PAM and CLARA that can deal with large datasets. We have also implemented Cluster Fanny, a fuzzy clustering algorithm. Except, K-Means, all unsupervised learning algorithms are implemented using the cluster library in R. The K-Means algorithm is implemented using the stats library in R. Hierarchical algorithms with well known distance based metrics like Euclidean and Chebychev available in MATLAB are implemented in the SPIRIT-ML platform.

For classification problems, the transformed data is distributed with a fixed percentage utilized for training (usually 70 %), validating (15 %) and testing purposes (15 %) prior to developing the learning models. This is part of all R and MATLAB codes integrated within SPIRIT-ML. Decision tree [8] algorithm using the rpart library and C5.0 algorithm [9] using the C50 library were implemented in R. These algorithms help convert the features into rules/decisions driven by the underlying data. Support Vector Machines (SVMs) [10] and Naïve Bayes algorithms [4] were implanted using the e1071 package in R. SVMs are useful to separate datasets using linear classifiers in a higher dimensional space. Independent features are best modeled using the Naïve Bayes classifier. Biologically inspired artificial neural networks [11] are able to approximate nonlinear functions and are referred to as nonlinear classifiers. MATLAB's neural network toolbox was utilized to implement this algorithm in SPIRIT-ML. Logistic regression i.e. multinomial log-linear model was implanted in R using the nnet library. These are best suited for classification problems where the class label is binary. Random Forests (RF [12]) implemented using the randomForests library in R is an ensemble of decision trees included in the suite of supervised learning algorithms.

SPIRIT-ML ranks features in decreasing order of their importance in building supervised learning models. For decision trees, the topmost node of the tree where maximum data instances are classified was used to identify the first rank. This process is iteratively applied on the remaining set of features. For SVMs, the root squared coefficients of the support vectors were used to rank all the features. For ANNs, the connection weights between the different layers were used to rank the features. For RF, the importance measure in the randomForest package in R was used to rank the features. For multinomial log-linear models, the exponential of logistic regression coefficients were used to rank the features.

For developing Bayesian networks from a given dataset, eight algorithms (Grow-Shrink, Hill-Climbing, Tabu Search, Restricted Maximization, Incremental Association, Max-Min Hill Climbing, Fast Incremental Association and Chow-Liu algorithms) have been implemented using the bnlearn library in R [13]. Hugin module within SPIRIT-ML can be utilized to create influence diagrams.

Multiple cross-validation methods [14] such as 5-fold, 10-fold as well as leave one out cross validation methods have been implemented. The outputs of the unsupervised models are clusters that may be visualized either as dendrograms or cluster plots. The performance of the supervised learning models are visualized using the Receiver Operating Characteristic curves (ROC). The results are summarized and made available as a pdf file. This file includes a side by side comparison of all the supervised learning model results obtained when solving a classification problem, the visualizations obtained from unsupervised learning models obtained when solving clustering problems and learning diagrams when constructing Bayesian network models.

3   Results

3.1   Predictive Model Building: Use Case 1

Fine needle aspiration (FNA) cytology characteristics of tumor cells differ between benign and malignant samples from breast cancer patients. Deterministic features measured by Dr. Wolberg and colleagues at University of Wisconsin

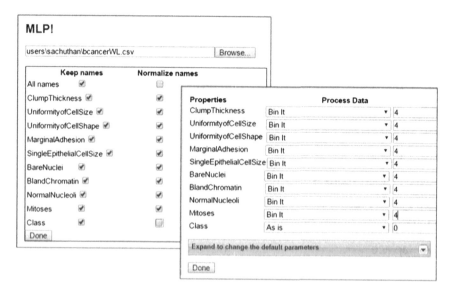

Fig. 4. Normalization and binning raw data

Hospitals from digitized image of aspirated cells [3,4] can be used to predict tumor malignancy. The dataset has been archived at UCI's machine learning repository and is referred to as the Wisconsin Breast Cancer dataset. This dataset contains 699 instances with each instance represented by a sample ID and 9 other numeric features. Supervised learning (classification) algorithms in SPIRIT-ML were utilized to predict tumor malignancy.

Figure 4 displays the features that were analyzed in the Wisconsin Breast Cancer dataset. The features assumed numeric values in the range of 1–10. The class labels were Benign as well as Malignant. In 16 instances, one of the nine features (BareNuclei) analyzed was missing a value. A random value between 1 and 10 was assigned for these instances. Since the nine features considered were continuous with values ranging between 1 and 10, we chose to normalize all of them. Each feature was then binned (4 bins with uniform width).

If the tab that indicates *Expand to change the default parameters* is selected, a drop down appears as a list of parameters (Fig. 5) for supervised learning models with editable values. For example, DT_minsplit, DT_CP and DT_minbucket refer to the minsplit, CP(Complexity Parameter) and minbucket parameters, respectively, expected by control option within the *rpart* command for the decision tree algorithm in R.

For the supervised learning task, SPIRIT-ML provides the results for all the algorithms side by side (Fig. 6). The first table compares the Accuracy of the seven supervised learning models based on the training dataset which in this case comprised of 70 % of the entire dataset. The second table in Fig. 6 compares the Precision, Recall, F_Measure and Specificity [15] across all the models. The final table in Fig. 6 ranks the top five features that led to the classification based

Expand to change the default parameters

DT_minsplit	2
DT_CP	0.001
DT_minbucket	1
C5_Winnow	TRUE ▼
SVM_kernel	'sigmoid' ▼
ANN_HiddenNeurons	10
ANN_HiddenLayers	1
LL_Hess	FALSE ▼
NB_laplace	0

Fig. 5. Default parameters that can be modified

Prediction Accuracy with Training Data (Static Learning)							
Data_Type	Decision Trees	C5 Trees	Support Vector Machines	Artificial Neural Networks	Random Forests	Log-Linear_Model	Naive Bayes
Correctly classified instances	488	475	472	478	339	475	473
Accuracy	99.796	97.137	96.524	98	69.325	97.137	96.728

Performance Comparison with Training Data							
Data_Type	Decision Trees	C5Trees	Support Vector Machines	Artificial Neural Networks	Random Forests	Log-linear Model	Naive Bayes
Precision	1	0.98	0.98	0.97	0.68	0.98	0.98
Recall	1	0.98	0.96	0.99	1	0.98	0.97
F_Measure	1	0.98	0.97	0.98	0.81	0.98	0.97
Specificity	0.99	0.96	0.97	0.95	0.11	0.96	0.97

Top 5 Relevant Features that led to Classification					
Decision Trees		Support Vector Machines	Artificial Neural Networks	Random Forests	Log-linear Model
BlandChromatin		Mitoses	Mitoses	BlandChromatin	UniformityofCellSize
UniformityofCellSize		MarginalAdhesion	ClumpThickness	ClumpThickness	NormalNucleoli
UniformityofCellShape		UniformityofCellShape	MarginalAdhesion	BareNuclei	SingleEpithelialCellSize
BareNuclei		SingleEpithelialCellSize	BareNuclei	UniformityofCellSize	BlandChromatin
SingleEpithelialCellSize		BlandChromatin	BlandChromatin	UniformityofCellShape	MarginalAdhesion

Fig. 6. Accuracy, Performance Measures and Feature Ranking based on training data

once on the training data. To combine the results of feature ranking we adopt the consensus polling method to determine the most important features. In our use case they were: BlandChromatin, UniformityofCellSize, ClumpThickness, MarginalAdhesion, UniformityofCellShape and BareNuclei.

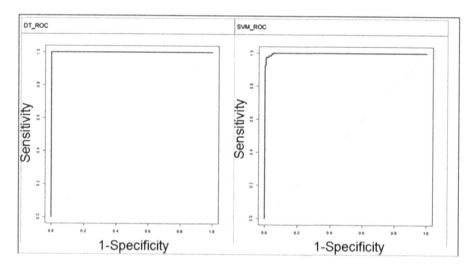

Fig. 7. ROC based on training data for two supervised learning algorithms

Prediction Accuracy with Test Data (Static Learning)							
Data_Type	Decision Trees	C5Trees	Support Vector Machines	Artificial Neural Networks	Random Forests	Log-linear Model	Naive Bayes
Correctly classified instances	101	100	100	100	71	99	101
Accuracy	96.19	95.238	95.238	95	67.619	94.286	96.19

Performance Comparison with Test Data							
Data_Type	Decision Trees	C5Trees	Support Vector Machines	Artificial Neural Networks	Random Forests	Log-linear Model	Naive Bayes
Precision	0.96	0.95	0.97	0.97	0.67	0.94	0.97
Recall	0.99	0.99	0.96	0.96	1	0.97	0.97
F_Measure	0.97	0.97	0.96	0.96	0.8	0.96	0.97
Specificity	0.91	0.89	0.94	0.94	0.03	0.89	0.94

Fig. 8. Accuracy, Performance Measures and Feature Ranking based on test data

The Receiver Operating Characteristic (ROC) curves based on the training data for two of the supervised learning models are shown in Fig. 7. They indicate that for the training data these models are quite good. To test these models, we used the test data against the models we created. The results for all the models are shown in Fig. 8. We found that the accuracy and performance on test data are greater than 94 % for all models except that obtained by Random Forests algorithm.

3.2   Clustering Dataset: Use Case 2

Identifying relevant patient characteristics in the case of complex diseases such as diabetes, cancer and dementia is quite challenging. Patient demographics, diagnosis and procedure information are usually captured in coded format within

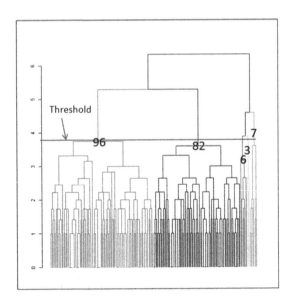

Fig. 9. Dendrogram depicting 5 clusters using Cluster DIANA

clinical databases. Patterns within the coded fields may reveal clinical characteristics across patients that would be difficult to determine manually. To automate this process, we developed a use case based on coded features derived from
MIMIC II dataset (http://mimic.physionet.org/), a publicly available clinical
database, using SPIRIT-ML.

Type II diabetic patients with certain types of cancer (Liver, Pancreatic,
Uterus, Colon, Bladder, Breast, Kidney, Esophageal and Ovarian) within MIMIC
II dataset were clustered using the clustering algorithms in SPIRIT-ML to reveal
clinical characteristics across patients. A total of 194 patients (instances) with
ten features (Age, Gender, Ethnicity, BMI, Congestive Heart Failure Yes/No,
Cardiac Arrthymias Yes/No, Hypertension Yes/No, Chronic Pulmonary Yes/No,
Renal Failure Yes/No and Liver Disease Yes/No) were analyzed.

Figure 9 is a dendrogram visualization of the five clusters obtained by Cluster
DIANA algorithm, one of the six clustering algorithms implemented in SPIRIT-
ML. The threshold decides the number of clusters identified. In this case, there
are two major clusters and three minor clusters. The numbers in Fig. 10 indicate
the number of patients in each cluster. The characteristics that decide the cluster
membership for each patient can be determined by converting the clustering
problem into a classification problem where the cluster membership is taken to
be the class label. Figure 8 depicts the cluster plot for the five clusters. These
plots are helpful in visualizing where the individual clusters lie in relation to other
clusters. The clusters with 3 and 7 patients seemed to be within the cluster with
96 patients. The cluster with 6 patients overlaps with the two major clusters.
This plot suggests that in reality there are only two main patient clusters.

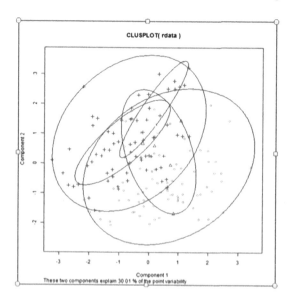

Fig. 10. Cluster plot using cluster DIANA

4   Future Work

The future development of platform will include vertical and horizontal integration to enable integrated research informatics. The horizontal integration currently planned include integration of SPIRIT-ML with the biomedical and clinical natural language processing component of SPIRIT (SPIRIT-NLP), image analysis and genomics computational pipelines being implemented at COH as part of SPIRIT platform.

The vertical integration of SPIRIT-ML with the n-tier SPIRIT platform is also being planned. This integration will include application integration using FUSION middleware, web services, common user interface components shared amongst other SPIRIT applications.

5   Conclusions

SPIRIT-ML is a functional machine learning platform that is used to discover and reveal patterns in biomedical datasets. SPIRIT-ML provides the following features: (a) Normalization and harmonization of input data (b) Clustering, classification and Bayesian network algorithms for deciphering relationships within a dataset (c) Various Validation methods (d) Integrated reporting system for comparative analysis of results. The underlying design of the platform is flexible enough to include machine learning models of choice, and facilitates comparison of results obtained by each model side by side. With the aid of SPIRIT-ML, the needs of multiple translational research projects that require data driven knowledge extraction can be addressed. We intend SPIRIT-ML to be an open source platform so that machine learning methods developed in other packages such as WEKA can be incorporated with minimal effort via Web Services.

Acknowledgments. The authors would like to thank Dr. Joyce Niland, Dr. Haiqing Li and Dr. Weizhong Zhu for their input and feedback.

References

1. Ross, M.E., Zhou, X., et al.: Classification of pediatric acute lymphoblastic leukemia by gene expression profiling. Blood **102**(8), 2951–2959 (2003)
2. Cleophas, T.J., Zwinderman, A.H.: Machine Learning in Medicine. Springer, Netherlands (2013)
3. Wolberg, W.H., Mangasarian, O.L.: Multisurface method of pattern separation for medical diagnosis applied to breast cytology. PNAS **87**, 9193–9196 (1990)
4. Zhang, J.: Selecting typical instances in instance-based learning. In: Proceedings of the Ninth International Machine Learning Conference, Aberdeen, Scotland, pp. 470–479. Morgan Kaufmann (1992)
5. Friedman, N., Geiger, D., Goldszmidt, M.: Bayesian network classifiers. Mach. Learn. **29**(2–3), 131–163 (1997)
6. Kaufman, L., Rousseeuw, P.J.: Finding Groups in Data: An Introduction to Cluster Analysis. Wiley, New York (1990)
7. Hartigan, J.A.: Clustering Algorithms. Wiley, New York (1975)
8. Breiman, L., Freidman, J., Stone, C.J., Olshen, R.A.: Classification and Regression Trees. Chapman and Hall/CRC, Boca Raton (1984)
9. Kuhn, M., Johnson, K.: Applied Predictive Modeling. Springer, New York (2013)
10. Cortes, C., Vapnik, V.: Support-vector network. Mach. Learn. **20**, 1–25 (1995)
11. Werbos, P.J.: Beyond Regression: New Tools for Prediction and Analysis in the Behavioral Sciences. Ph.D. thesis, Harvard University (1974)
12. Breiman, L.: Random forests. Mach. Learn. **45**(1), 5–32 (2001)
13. Nagarajan, R., Scutari, M., Lebre, S.: Bayesian Networks in R: with Applications in Systems Biology. Springer, New York (2013)
14. Kohavi, R.: A study of cross-validation and bootstrap for accuracy estimation and model selection. In: Proceedings of the Fourteenth International Joint Conference on Artificial Intelliegence, vol. 2(12), pp. 1137–1143 (1995)
15. Powers, D.M.W.: Evaluation: from precision, recall and F-measure to ROC, informedness, markedness and correlation. J. Mach. Learn. Technol. **2**(1), 37–63 (2011)
16. Amazon Web Services Machine Learning. http://aws.amazon.com/machine-learning/
17. H2O - the open source predictive analytics platform. http://0xdata.com/product/
18. The Apache Mahout. http://mahout.apache.org/
19. Waikato Environment for Knowledge Analysis (WEKA). http://www.cs.waikato.ac.nz/ml/weka/
20. Pipeline Pilot platform. http://accelrys.com/products/pipeline-pilot/
21. Hugin, the decision support tool. http://www.hugin.com/productsservices/products/academic/researcher

Demonstration: Mining Sentence and Annotation Evidence for a Cross Genome Study of the Plant Hormone Ethylene

Nick Becker[2], Caren Chang[1], Louiqa Raschid[1(✉)], Padmini Srinivasan[2],
Bram Van de Poel[3], Xiao-Ning Zhang[4], and Elena Zotkina[1]

[1] University of Maryland, College Park, USA
carenc@umd.edu, {louiqa,ezotkina}@umiacs.umd.edu
[2] University of Iowa, Iowa City, USA
becker.nick.a@gmail.com, padmini-srinivasan@uiowa.edu
[3] Ghent University, Ghent, Belgium
bram.vandepoel@ugent.be
[4] St. Bonaventure University, New York, USA
xzhang@sbu.edu

1 Introduction

This demonstration paper will illustrate the use of two tools, Ferret and semEP, to mine the sentence evidence and the annotation evidence, respectively, for cross genome gene function discovery. A case study of the plant hormone ethylene across the genomes of a plant, Arabidopsis thaliana and an alga, Spirogyra pratensis, will use the annotation evidence and sentences from the literature to showcase our discovery process and tools.

2 Background on a Cross Genome Discovery Case Study

Co-authors Chang and Van de Poel are investigating the evolution of the plant hormone ethylene. Chang is an expert on ethylene signaling in Arabidopsis thaliana. They are now studying Spirogyra pratensis, a freshwater alga [3]. As the closest living relative of land plants, this algal group is very valuable for studying the evolution of plants and their transition to land. One of their goals is to identify the genes and pathways that are regulated by ethylene. Since the growth and development of plants is regulated by signaling from plant hormones, a well known approach for such research would first identify evidence of hormonal crosstalk that involves ethylene. This can eventually lead to the identification of relevant genes and pathways. They carried out a time-course RNA-seq experiment to see which genes are differentially expressed upon ethylene treatment of Spirogyra and air (as a control), with samples taken at different time points. For this case, they provided us with a set of 569 genes that were up- or down-regulated by ethylene, and the corresponding Arabidopsis AT numbers.

© Springer International Publishing Switzerland 2015
N. Ashish and J.-L. Ambite (Eds.): DILS 2015, LNBI 9162, pp. 251–255, 2015.
DOI: 10.1007/978-3-319-21843-4_20

3   Mining the Sentence Evidence Using Ferret

Ferret is a system for sentence-based scanning of the literature [6]. It has a focus on gene-centric relationships and supports multi-species searches. The system takes as input a list of one or more genes of interest and an optional list of keywords. Keywords may be a combination of phenotypes, treatments, drugs, function verbs, etc. Ferret employs document filters and gene ambiguity detection and resolution strategies, and measures of sentence interestingness. Sentences are selected if they are likely to show a relationship between two genes or between a gene and a keyword. Ferret outputs a set of ranked sentences with links to the associated documents.

Ferret supports the bio scientist with varying literature-tracking goals. A scientist may want to find out all that is known about two interacting genes, or to explore possible functions and phenotypes of a newly encountered gene, or find explanations for observed empirical results.

We summarize the results of a Ferret search for sentence evidence for this case; details are reported in [6]. The scientists used a gene functional annotation tool, DAVID [2], to identify GO terms that were enriched for the 569 genes. This resulted in the following Top K keywords: ethylene, abscisic acid (ABA), auxin, cytokinin, gibberellin and brassinosteroid. Note that these five terms are hormones. Ferret then performed a search using the 569 genes and these six keywords. Of 167,286 searches, 722 retrieved 1 or more sentences from 3,690 documents. The researchers rated 1,668 sentences (from 1011 documents); they found 1073 sentences (530 documents) to be relevant and 595 sentences (481 documents) to be non relevant. This reflects that Ferret was used to quickly scan 1000+ documents via 1600+ sentences and found 52 % of the documents and 64 % (1073/1668) of the sentences to be relevant. Specific insights from the study are reported in [6].

4   Finding Patterns in Bipartite Annotation Graphs Using semEP

The semEP methodology to discover patterns in the annotation evidence will focus on a labeled (typed) bipartite graph, i.e., where all nodes and edges are associated with a type. Consider a labeled bipartite graph, $BG = (Gene \cup GO, HasAnnotation)$, where $Gene$ represents a set of genes (nodes), GO represents a set of Gene Ontology (GO) terms (nodes), and $HasAnnotation$ represents an annotation (edge) of a gene with a GO term. We used the results of the Ferret retrieval mentioned in the previous section to create an annotation dataset for semEP using the following protocol:

- A search was completed by Ferret using the keyword Ethylene and the 569 genes circa October 2014.
- Co-authors Chang and Van de Poel rated the retrieved sentences. From sentences ranked to be *relevant* and/or *interesting*, we obtained 21 genes.

– 221 GO annotations were then retrieved from TAIR (https://www.arabidopsis.org) for the 21 genes, and were used to create three bipartite graph corresponding to the three branches - Biological Process (BP), Molecular Function (MF) and Cellular Component (CC), of GO.
– A normalized BLAST similarity score was used to compute the *semantic distance* between a pair of genes. A topological similarity metric was used to compute the semantic distance between a pair of GO terms. Details are in [5].

Our methodology relies on a semantics based edge partitioning (semEP) solution; semEP is a variant of community detection. Details of semEP are in [1,4]. For ease of understanding, we skip the technical details and use Fig. 1 to illustrate the application of semEP, to the three bipartite graphs BP, MF and CC, to create clusters. Each cluster would favor groups of genes that were similar to each other, as well as groups of genes that shared a neighborhood of GO terms. Each cluster also included a group of related GO terms reflecting some concept captured by GO. Genes could be placed in multiple clusters to reflect a diversity of gene function. In contrast, a GO term would typically be associated with a single concept and placed in a single cluster. A GO term would be placed in multiple clusters if it annotated a pair of genes that had low sequence based similarity and did not share any other GO terms.

5   Results of Ferret Sentence Retrieval for semEP Clusters

We first highlight some insights from the sentence from Ferret, across the 569 genes and six search terms. We then discuss Ferret retrieval applied to semEP clusters.

Ferret sentence evidence highlights potential complex hormonal crosstalk with ethylene in Spirogyra. Sentences retrieved for AT4G26080 (ABI2), a gene involved in ABA signaling, indicated that this gene might be a key gene for hormonal crosstalk between ethylene and ABA in Spirogyra. Other ABA signaling, transport and biosynthesis genes including the following four: AT4G33950 (OST1), AT5G05440 (PYL5), AT5G13630 (ABAR) and AT5G67030 (ABA1), were found to have many (>80) matching sentences. Similarly, AT5G35750 (AHK2) and AT1G27320 (AHK3), two cytokinin receptor homologs were used to retrieve many (>60) sentences and might indicate hormonal crosstalk between ethylene and cytokinin in Spirogyra. For the other plant hormones (auxins, brassinosteroids and gibberellins) no significant sentences were retrieved.

After applying semEP clustering to the set of 21 genes and their 221 GO annotations, we selected several clusters in which three histidine kinase genes, AHK2 (AT5G35750), AHK3 (AT1G27320) and AHK4 (AT2G01830) participate. Figure 1 shows a partial view of the clusters; the large number of genes and GO terms in some semEP clusters prevents a complete visualization. Ferret retrieved sentences for the three genes, AHK2, AHK3 and AHK4 and the following keywords (corresponding to the GO terms in the clusters): cytokinin, phosphorelay, ABA, circadian rhythm and anthocyanin.

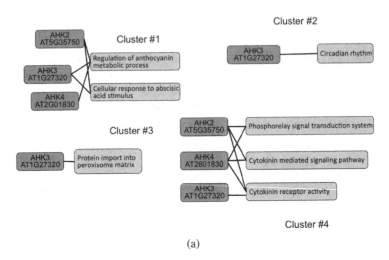

(a)

Fig. 1. Several clusters for genes AHK2, AHK3 and AHK4

As expected, there was excellent evidence for cytokinin including 90 sentences for AHK4 and 20 sentences each for AHK2 and AHK3.

There was no sentence evidence retrieved for the keyword circadian rhythm which is associated with AHK3 in the semEP clusters. An examination of the annotation details for AHK3 reveals that this annotation has evidence code *inferred from reviewed computational analysis*. Three sentences were retrieved for phosphorelay and AHK4; 2 of these sentences also mention AHK2 and AHK3. One sentence associating ABA with AHK2 and AHK3 was also retrieved by ferret.

6   Summary

We demonstrate the use of Ferret and semEP to explore the sentence and annotation evidence for gene function discovery. To summarize the case, using Ferret alone, sentence evidence for hormonal crosstalk between ethylene and the plant hormones ABA and cytokinin was obtained. Using a workflow of Ferret retrieval, followed by semEP clustering, followed by Ferret retrieval, a combination of the sentence and annotation evidence was used to target three genes, AHK2, AHK3 and AHK4. An additional GO term related to phosphorelay signal transduction was identified as well as some evidence for ABA signaling. Finally, semEP identified (inferred) annotation evidence to associate AHK3 with circadian rhythm.

References

1. Anderson, P., Thor, A., Benik, J., Raschid, L., Vidal, M.E.: Pang - finding patterns in annotation graphs. In: Proceedings of the ACM Conference on the Management of Data (SIGMOD) (2012)

2. Huang, D., Sherman, B., Lempicki, R.: Bioinformatics enrichment tools: paths toward the comprehensive functional analysis of large gene lists. Nucleic Acids Res. **37**(1), 1–13 (2009)
3. Ju, C., de Poel, B.V., Cooper, E., Thierer, J., Gibbons, T., Delwiche, C., Chang, C.: Conservation of ethylene as a plant hormone over 450 million years of evolution. Nat. Plants **1**(1), 1–7 (2015)
4. Palma, G., Vidal, M.-E., Raschid, L.: Drug-target interaction prediction using semantic similarity and edge partitioning. In: Mika, P., et al. (eds.) ISWC 2014, Part I. LNCS, vol. 8796, pp. 131–146. Springer, Heidelberg (2014)
5. Palma, G., Vidal, M.-E., Haag, E., Raschid, L., Thor, A.: Determining similarity of scientific entities in annotation datasets. Database J. Biol. Databases Curation (2015)
6. Srinivasan, P., Zhang, X., Bouten, R., Chang, C.: Ferret: a sentence-based literature scanning system. BMC Bioinf. (2015, to appear)

Graduate Student Consortium

GAAIN Virtual Appliances: Virtual Machine Technology for Scientific Data Analysis

Arihant Patawari[✉]

Laboratory of Neuroimaging, Keck School of Medicine of USC, Institute
for Neuroimaging and Informatics, University of Southern California,
2001 N Soto Street, Los Angeles, USA
patawari@usc.edu

Abstract. We present our experience with technology for developing virtual machines and virtual appliances. Our goal is to facilitate scientific workflow sharing and analysis for scientific investigation using virtual machine technology. Our work is in the context of a larger effort on building an efficient data sharing and analysis network for data providers as well as scientific investigators in the domain of Alzheimer's Disease (AD) research.

1 Introduction

This student abstract discusses our work in progress on virtual machine technology for scientific workflows sharing and analysis. The overall context of our work is an effort for "GAAIN" which stands for the Global Alzheimer's Association Interactive Network ([1]GAAIN 2014), which is a federated network of Alzheimer's disease organisations from around the globe. The aim of GAAIN is to provide harmonised data across multiple, independently created Alzheimer's datasets from data providers around the globe to the investigators. GAAIN also aims to provide computational and analytical resources, storage and other capabilities to any investigator on the network, by leveraging it anywhere on the shared network. As a part of this network infrastructure, we aim to provide the capability of independently developing and sharing scientific workflows and analysis amongst the investigators and data providers. This work reports our experience with the same.

The technology for medical (or generally scientific) analysis and workflow management is well developed. In the recent years, scientific workflow frameworks are being developed for more dynamic and flexible computing environments such as grids or cloud environments [1]. For instance, the [2]LONI Pipeline is a robust and widely adopted workflow system in the Neuroimaging and Informatics domain [2]. Other popular workflow frameworks including Taverna, Pegasus are highly used in Bio-Informatics [3–5]. The utility based resources available through cloud computing has several benefits, such as, the pay-as-you-go model for access to high-end data storage and computing, outsourcing of computation and data management to the cloud, and enhanced collabo-

---

[1] www.gaain.org.
[2] www.loni.usc.edu/Software/Pipeline.

© Springer International Publishing Switzerland 2015
N. Ashish and J.-L. Ambite (Eds.): DILS 2015, LNBI 9162, pp. 259–264, 2015.
DOI: 10.1007/978-3-319-21843-4_21

ration capability, has motivated researchers to develop scientific workflow systems for cloud based frameworks such as for [3]Amazon-EC2 [4, 6, 10].

Such paradigms and frameworks have brought significant utility to the investigators and can indeed be credited for making high end and often expensive computation and storage resources readily and widely accessible to a larger pool of investigators. Such frameworks, however, are not suitable for the analysis of sensitive data. For example, in the Alzheimer's disease domain, organisations typically have data comprising of demographics, imaging, genetics and phenotypic details for each subject and should be carefully handled. Data owners are highly sensitive with regard to the distribution of such data given the scientific value and also resources committed towards creating and assembling such data. In many cases, the data also contains identity details and hence, data owners are under legal and ethical obligation to not to distribute the data indiscriminately. As a result, cloud or grid-based workflow environment is not suitable for shared data analysis, as the risk of data exposure exists. Also data transfer over a network is a matter of concern. In the Alzheimer's disease domain the size of data for every subject is often huge [7] and is in GBs. The data transfer time has in fact motivated the development of tools such as GridFTP to optimise and manage the transfer of large volumes of biomedical data over a network or grid [8]. On the other hand, the merits of medical workflow analysis and data sharing, with in-built collaboration capability are well acknowledged, and hence, motivates the need for the data owner to provide the sensitive data for research and analysis. Our approach to address the above is simple, which is, instead of sending data to where the processing (workflow) is, we 'ship' the processing workflow to the place where the data resides. We achieve this via the concept of a 'Virtual Appliance' (VA), a virtual computing machine, i.e., a software footprint that can be sent to the data provider.

2   Virtual Machines and Appliances

A Virtual Machine (VM) is defined as *"a software-based computer that provides operating systems and applications with 'virtual' access to hardware resources such as CPU, RAM, networking and storage."* ([4]VMWare 2014). The VM encapsulates and provides all the capabilities of a 'regular' computing machine, such as a PC, and also has several advantages such as, user may not have to obtain or maintain the computing hardware, ability to share a Virtual Machine (remotely) to multiple users, if required, and the ability to use the resources on pay-as-you-go basis. Virtual *Appliances*, like virtual machines, incorporate an application, operating system and virtual hardware. However, virtual appliances differ from virtual machines in a way that they are delivered to customers as preconfigured "turnkey" solutions that simplify deployment for customers by eliminating the need for manual configuration of the virtual machines and operating systems used to run the appliance.

---

[3] www.aws.amazon.com/ec2/.

[4] www.vmware.com.

Popular frameworks for hosted Virtual Machines on the cloud includes the likes of [5]Amazon EC2 (EC2 2014) and [6]Microsoft Azure (Azure 2014). Many frameworks are now available for developers to create their own virtual machines on a virtual environment that they can enable on their desktop or on dedicated hardware. Some of these frameworks include VMWare (VMWare 2014), [7]SUSE Studio (SUSE 2014), [8]Oracle VirtualBox (VirtualBox 2014), [9]Citrix XenServer (XenSever 2014), Microsoft Hyper-V (HyperV 2014), [10]Virtual Bridges (Bridges 2014), [11]Proxmox (Proxmox 2014), [12]Parallels (Parallels 2014) and [13]IBM z/VM (IBM VM 2014). These frameworks provide easy to use desktop capabilities to developers to create, use and share virtual machines. An example of a virtual machine, and the virtual machine framework desktop manager, using the Oracle VirtualBox framework is illustrated in Fig. 1. We have adopted Oracle VirtualBox as one of the primary frameworks for GAAIN virtual machines given that it is robust, easy and intuitive to use, and is also an open-source technology.

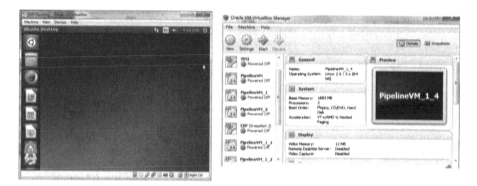

Fig. 1. A virtual machine, and a virtual machine manager console

A very recent framework, Docker[14], is significantly more light-weight framework for developing virtualised and packaged applications. Docker is an open platform for developers and administrators to develop, ship, and execute distributed applications. At the core of Docker is the Docker Engine, a portable, lightweight runtime tool that supports the encapsulation and exaction of applications. And also The Docker Hub, a cloud-based service for sharing applications and managing access control. The key

[5] www.aws.amazon.com.
[6] www.azure.microsoft.com.
[7] www.susestudio.com.
[8] www.oracle.com.
[9] www.citrix.com.
[10] www.vbridge.com.
[11] www.proxmox.com.
[12] www.parallels.com.
[13] www.ibm.com.
[14] www.docker.com.

differentiator between Docker and a "regular" virtual machine is that while a virtual machine typically include a complete operating system, a Docker image typically has a very minimal layer for application support. Developers add utilities only to the extent required to be able to run their specific applications which helps in keeping overall image size to minimum.

Table 1 provides the information on key aspects of the VirtualBox and Docker frameworks based on our experience with building virtual appliances with them.

Table 1. VirtualBox and Docker

Aspects	VirtualBox	Docker
Virtual image type (formats)	The open-virtual-format as '.OVF' and '.OVA' files	Proprietary Docker image format
Requirements	Any virtualization hypervisor that can run the open virtualization format images	Docker shell
Architecture	Typically the core virtual image contains a complete operating system of choice	Minimal system layer is provided and components are added only as required
'Typical' image sizes	Encapsulating a simple application (for instance a single workflow) results in a machine of size ~1.5 GB. However options are recently becoming available for including only a liminal operating system layer.	Typically only a few hundred MB for the same applications
Management and sharing	No specific capabilities provided	Docker Hub for centralized Docker image storage, tagging, and sharing
Access control	No specific capabilities provided	Docker Hub provides account management and access control
Network access	Can provide network access between Virtual Box VM and external machines/ networks.	External network access to Docker image can be provided but with limitations
Host folder mounting	Possible but with some additional software installation	Host folder mounting can be done more easily with a single command

3 Challenges

Software Execution in VM: Some minor technical issues with the execution of software within the VM environment are encountered. For instance, one of the issue is that the workflow analysis in VA starts it's execution *before* the data from the host machine actually gets mounted. However, this can be addressed by initial configuration of the virtual appliance after installation to ensure that the shared folder mounting happens before any packaged analysis workflow starts it's execution on the VM [9].

VA Size: The size of the VAs is a concern. Generally, for a VA to run complex workflows, the underlying VM must be provided with sufficient memory and virtual disk resources, which causes the size of the VM image to be quite large (size ranges in single digit GB). Thus, the time to transfer VM images over the network is large. Conventional file compression techniques do not apply to compressing virtual machine images as the machine image is not the data that can be compressed, rather it encapsulates resources such as virtual disks and memory for a machine. We have investigated techniques and softwares that are built specifically for virtual machine image compression. An example is the [15]Parallels Compressor which (1) defragments virtual disks and cleans up unused space, and (2) compacts virtual disks on the virtual machine, to compress the VM image.

Interoperability: It is important for the GAAIN VAs to be able to run across multiple VM frameworks. This is because partners on the network can already be committed to or may be using any specific virtualisation framework at their end. For instance, NeuGRID uses XenServer (XenServer 2014) for its overall computing environment, so it is an advantage if the GAAIN VAs can execute seamlessly on the XenServer environment, as there are no additional virtualisation requirements at the NeuGRID end. Similarly, vSphere (VMWare 2014) is another common virtualisation environment included in Alzheimer's and other medical informatics computing and data management facilities. We are thus exploring interoperability with multiple virtualisation frameworks to ensure that GAAIN VMs can run seamlessly on a wide variety of frameworks.

Execution Validation: The virtual appliance is created by one organisation but typically executes in the execution environment of another. It is important to try and ensure that the VA is only conducting legitimate and permissible analysis operations and data transfer at and from the environment it runs in. We are working on adding logging capabilities and other heuristic checks on data transferred (out) by the VA in this regard.

4   Conclusions and Future Work

We have reported our experience with the "initial design and implementation" of a virtual appliances based solution for medical data analysis in environments where data ownership is of paramount concern. Currently, we are working on scaling the solution to operate on a larger scale within the GAAIN network. By this, we envision a virtual appliances environment wherein a large number of investigators from across the globe can contribute in data analysis workflows. And also the other investigators can select and use (or build upon) such pre-packaged workflows from a large library of virtual appliances with pre-packaged workflows. Our model also incorporates abstraction of data from the investigator.

---

[15] www.parallels.com.

An important element here becomes the *provenance* associated with each VA i.e., a meta-data description of the virtual appliance and the workflow(s) it contains. The virtual machine image itself has been identified as a source of provenance for a virtual appliance or machine [11, 12], however the provenance needs to be extended to meaningful descriptions and terms that investigators would use to both describe their workflows as well as when trying to locate them for their use.

References

1. Foster, I., Kesselman, C., Tuecke, S.: The anatomy of the grid: enabling scalable virtual organisations. Int. J. High Perform. Comput. Appl. **15**(3), 200–222 (2001)
2. Dinov, I., et al.: Neuroimaging study designs, computational analyses and data provenance using the LONI pipeline. PloS one **5**(9), e13070 (2010)
3. Wolstencroft, K., Haines, R., Fellows, D., Williams, A., Withers, D., Owen, S., Soiland-Reyes, S., Dunlop, I., Nenadic, A., Fisher, P., Bhagat, J., Belhajjame, K., Bacall, F., Hardisty, A., Nieva de la Hidalga, A., Balcazar Vargas, M.P., Sufi, S., Goble, C.: The Taverna workflowsuite: designing and executing workflows of Web Services on the desktop, web or in the cloud. Nucleic Acids Res. **41**(W1), W557–W561 (2013)
4. Deelman, E., Gil, Y.: Managing large-scale scientific workflows in distributed environments: experiences and challenges. In: E-Science 2006: Proceedings of the Second IEEE International Conference on e-Science and Grid Computing, p. 144. IEEE Computer Society, Washington, DC (2006)
5. Barseghian, D., et al.: Workflows and extensions to the Kepler scientific workflow system to support environmental sensor data access and analysis. Ecol. Inform. **5**(1), 42–50 (2010)
6. Singh, M.P., Vouk, M.A.: Scientific workflows: scientific computing meets transactional workflows. In: NSF Workshop on Workflow and Process Automation in Information Systems: State of the Art and Future Directions (1996)
7. Bresnahan, J., et al.: Globus GridFTP: what's new in 2007. In: Proceedings of the First International Conference on Networks for Grid Applications. ICST (Institute for ComputerSciences, Social-Informatics and Telecommunications Engineering) (2007)
8. Neu, S.C., Crawford, K.L., Toga, A.W.: Practical management of heterogeneous neuroimaging metadata by global neuroimaging data repositories. Front. Neuroinformatics **6**, 8 (2012). PMCID: 3311229
9. Van Steen, M., Homburg, P., Andrew, S.T.: Globe: a wide-area distributed system. IEEE Concurrency **7**(1), 70–78 (1999)
10. Juve, G., Deelman, E.: Scientific workflows and clouds. Crossroads **16**(3), 14–18 (2010)
11. Taylor, I.J., et al.: Workflows for E-Science: Scientific Workflows for Grids. Springer, London (2014)
12. Lampoudi, S.: The Path to Virtual Machine Images as First Class Provenance. Age, USA (2011)

The GAAIN Entity Mapper: Towards Practical Medical Informatics Application

Peehoo Dewan[✉]

Laboratory of NeuroImaging, Keck School of Medicine of USC, Institute for Neuroimaging and Informatics, University of Southern California, 2001 N Soto Street, Los Angeles, USA
pdewan@usc.edu

Abstract. We discuss our work in progress towards the practical application of a system we have developed for automated schema mapping of medical datasets. While starting with a purely knowledge-driven approach to the schema mapping problem, based on information in data dictionaries, we are now incorporating machine-learning classification for determining mappings. We are further integrating the mapping system into a production medical informatics environment. We discuss our ongoing approach and progress in these areas, as well as current challenges.

1 Introduction and Motivation

This student abstract discusses our in progress work on a system for automated schema mapping of medical datasets. In particular, we discuss the work on practical application of the system for medical data management and integration tasks. The overall context of our work is a system call the GAAIN Entity Mapper or "GEM" [2] which we have developed for automated mapping of data elements from datasets of Alzheimer's disease research data. GAAIN itself stands for the Global Alzheimer's Association Interactive Network,[1] a data sharing federated network of Alzheimer's disease datasets from around the globe. The aim of GAAIN is to create a network of Alzheimer's disease data, researchers, analytical tools and computational resources to better our understanding of this disease. A key capability of this network is also to provide investigators with access to harmonized data across multiple, independently created Alzheimer's datasets. For the harmonization of data, GAAIN employs a common data model approach where any Alzheimer's disease dataset in the GAAIN network is mapped to a common data model. By mapping we mean establishing a correspondence and transformation between individual data elements in any dataset and data elements in the common data model. Such data mappings are typically done manually, which is an effort, time and resource intensive process. We are thus developing the GEM automated data mapping tool that we envision as being an intelligent software assistant utility to data analysts conducting data mapping tasks.

We have completed a first version of the GEM system [1] where we have taken a knowledge driven approach. We exploit the detailed information provided in descriptive

---

[1] http://www.gaain.org

© Springer International Publishing Switzerland 2015
N. Ashish and J.-L. Ambite (Eds.): DILS 2015, LNBI 9162, pp. 265–270, 2015.
DOI: 10.1007/978-3-319-21843-4_22

data dictionaries with each dataset. This work discusses our ongoing work as we begin to apply the GEM system to actual data mapping tasks in the GAAIN project as well as related data or schema mapping tasks in other medical informatics efforts. Specifically, we focus on two problems:

(1) Adding active-learning [3] capabilities and machine-learning techniques to improve data mapping in the GEM system. Further, the system can learn and improve from 'feedback' provided by users as they conduct mapping tasks.
(2) Providing a usable schema mapping library to data analysts for a variety of data design and integration tasks.

2   Methods

2.1   Active Learning and Machine-Learning Incorporation

Our motivation for the incorporation of machine-learning based classification techniques for schema mapping is two-fold. First, in the existing GEM system we try and map data elements across different datasets using multiple indicators associated with the data elements. These indicators include the similarity of two data element names, the text similarity of the element descriptions using two different algorithms namely a text similarity match based on topic modeling and also TFIDF based text similarity match. To optimally combine such and other indicators for determining mappings we need a feature based classifier approach. Next, the GEM system is intended to operate as an intelligent software assistant that suggests data mappings to human data analysts and data integration developers. As such analysts and developers "select" correct matches (from alternatives provided by the system), they implicitly provide training data to the system in terms of labeled data mapping examples. The system must incorporate this training data and improve the data mapping by leveraging the new knowledge.

Given a pair of *data elements* from different sources, our system uses a combination of both supervised and unsupervised machine learning approaches to classify the pair as matching or not. For each pair of data elements, we generate various features from the metadata information extracted from the data dictionaries. In particular, we extract the following features

1. **TFIDF Similarity.** We calculate the similarity score of the text descriptions based on TFIDF similarity [4] of the two data elements present in their respective data dictionaries.
2. **Topic Modeling Similarity Score.** We build a topic model [1, 5] from the column descriptions of all the data elements of the two sources. We then calculate a similarity score based on the cosine similarity of the topic distributions of the two data elements.
3. **TFIDF Rank.** Sometimes the TFIDF and topic modeling score for an element may not be high, however the score maybe relatively higher than other data elements in the second source. To counter the situation, given a data element e1 from source s1, we get the list of all data elements from source2 sorted by their TFIDF score

and calculate the rank of element e2 among the sorted list. We use the rank as one of the features.

4. **Topic Modeling Rank.** Similar to 3.
5. **Name Match.** Data element names in medical data are cryptic and/or composite. We have developed a classifier for computing name similarity across two element names that takes into account common abbreviations, prefixes and other qualifiers (such as year or visit number) in the element names. This feature is set to true if a name match exist, and is false by default.
6. **Name Matching Score.** This feature stores the confidence score for the previous feature. A high value of this score along with the "true" label for the previous feature is a very strong indication of a good name match. Similarly, a high value of this score along with the "false" label for the previous feature is a very strong indication of not a good name match.
7. **Cardinality.** We extract the cardinality of the two data elements from the data dictionaries and use them as features.
8. **Range.** We extract the range (min and max) of the two data elements from the data dictionaries and use them as features.
9. **Edit Distance.** We calculate the edit distance (word based) between the source and the destination.
10. **Table Names.** Data elements in a dataset are typically clustered into several distinct groups such as elements related to family history, physical examination, neurological assessments etc. The previous system considered elements individually when mapping. We have tried to leverage inter element associations during mapping. Hence we use table names of the two data elements as reference of locality.

We then use the feature vector of all the training examples for training a classifier that classifies a given pair of data elements as matching or non-matching. We have conducted preliminary experimental evaluations by employing the above kinds of features and evaluating multiple classifiers for determining mappings. We used four of the data sources of Alzheimer's disease data that we have in GAAIN namely ADNI [6, 7], NACC [8], INDD [9] and LAADC [10]. Our experimental setup consists of a manually curated goldset of true mappings between above sources. We generate features for the examples in the goldset and use them as positive training examples. For each example in the goldset we also randomly select 20 non-matches and use them as negative training examples. The number of positive and negative

Table 1. Preliminary results

Dataset/schema pairs	Precision	Recall	F-Score	Positive examples	Negative examples
LAADC-ADNI	0.944	0.895	0.919	38	798
INDD-ADNI	1	0.886	0.939	35	735
NACC-ADNI	0.944	0.905	0.924	74	1554

examples used for training is mentioned in the table. Below are the results that we obtained using a Simple Logistic Regression classifier with 10-fold cross validation.

Overall the preliminary results, conducted for various pairs of GAAIN datasets as shown in Table 1, look promising. We see that using a supervised approach on top of our unsupervised model has improved our F-Score by almost 5 %.

Figure 1 illustrates the active learning capability where Fig. 1(a) is a schematic representation of the active-learning architecture and Fig. 1(b) illustrates the graphical interface to the GEM schema-mapping system. As illustrated, the user is provided multiple alternative proposed matches for a given data element and he/she can select and identify the correct match.

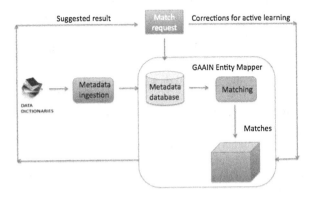

(a) Active-Learning Workflow

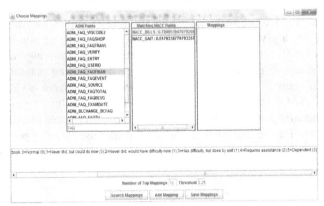

(b) Schema Mapping Interface

Fig. 1. GEM active learning

2.2   Library for Data Analysts

As mentioned earlier, any dataset to be integrated into the GAAIN network is transformed to the GAAIN common data model. This transformation is done by a software system called the GAAIN Transformation Tool. The data mappings in this tool are currently provided manually, using a graphical user interface, where a developer manually established data correspondence between the dataset data elements and the common model elements. We are currently integration the GEM system with this transformation tool. We are providing a packaged library of generic mapping functions that can further be called by the transformation tool. The transformation tool will also provide graphical browsing and querying for a developer to browse suggested data mappings.

Another practical use of our tool has been in *model discovery* i.e., identifying data elements for a common data model over a collection of multiple, disparate datasets. Common data model design in medical data domains and in general is a complex problem with multiple considerations that must be made towards an "optimal" common model. The optimality of a common data model depends not only on the constituent data sources it must encompass, but also the data retrieval application(s) the common model must serve in the first place. Both top-down as well as bottom-up methodologies have a role in this process. A system such as GEM can aid significantly in the bottom-up aspect of common model design by identifying the characteristics of various data elements based upon mappings. For instance it may help a data analyst to know for all data elements in a particular dataset or source, what are the mappings to the element i.e., corresponding data elements in *all other* datasets in a collection. It would help to know the 'coverage' i.e., fraction of sources a particular data element is present in.

We are currently developing such utilities over the GEM core mapping functionalities, where we aim to provide the above kinds of aggregated mappings and statistics to data analysts over a large collection of datasets. Such information would be valuable in identifying good candidate common model elements.

3   Challenges

The following are the current research and technical challenges in our work.

Feature Engineering and Classifiers. We are in the process of identifying optimal feature sets and applicable classifiers to the machine learning classification problem. We identified the table name as one of the features. However we have encountered datasets where the data dictionary does not provide any tables associated with the data elements, rather the data elements are (at best) grouped into broad categories such as 'Patient Demographic', 'Clinical Assessments' etc., We are exploring ways to represent and leverage such grouping information as well, in the absence of table associations.

Data Dictionary Format. Currently we require the users to provide data dictionaries in a specified Excel format. However this may be restrictive in certain environments as we are putting the burden of translating a data dictionary in its native format to our specified format. We will consider incorporating some utilities to assist with this process.

There are two problems to be addressed. First, the native data dictionary may be in a non-Excel format for instance as an MSWord or PDF document, in which case we need to be able to extract the data dictionary (element) details in a structured manner. Next we must ensure that the data dictionary information (per element) is formatted to our expected format.

Model Discovery. The functionality and specific capabilities that can be provided by a schema mapping system such as ours to help in data model design and discovery are best determined by developers and analysts that actual conduct such model design. We are thus working closely with such developers in the GAAIN project and other efforts to understand and provide mapping capabilities and functions for their needs.

References

1. Ashish, N., Dewan, P., Ambite, J., Toga, A.: GEM: The GAAIN entity mapper. 11th DILS (2015)
2. Dewan, P., Ashish, N., Toga, A.: A schema-matching tool for Alzheimer's disease data integration. In: 5th ACM BCB (2014)
3. Rubens, N., Kaplan, D., Sugiyama, M.: Recommender Systems Handbook. Springer, US (2011)
4. Tata, S., Patel, J.: Estimating the selectivity of tf-idf based cosine similarity predicates. Sigmod Rec. **36**(2), 75–80 (2007)
5. Blei, D.M.: Probabilistic topic models. Commun. ACM **55**(4), 77–84 (2012). doi: 10.1145/2133806.2133826
6. Mueller, S.G., Weiner, M.W., Thal, L.J., Peterson, R.C., Jack, C., Jagust, W., Trojanowski, J.Q., Toga, A.W., Beckett, L.: Alzheimer's disease neuroimaging initiative. Neuroimaging Clin. N. Am. **15**(4), 869–877 (2008)
7. Shen, L., Thompson, P.M., Potkin, S.G., Bertram, L., Farrer, L.A., Foroud, T.M., Green, R.C., Hu, X., Huentelman, M.J., Kim, S., Kauwe, J.S., Li, Q., Liu, E., Macciardi, F., Moore, J.H., Munsie, L., Nho, K., Ramanan, V.K., Risacher, S.L., Stone, D.J., Swaminathan, S., Toga, A.W., Weiner, M.W., Saykin, A.J.: Generic analysis of quantitative phenotypes in AD and MCI: imaging, cognition and biomarkers. Brain Imaging Beh. **8**(2), 183–207 (2014)
8. Beekly, D.L., Ramos, E.M., Lee, W.W., et al.: The National Alzheimer's Coordinating Center (NACC) database: The uniform data set. Alzheimer Dis. Assoc. Disord. **21**, 249–258 (2007)
9. Xie, S.X., Baek, Y., Grossman, M., Arnold, S.E., Karlawish, J., Siderowf, A., Hurtig, H., Elman, L., McCluskey, L., Van Deerlin, V., Lee, V.M., Trojanowski, J.Q.: Building an integrated neurodegenerative disease database at an academic health center. Alzheimer's Dement. **7**, e84–e93 (2011). doi:10.1016/j.jalz.2010.08
10. Wu, X., Li, J., Ayutyanont, N., Protas, H., Jagust, W., Fleisher, A., Reiman, E., Yao, L., Chen, K.: The receiver operational characteristic for binary classification with multiple indices and its application to the neuroimaging study of Alzheimer's disease. IEEE/ACM Trans. Comput. Biol. Bioinform. **10**, 173–180 (2013)

Efficient Management of Cached Data in the Global Alzheimer's Association Interactive Network

Swapnil Kothari[✉]

Laboratory of Neuro Imaging, USC Stevens Neuroimaging and Informatics Institute, Keck School of Medicine of USC, University of Southern California, 2001 N Soto Street, Los Angeles, USA
swapnil.kothari@usc.edu

Abstract. A key tenet of the Global Alzheimer's Association Interactive Network (GAAIN) is to protect the data ownership rights of its members. This prohibits data shared by its federated data repositories from being copied to any GAAIN disk drive and requires all GAAIN server caches to be managed in memory only. Further, the different data repositories collect different attributes for their subjects, and often there are different amounts of data collected for the subjects within the same data repository. We present a relational database design to manage this sparse cached data using elementary bit operators to perform queries and extract results from compact value representations.

Keywords: Relational database · Sparse data · Query optimization

1   Introduction

The Global Alzheimer's Association Interactive Network (GAAIN) is consolidating the efforts of independent Alzheimer's disease data repositories around the world with the goals of revealing more insights into the causes of Alzheimer's disease, improving treatments, and designing preventative measures that delay the onset of physical symptoms. As participation in GAAIN is voluntary, the needs and concerns of the participants must be properly addressed. One essential requirement is that the data ownership rights of its members must be protected. To this end, GAAIN has implemented a policy that prevents any data from the repositories it federates to be stored on any GAAIN server disk drive. In order to optimize performance, all data managed by GAAIN servers must then be cached in memory. The cache temporarily holds the results of recent queries that are accumulated from the GAAIN clients that are installed at each data repository.

Each data repository in GAAIN collects information (e.g., demographics, cognitive assessments, family history) on subjects who have volunteered to be studied. We define each recorded field as an *attribute*; for example, a gender attribute is used for collecting the *attribute values* "male" or "female" for each subject. This information is collected at different points in time in which each subject is contacted at predefined intervals after they first enter the study. Each time point is called a *visit* and the time between visits in GAAIN usually occurs in 6 month or 1 year intervals. Some attributes will change over time (e.g., subject's age) and others will not (e.g., subject's genotype).

© Springer International Publishing Switzerland 2015
N. Ashish and J.-L. Ambite (Eds.): DILS 2015, LNBI 9162, pp. 271–275, 2015.
DOI: 10.1007/978-3-319-21843-4_23

One important characteristic of the attribute data in GAAIN is that it is sparse. Different data repositories collect different attributes for their subjects, and often there are different amounts of data collected for the subjects within the same data repository. So for any given subject, the number of attributes for which data was collected is small. The requirements for our database design are: (1) the cache must efficiently manage sparse data, (2) cache queries must be optimal, and (3) the cache must reside entirely in computer memory.

Previous work on managing sparse data in Relational Database Management Systems (RDBMS) has involved different strategies to reorganize the data into data structures that require less storage space. One approach [1, 2] is to modify existing database source code. A disadvantage to this is that the modified code must be maintained for each new database version and it is not readily extendible between different database implementations. Other schemes [3, 4] attempt to create multiple tables that depend upon the sparseness characteristics of the data. Clustering algorithms [4] and correlation coefficients [3] are computed for each data set and used to determine the number of database tables to create as well as how the data is distributed in the tables. However, this approach is not optimal for managing sparse data in a cache where the data varies depending upon the results of the most recent queries. As the data is updated, the cache would have to be reexamined which may result in needing to reorganize the data frequently. Although sparse data can be managed in NoSQL databases using less storage than in RDBMS, to our knowledge there are no NoSQL database implementations that support storage entirely in memory. Our approach is similar to the bit-cube algorithms used in RDF storage engines [5] that first prune candidates using bit-vectors and then generate results from those candidates. Because our data model is simple and does not require a rich description framework for its description, we chose to pursue a simpler RDBMS implementation instead of using RDF.

In what follows, we present a strategy for efficiently managing sparse GAAIN data in an unmodified RDBMS using compact interpreted records [1] that store multiple values together in a *tuple*. Because each tuple is managed as a single item by the database, we introduce a scheme that makes use of simple bit operators to extract values from each tuple for use in basic SQL queries.

2   Methods

We divide each database query into two parts. First we find all the attributes referenced in the restriction of the query and then we use those to determine all the subjects that have non-null values for those attributes. Next, we use that subject list to locate and find the attribute values and perform the query. In our approach, we make use of long strings of bits (blob types) to keep track of subjects and attribute values and we perform bit operations such as bitwise AND's, bit shifts, and bit counts to manipulate sets of subjects and extract attribute values from stored tuples.

The number N of subjects in GAAIN is the total number of subjects from all the federated data repositories, and we assign each subject a unique number $(0, 1, \ldots, N-1)$. We also enumerate the attributes along with their visits by assigning each attribute/visit pair an attribute number (1, 2, …). We create a table that has two columns as shown in Table 1. For each attribute, we store a bit string of length N that records whether or not each subject has a non-null value for that attribute. A "1" in the bit string signifies that a subject has a non-null value for the attribute; for example, a bit string of "011" indicates that subject #0 has a null value of the attribute and subjects #1 and #2 have non-null values.

Table 1. Example of the table for recording non-null attribute values for each subject.

Attribute_number	Subject bit string
1	101….
2	100….
3	010….

At the beginning of a GAAIN query, we find all attributes referenced in the restriction of the query (WHERE clause) and get the subject bit strings for each of those attributes. We then perform a bitwise AND of all bit strings in this set. The result of this operation is a bit string of the subjects in the result set of the query. Because the data is sparse, this step can eliminate many unnecessary attribute table searches by quickly determining the subjects whose data need be searched. It is also worth noting that this table can be stored on disk because GAAIN requires only that attribute values be cached in computer memory.

If the subject bit string resulting from the bitwise AND's is S and there is a table with a column *subject_number* that stores the number of each subject, we can use it in the WHERE clause of an SQL query to restrict the results to the subjects in the bit string:

$$\text{WHERE } (((S >> subject\_number-1) \text{ \& } 1) == 1).$$

We note that in order to make efficient use of storage space, we can map finite sets of attribute values to a set of integers. For example, the values of a gender attribute ("male" and "female") can be numbered (0, 1) and stored using one bit. In the case of floating point numbers, we can limit the precision of each value and store instead integer values (e.g., "3.1415" might be rounded to "3.14" and stored as "314" using 9 bits).

We store the non-null attribute values for each subject in the compact form in shown in Table 2. A table is defined for all attribute values that are stored using the same number of bits per value. Table 2 shows values that can be stored using 3 bits, and we call this a 3-bit table. In these tables there is a row for each subject that has at least one non-null attribute value stored in the table. After determining the attributes whose values are stored in the table, we assign each of them a number (1, 2,…). The attribute values for each subject are concatenated and stored in the *tuple* column of the table. A bit string is constructed that indexes the values in the tuple and it is stored in a separate column. Because the data is sparse, the tuple representation of the attributes values is an efficient way to store the data values.

Table 2. Example of a table that stores 3 bit attribute values for each subject.

Subject_number	Index bit string	Tuple
1	1000	110
2	1010	001110
3	1101	110101111

In the example shown in Table 2, there are 4 attributes that have values that can be stored using 3 bits. A "1" in an index bit string signifies that there is a value stored for an attribute. The index bit string in the first row is "1000," which indicates that subject #1 has a value ("110") for only the first attribute. There are two attributes values stored in the *tuple* in the second row, one for the first attribute and one for the third attribute (as denoted in that row's index bit string "1010"). The value for the first attribute is "001" and the value for the third attribute is "110."

We can extract a value from a *tuple* using the following bit operations. If we want the 4th attribute value in the *tuple* that is indexed by an index bit string A in a 3-bit table, we first construct a string of 1's that has a length of 4 ("1111"). The index of the value is computed using:

$$index = \textbf{BIT\_COUNT}\,(A\&1111) - 1.$$

To extract the value, we need to bit shift the *tuple* to the value:

$$Value = (tuple >> 3 * index)\&111$$

where we have made use of the fact that each value is 3 bits.

3   Discussion

Our use of elementary bit operators (bitwise AND, bit shift, and bit count) provides a simple, non-database specific method of managing sparse data sets in a relational database.

We are using MySQL[1] in our test implementation, which is limited to 64-bit operations, and although it defines the bit operators we need, it does not implement those functions for blob types greater than 64 bits. Creating stored functions was found to be inefficient because of the buffering MySQL uses when managing the inputs and outputs of the functions. It resulted in slowness due to unwanted copying. MySQL's implicit string casting has also added to unwanted type conversions. We have overcome many of these limitations using MySQL's User Defined Functions (UDF) but this restricts generalization to other RDBMS.

We note that we could compress bit strings and tuples before storing to save even more space. Since this will result in slower query times as these quantities need to be uncompressed, we plan on evaluating this approach to see if it is worthwhile.

---

[1] http://www.mysql.com

Acknowledgments. We would like to thank Dr. Arthur Toga, Dr. Scott Neu, Karen Crawford, and the reviewers of this paper for their insightful feedback on an earlier draft of this paper. This work was supported by the Global Alzheimer's Association Interactive Network (GAAIN) initiative of the Alzheimer's Association and by National Institutes of Health grants 5P41 EB015922-16 and 1U54EB020406-01.

References

1. Beckmann, J.L., et al.: Extending RDBMSs to support sparse datasets using an interpreted attribute storage format. In: Proceedings of the 22nd International Conference on Data Engineering, ICDE 2006. IEEE (2006)
2. Corwin, J., et al.: Dynamic tables: an architecture for managing evolving, heterogeneous biomedical data in relational database management systems. J. Am. Med. Inform. Assoc. **14**(1), 86–93 (2007)
3. Cui, B., Zhao, J., Yang, D.: Exploring correlated subspaces for efficient query processing in sparse databases. IEEE Trans. Knowl. Data Eng. **22**(2), 219–233 (2010)
4. Cui, B., Zhao, J., Cong, G.: ISIS: a new approach for efficient similarity search in sparse databases. In: Kitagawa, H., Ishikawa, Y., Li, Q., Watanabe, C. (eds.) DASFAA 2010. LNCS, vol. 5982, pp. 231–245. Springer, Heidelberg (2010)
5. Atre, M., et al.: Matrix bit loaded: a scalable lightweight join query processor for RDF data. In: Proceedings of the 19th International Conference on World Wide Web. ACM (2010)
6. Golubchik, S., Hutchings, A.: MySQL 5.1 Plugin Development. Packt Publications, UK (2010)

Domain Specific Document Retrieval Framework for Real-Time Social Health Data

Swapnil Soni[✉]

Kno.e.sis center, Wright State University, Dayton, OH, USA
swapnil@knoesis.org

Abstract. With the advent of the web search and microblogging, the percentage of Online Health Information Seekers (OHIS) using these online services to share and seek health real-time information has increased exponentially. OHIS use web search engines or microblogging search services to seek out latest, relevant as well as reliable health information. When OHIS turn to microblogging search services to search real-time content, trends and breaking news, etc. the search results are not promising. Two major challenges exist in the current microblogging search engines are keyword based techniques and results do not contain real-time information. To address these challenges, we developed an approach to search near real-time and reliable content from Twitter, based on triple-pattern mining, near real-time retrieval, and ranking considering popularity and relevancy of the results.

Keywords: Twitter · Data mining · Triple pattern · Real-time · Health · Chronic disease · Social media analysis · Text mining

1 Introduction

Over the past ten years, percentage of social media users has increased exponentially. In the U.S, 72 % of online users use social media and its popularity grown by 64 % since 2005 [1]. Social media has become primary mode for users to share and find information on different topics, including health information. According to a consumer survey, one-third of the consumers now use social media for seeking medical, tracking and sharing health information [2]. A popular service, Twitter, allows users to create tweets and optionally include links in the tweets to share health information publicly. This health information can be useful for others to learn from the shared information. On the Twitter, more than 75 K worldwide healthcare professionals post 152 K tweets every day [6]. In our study, we have used Twitter as a data source and one of the most common chronic diseases, diabetes, as a use case.

1.1 Background and Motivation

OHIS have different preferences when it comes to find out information related to health conditions through social media search [3]. Some OHIS prefer real-time (latest) information, breaking news (articles), while others prefer facts and

© Springer International Publishing Switzerland 2015
N. Ashish and J.-L. Ambite (Eds.): DILS 2015, LNBI 9162, pp. 276–280, 2015.
DOI: 10.1007/978-3-319-21843-4_24

the information that contributes to general understanding of a health condition [3,4], etc. OHIS have many options on the Internet for health information seeking in real-time such as Google time-bound search, Twitter search, etc. But search results from these venues possess some significant challenges: the results are not real-time, search results are based on keyword-based techniques, and ranking of the results based on a relevance to each individual keyword in the query. A leading microblog search service such as Twitter use keyword-based approach, and since the Twitter is overloaded with information, and merely matching query keywords with tweets to locate relevant set of documents of information is inappropriate. Also, we observed that in Twitter search the results are not near real-time due to the keyword-based relevancy algorithm. Furthermore, Twitter search does not use domain knowledge and reliability factors to rank the results.

The objective of this research is to build a system for users to ask health-related questions to obtain reliable, and relevant health information shared on social media in near real-time. But, how to extract near real-time, reliable and relevant documents from the health information shared on a Twitter for a given user query? To extract relevant documents from a Twitter in near real-time based on a given user query, we have to deal with real-time tweets, information overload, and noisy data.

2   Related Work

2.1   Microblog Retrieval Method

The amount of conversation on Twitter has increased exponentially over last decade. To address the Twitter's information overload challenge, many researchers use microblogging services like Twitter to find out health information;however, extracting useful information is challenging given its volume, inconsistent writing, and noise. To extract useful information from a Twitter, many researchers worked on various retrieval models such as a user-based tree model, term-based, and pattern-based approaches. A Twitter based social media analytics system, Twitris uses Spatio-Temporal-Thematic (STT) processing of the Twitter data [9, 10]. However, many researches favor term-based extraction model also known as keyword based extraction. The keyword based model extract information based on keyword matching of users query. Its possible to extract undesired results based on a user query due to keyword based model extraction.

Magnani et al. proposed a term-based model for retrieving conversations from microblogs [5]. In this study, the concept of conversation retrieval from Twitter, a preliminary version of the concept presented by Magnani et al., proposes a user-based tree model to retrieve conversations from microblogs [5]. In this research, the whole conversation of users are represented as a tree, and its message and reply are represented as nodes. These conversations are stored in IR engine Lucene for indexing the text which can help the system to retrieve the relevant conversation documents based on the query. After finding the relevant conversation, the system ranks the relevant conversations based on text relevance, popularity, timeliness, audience, and density features.

3   Data Collection and Feature Extraction

In this study, we have used tweets (messages shared on Twitter) and URLs content (for URL(s) mentioned in the tweets) as the data sources to extract relevant information for a given user query. To extract features from real-time tweets, the first challenge is to create a infrastructure to collect real-time tweets. In our research, we have used Apache Storm to collect the real-time tweets using the public Twitter streaming API while also performing meta-data extraction. Apache storm is, open source software, used for real-time, distributed computing. Spouts and Bolts are the basic components in the storm for real-time processing of the data. The bolts contain computation logic to perform features extraction logic in real-time.

A tweet has many features, such as text, short url, latitude or longitude, re-tweet count, etc. All these features are useful for finding out useful information. To extract theses features from the tweets in real-time, we have used bolts (a Apache storm's components) to implement the logic. This process is also known as a pre-processing pipeline in our system.

4   Extraction of Relevant Documents

The objective of this research is to build a system to ask health-related questions on Twitter data. Hence, we have divided users questions into two categories: static and dynamic. The static questions are preselected frequently asked questions collected from the different sources. Also, the dynamic questions are typed by the user on the fly, which is not the case with the static queries. We proposed a novel approach by extracting real-time tweets, pattern-mining, incorporating domain knowledge, and including popularity measures of the content (tweets + URLs) in ranking of the results.

To make the system near real-time, the search results are divided into intervals of six hours. The near real-time process of extracting relevant documents is depends on static and dynamic questions are different. In the case of static questions, we extract documents every six hours, while in dynamic questions, we extract documents from that moment to last six hours data. To extract document, we have used triple based pattern (subject, predicate, and object) mining technique to extracts triple patterns from microblog messages–related with chronic health conditions. The triple pattern is defined in the initial question. To extract information or documents we have used the IBM text analytic tool AQL (Annotated Query Language). AQL is a query language to help developers to build queries that extract structured information from unstructured or semi-structured text. We have used an AQL tool to construct triple-patterns, and for faster processing we implemented it on Apache Hadoop Map-Reduce framework. To expand the query (or triple), we have Incorporated the domain knowledge using UMLS-Metathesaurus (Unified Medical Language System) and WordNet. UMLS is used to collect authentic and reliable vocabularies related to health and biomedical. Similarly, we used the WordNet to get the synonyms of the tokens (non medical term). Furthermore, in addition to tweets, we use URLs (mentioned in the tweet) content as the data source.

5   Ranking

To simply receiving results, users want the results to be good quality, reliable and well-ordered. Existing microblog search engines (e.g., Twitter) focused on ranking algorithms to order the results based on relevance to each individual keyword in the query. We have used the following features to rank the results are: popularity, relevancy, and reliability. To check the popularity of URLs through social media (e.g., a Twitter and a Facebook) share and like counts. Similarly, for reliability we use the URLs Google domain pagerank (filtration criteria is pagerank greater than 4). Also, we have used the relevance of the documents based on the similarity score. In our approach, we have used a TF-IDF cosine similarity algorithm. Once all the features are extracted, we have evaluated many machine learning algorithms and selected one of them based on an evaluation matrix (Normalized discounted cumulative gain). The algorithm we have chosen is the "Random Forest" algorithm.

6   Evaluation

As our research is focused on extracting near real-time health information based on users search queries, we have made the decision to evaluate our systems results with existing real-time search engine is a Twitter. We have selected reliability, relevancy, and real-time factors to measure our results with Twitter. To evaluate the reliable source, we compared a Google domain pagerank of our top 10 results with the Twitter's top 10 results. Also, for real-time we have compared the Twitter search results with our system's search results. We found that Twitter search results are not real-time as compared to our results (which is six hours of data). Similarly, we conducted three surveys to check the relevance of the results in which we selected three questions dealing with the chronic disease diabetes. The questions are "How to control diabetes?", "What are the causes of diabetes?", "What are the symptoms of diabetes?". Upon completion of the surveys, for all the queries 50 %, 60 % and 50 % of users ranked the quality of our results as "very good", whereas the results were 40 %, 10 % and 40 % for a Twitter search results.

7   Discussion and Conclusion

To find useful health information in real-time from Twitter, there are many challenges such as the real-time nature of Twitter, information overload and noisy data. We have dealt with each of the challenges by using state-of-the-arts technologies and a novel approach in our system. Also, we have used URL's content for finding information because the tweets contains less information. However, the system does not extract factual answers of a user questions. In this thesis, I am extracting relevant documents based on a user query in near real-time. We want to extend this thesis further by including semantic categorisation in which the results will be categorised (drug, medication, symptom, etc.) using prior work [7,8].

Twitter has changed the traditional way of sharing and seeking health information by health-care professionals and the general users. All kinds of information are available on the Internet for each type of user. We have tried to resolve the challenges for those who want the latest information. Our system provides a platform to users to use Twitter for finding relevant documents based on a user's question in near real-time.

Acknowledgement. I would also like to thank my thesis advisor Prof. Amit Sheth from Kno.e.sis center, Wright State University and my mentor Mr. Ashutosh Jadhav for their support and guidance.

References

1. Brenner, J., Smith, A.: Online Adults are Social Networking Site User, Pew Research Center Internet (2013)
2. Ottenhoff: Infographic, Rising Use of Social and Mobile in Healthcare, The Spark Report (2012)
3. Choudhury, M.D., et al.: Seeking and sharing health information online: Comparing search engines and social media, ACM (2014)
4. Teevan, J., et al.: # TwitterSearch: a comparison of microblog search and web search. ACM, The Spark Report (2011)
5. Magnani et al.: Advances in Information Retrieval, Springer (2011)
6. MacDonald, I.: Healthcare professionals flock to Twitter, FierceHealthcare
7. Jadhav, A., Sheth, A., Pathak, J.: Analysis of online information searching for cardiovascular diseases on a consumer health information portal. AMIA Annu. Symp. (2014)
8. Jadhav, A., Wu, S., Sheth, A., Pathak, J.: Online Information Seeking for Cardiovascular Diseases: A Case Study from Mayo Clinic at 25th European Medical Informatics Conference (2014)
9. Sheth, A., Jadhav, A., Kapanipathi, P., Lu, C., Purohit, H., Smith, G.A., Wang, W.: Twitris- a system for collective social intelligence. Encyclopedia of Social Network Analysis and Mining (ESNAM) (2014)
10. Jadhav, A., Purohit, H., Kapanipathi, P., Ananthram, P., Ranabahu, A., Nguyen, V., Mendes, P., Smith, A.G., Cooney, M., Sheth, A.: Twitris 2.0: Semantically Empowered System for Understanding Perceptions From Social Data, Semantic Web Application Challenge at ISWC (2010)

Author Index

Printed in the United States
By Bookmasters